When Pregnancy
Isn't Perfect

When Pregnancy *Isn't* Perfect

—-—

A Layperson's Guide to Complications in Pregnancy

—-—

LAURIE A. RICH

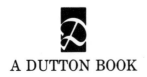

A DUTTON BOOK

DUTTON
Published by the Penguin Group
Penguin Books USA Inc., 375 Hudson Street, New York, New York 10014, U.S.A.
Penguin Books Ltd, 27 Wrights Lane, London W8 5TZ, England
Penguin Books Australia Ltd, Ringwood, Victoria, Australia
Penguin Books Canada Ltd, 2801 John Street, Markham, Ontario, Canada L3R 1B4
Penguin Books (N.Z.) Ltd, 182-190 Wairau Road, Auckland 10, New Zealand

Penguin Books Ltd, Registered Offices: Harmondsworth, Middlesex, England

First published by Dutton, an imprint of New American Library,
a division of Penguin Books USA Inc.
Distributed in Canada by McClelland & Stewart Inc.

First Printing, March, 1991
10 9 8 7 6 5 4 3 2 1

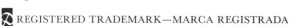 REGISTERED TRADEMARK—MARCA REGISTRADA

LIBRARY OF CONGRESS CATALOGING-IN-PUBLICATION DATA:
Rich, Laurie A.
    When pregnancy isn't perfect : a layperson's guide to
complications in pregnancy / Laurie A. Rich.
        p.   cm.
    Includes bibliographical references and index.
    1. Pregnancy, Complications of—Popular works.   I. Title.
RG572.R53   1991
618.3—dc20   90-46190
                                                                     CIP
0-525-24961-3

Printed in the United States of America
Set in Baskerville
Designed by Eve L. Kirch

NOTE TO THE READER:

The ideas, procedures, and suggestions contained in this book are not intended as a substitute for consulting with your physician. All matters regarding your health require medical supervision.

For Jenny

ACKNOWLEDGMENTS

To the hundreds of women (and the men) who shared the intimate details of their pregnancy experience with me, a perfect stranger, for the sole purpose of helping others whose pregnancies are not perfect, my thanks, and my respect for your bravery and selflessness.

My deepest thanks to the helping professionals and organization leaders who gave generously of their time, knowledge and experience to help make this book as complete as possible:

Rev. James Cunningham, Fairview General Hospital, Cleveland, OH
Ellen M. Ebert, Perinatal Consultant and Childbirth Education Specialist, Philadelphia, PA
Connie Furrh, R.N., Founder, PRIDE, Oklahoma City, OK
Janice Heil, M.Ed., Executive Director, UNITE, Philadelphia, PA
Judith Howard, Founder, The Confinement Line, Alexandria, VA
Caryn R. Johnson, O.T.R./L., President, Occupational Therapy Associates; Clinical Assistant Professor, Department of Occupational Therapy, Thomas Jefferson University, Philadelphia, PA
Jean Kollantai, Founder, Our Newsletter Network, Palmer, AK
Sister Jane Marie Lamb, Founder, SHARE
Jan Litkin, American Diabetes Association
Nancy E. Malcolm, R.N., Administrative Director of Nursing Education and Research/Special Projects, Toronto Women's Hospital, Canada
Lennette Moses, Founder, Intensive Caring Unlimited, Philadelphia, PA
Michele Mowry, Office Manager, TWINLINE, Berkeley, CA

Kate T. Ruddon, Public Information Assistant at the American College of Obstetricians and Gynecologists

Mark S. Simmons, D.D.S., M.A., Director of the General Practice Residency Program at the University of Minnesota School of Dentistry

Patricia Smith, High Risk Moms, Inc., Naperville, IL

Nancy Young-Diaz, R.N., Parent Care, Inc., Alexandria, VA

Thomas Zerbel, Funeral Director, Escanaba, MI; Proprietor, Bay Memorials-Burial Cradle Baby Casket Products

My sincere appreciation to the physicians and other helping professionals who took the time to review portions of my manuscript for medical and factual accuracy:

Janet L. Bleyl, President, The Triplet Connection, Stockton, CA

Sharon N. Covington, M.S.W., L.C.S.W., infertility and perinatal loss counseling specialist, Rockville, MD

Marie L. Epling, M.S.W., Perinatal Social Services Manager, Healthdyne Perinatal Services, Rockford, IL

John W. Hare, M.D., Joslin Clinic, Boston, MA

Sherokee Ilse, bereaved mother and author, *Empty Arms: Coping with Miscarriage, Stillbirth and Infant Death,* co-author *Miscarriage: A Shattered Dream,* Founder and President, Pregnancy and Infant Loss Center, Wayzata, MN

Julie R. Ingelfinger, M.D., Co-Director, Pediatric Nephrology Unit, Massachusetts General Hospital, Boston, MA

Michael Katz, M.D., Chief, Perinatal Service, Children's Hospital of San Francisco, and author, *Preventing Preterm Birth: A Parent's Guide*

Rana K. Limbo, R.N., M.S., Director, Resolve Through Sharing

Carol Livoti, M.D.

Judith L. M. McCoyd, A.C.S.W., L.S.W., private clinical practice (therapy and counselling)

Albert Sassoon, M.D.

Sara Rich Wheeler, R.N., M.S.N., Director of Education, Resolve Through Sharing

And finally, to the three people without whom I could not have written this book:

My husband, who read and edited every page.

My assistant, Diane Brown, who painstakingly indexed, catalogued and made order out of the chaos that is my office.

And my son, who, from the instant of his birth made every moment of my complicated pregnancy and the forever-after part worthwhile.

I love you.

Laurie

CONTENTS

FOREWORD

For the average woman planning to have a baby, there are no great surprises. Her pregnancy progresses in an ordinary manner without complications. But for an unfortunate few, complications do arise. This book is addressed to those few.

Laurie has been a patient of ours for many years. She has been and continues to be a healthy woman. Our initial concern was her previous ectopic pregnancy which ultimately caused no problems. Unfortunately, Laurie's pregnancy became a textbook example of pregnancy-related complications—she was carrying twins, and she experienced prolonged bleeding, hypertension, diabetes, intrauterine growth retardation, premature ruptured membranes, premature labor, and placental abruption—all leading to premature delivery and her babies' treatment in the neonatal intensive care unit. Through all of these problems, Laurie asked intelligent questions and was responsive to all recommendations. In the course of her pregnancy, during long hours of strict bedrest, Laurie decided to write this book. Not only was writing this book good therapy for her, but the book she produced will be a source of solid information for any woman whose pregnancy isn't perfect.

It is important to emphasize that no pregnancy is *absolutely* perfect. In the course of nine months, some problems are bound to arise. These problems are almost always minor in nature and can be readily corrected by alterations of lifestyle, diet, and/or medication. Furthermore, some ''complications'' are not complications at all, but rather, normal symptoms of pregnancy.

Your obstetrician is your guide through pregnancy. He or she should be your primary source of information. Your doctor is the expert to whom you should turn if things do not seem to be going well, and he or she should be available for problems twenty-four hours a day. In return, to make the relationship totally effective and beneficial, you should have faith in his or her advice and recommendations. Without mutual trust and respect, the critical doctor-patient relationship is flawed. If you feel uncomfortable with your obstetrician, you will be doing both you and your doctor a favor by voicing your discomfort.

As we all know, "A little knowledge is a dangerous thing." No one is asking you to be your own obstetrician: The worst thing you can do is attempt to manage your own pregnancy and delivery. An informed patient, on the other hand, facilitates communication. She understands the nature of the problem, what steps need to be taken, and when to defer to her obstetrician's judgment. There is a fine line between being well informed and becoming overly concerned about every small problem that may arise. Pregnancy, after all, should be a joyful time.

When Pregnancy Isn't *Perfect* strikes a fine balance for the concerned pregnant woman. Laurie discusses many of the potential complications of pregnancy in a clear, nonthreatening manner. If one of these complications arises, this book can provide a basis for important communication and informed decision making between you and your doctor. We are obstetricians who deliver hundreds of babies every year. Our practice crosses all walks of life and covers every age group. It is a rare woman who wouldn't refer to this book at least once during her pregnancy. We feel that *When Pregnancy* Isn't *Perfect* will be a worthy addition to any home library and an excellent reference for any obstetrical patient. However, above all, *we urge you to communicate with your doctor.*

—Carol Livoti, M.D.
Al Sassoon, M.D.

PREFACE
Why I Wrote This Book

By the time I was thirteen weeks' pregnant, I had already been bleeding off and on, and in bed, for ten weeks. After trying for a long time, I was finally pregnant—with twins. My job now was to stay prone and quiet in order to keep the bleeding to a minimum. It seemed logical to me, so I didn't ask too many questions, even though I was scared out of my wits.

But my "let them handle it" phase didn't last for long. It ended when my OB told me I'd be in bed for at least another two months. "At least!" I cried to myself, "I've got to understand this thing." In my case the "thing" was *placenta previa:* My lower twin's placenta had developed abnormally low in my uterus, so I would be in bed until it migrated out of the way—if it ever did! And that's when I asked my husband, "Honey, would you get me the book that tells all about placenta previa?" But he came back empty-handed.

You might call "Honey, would you get me a book about . . ." one of the themes of my pregnancy. In all, I had ten major complications (not including an emergency c-section). I was on bedrest for thirty of my thirty-three and a half weeks of pregnancy, and the last five and a half of those I spent in the hospital.

Each time my doctors gave me a new diagnosis, I'd ask my husband, "Honey, could you get me the book . . ." And each time, he could find nothing more than a paragraph to a couple of pages in a "well pregnancy" book. There were no books available for women like me, women who wanted comprehensive, understandable information about complications like gestational diabetes, placenta previa, and intrauterine growth retardation (to name just three of my own).

I was offended and frustrated. I had spent years as a science journalist writing about complex environmental and technical subjects. It was my job to make these topics understandable to nonscientists—to lay readers like myself. Now, when I needed to have something explained to me in layman's terms, nothing was available. Even though 875,000 women a year suffer one or more of the problems I was having, my only choices were to wade through hard-to-comprehend medical texts while flat on my back or to remain uninformed.

I never did find the material I wanted. Not for my whole pregnancy. And for me, pregnancy became a long nightmare of fear and inability to really grasp what was happening. Without the information I needed, I felt helpless, victimized, and unhappy.

When it was all over, and I'd recovered enough to try to make sense out of what had happened to me, I decided to do something about that. "I have the skills. I can write that book," I thought. "I'll write the book I wished I'd had to read while I was pregnant." A book with full information about each complication, in lay language, explaining every medical term. A book that emphasizes the positive without skipping over the negative, written from the woman's perspective, with information on how to cope. And, finally, a book that would counter fear and isolation, by giving the reader a true sense of what to expect.

This is that book. Knowing what I know now, from my research, and my experience, I am certain that my next pregnancy will be very different for me—easier, and less stressful, no matter how many complications I have (if any!)—because I have the information.

And by reading this book, so will you. I wrote it so that no woman would ever have to go through what I experienced without the means to be well-informed. My goal was to give you the tools to understand what's happening to you and your baby, so that you can take an active role in your care and make informed choices. If I help just one of you, I'll be satisfied that I have done my job.

—Laurie A. Rich

When Pregnancy
Isn't Perfect

1

What's Here for You (How to Use This Book)

I knew what it would be like to be pregnant and have a baby: I'd feel great, energetic, and proud. I'd work right up until I delivered, using my evenings and weekends to decorate the nursery, buy infant clothes, and shop for furniture. My friends would throw me a lovely baby shower, and everyone would tell me how radiant I looked. My husband would take me out all the time to show off my big belly. We'd go on a long, last, just-the-two-of-us vacation, and sex would be fabulous. Finally, when the time came, I'd have a vaginal delivery in a homey birthing room, with no monitors or medical intervention in sight. Yes, my pregnancy would certainly be perfect.

It was December 1986, almost the end of the year. I would soon be thirty-three, and I was certain I was pregnant. I had taken fertility drugs for the first time that month (we'd been trying on our own for over a year), and I had all the symptoms: I was nauseated, my breasts were large and tender, and I was sleepy almost all the time. On December 22, I arranged to have a pregnancy test the very next day, so I'd be able to give my husband our news as a Christmas present. I was so excited!

Then I started bleeding. I was heartbroken. I'd been so sure. But the next morning the bleeding stopped; I just stained a little bit. That wasn't the way my period usually went. I called my OB from my office to ask if this was common after taking fertility drugs.

"Laurie, what are you doing at work?" the nurse admonished me. "Get up here right now and have a pregnancy test. You may very well be pregnant!"

The test gave me the joyous news I'd waited so long to hear. I *was* pregnant! But my OB gave me orders to go home immediately, where I was to stay in bed until forty-eight hours after I stopped staining. "Is this normal?" I asked. "How many women does this happen to?" Oh, about one in five, the nurse replied. But I'd probably be up and around in no time. Even so, this wasn't starting out at all like the pregnancy I'd planned.

And unfortunately, that was as perfect as my pregnancy ever got. With the exception of four days during my eighth week, when I got to go back to work and act normally, I never left my bed again. I bled off and on until my twentieth week, first because of implantation bleeding (when the fertilized egg burrows into the lining of the uterus); then because my son's placenta was too low in my uterus (called *placenta previa*). At twenty weeks, my daughter—oh yes, I was carrying twins— began to show signs of abnormally slow growth, so they kept me in bed to assure that she'd get more of my oxygen supply and better nutrition.

I developed insulin-dependent gestational diabetes in my twenty-sixth week, so I was hospitalized for five days while I learned how to inject myself and bring my blood sugar under control. At twenty-nine weeks, my daughter's water broke, sending me into labor. I never left the hospital again until I delivered, prematurely and by cesarean, at thirty-three and a half weeks.

I brought my healthy, normal son home two weeks later. Jenny died eighteen hours after birth, because of complications from her prematurity and the severely premature rupture of her amniotic sac.

While all this was happening to me, I was a study in terror, sadness and anger. I found no books that dealt with complications in depth, and I didn't know how to ask the right questions of my doctors. Also, I didn't know another soul who was or had ever been on bedrest for her whole pregnancy.

Since I didn't know what to expect, I couldn't judge what was happening: Everything frightened me, especially the possibility of losing the babies. I was devastated and angry about losing my perfect pregnancy. I cried a lot. I was moody. I was bored, even though I continued working from my bed, via computer, until my twenty-ninth week. And I was starved for companionship. As the weeks dragged on, most of my friends seemed to have trouble dealing with my situation, so they just stopped visiting. Because of the trappings, I kept losing sight of the fact that I was pregnant, not sick. Often I became so self-absorbed I'd forget my husband was having a bad time, too. And I can't tell you how many times I thought I was going crazy.

But I wasn't. Some version of what I experienced is what happens to any woman with serious pregnancy complications. What happened to me was normal and natural under the circumstances.

AT LEAST 20 PERCENT OF ALL WOMEN WHO GIVE BIRTH EACH YEAR HAVE ONE OR MORE COMPLICATIONS OF PREGNANCY.

Right now I may be the only woman you've heard of who's had a complicated pregnancy, other than yourself. But I'm not the only one. Not by a long shot.

Of the approximately 3.9 million women who give birth in the United States each year, almost 25 percent (975,000) have one or more complications of pregnancy.* Even if you've got one of the rarer complications—with an incidence of only 1 percent—that means that there are at least 39,000 other women who will have your problem this year. On the following page are some examples of the company you'll keep.

And the numbers are on the rise for many of these complications, as more and more of us put off childbearing until we're thirty-something. Studies released in 1990 show that although delaying childbearing into one's thirties does not significantly increase the chances of having a low-birth-weight or premature infant, it does increase the risk of having certain complications, including diabetes, hypertension, uterine bleeding, and fetal distress during labor.

BUT JUST BECAUSE YOU HAVE A COMPLICATION DOESN'T MEAN YOU'LL LOSE YOUR BABY.

As more and more women decide to have children later in life, the practices of high-risk obstetrics and neonatal (newborn) intensive care are becoming increasingly sophisticated. High-risk care has now progressed to the point where the vast majority of complicated pregnancies can be extended to term, or almost. In general, that means no matter which complication(s) you have, the odds are excellent that you'll end your pregnancy with a healthy, normal baby.

Of course, there are a few sad exceptions where nothing can be done to save a pregnancy. These are:

---

*This number doesn't include c-sections, which comprise 24.7 percent of all births (about 965,000/year), or miscarriages, which are thought to account for 33 percent (over two million) of all pregnancies.

- when the embryo implants outside the uterus (ectopic pregnancy)
- miscarriage
- preterm birth before twenty-three weeks' gestation
- when only a placenta but no fetus forms (hydatidiform mole and blighted ovum)
- when the placenta shears completely loose from the uterus before the baby is born (total placental abruption)

But other than miscarriage (again, one-third of all pregnancies end in miscarriage, 80 percent before the end of the first trimester), these complications rarely happen. That means that you have every chance of beating your problem and having a healthy baby.

YOU ARE NOT ALONE:
SOME EXAMPLES OF THE COMPANY YOU KEEP

Hundreds of thousands of women have pregnancy complications every year. Did you know that in bearing the 3.9 million babies that will be born in the U.S. this year:

1,600,000	women will have placentas that form too low in the uterus 17,500 of which will remain too low and force operative delivery
975,000	women will develop a hypertensive disorder. Of these, 234,000–273,000 will have preeclampsia and 13,650 will have eclamptic seizures
965,600	women will give birth by cesarean section
390,000–780,000	will experience abnormal bleeding
350,000	will go into labor too early
195,000	will come down with viral infections
127,000–390,000	women will have babies with intrauterine growth retardation (IUGR)
117,000–468,000	will have gestational diabetes
78,000–429,000	will get urinary tract infections
39,000	will have too much amniotic fluid surrounding the baby
19,500–39,000	will have placentas that abrupt—separate from the uterus too soon
3,900–11,700	will vomit so severely they will need hospitalization

And finally, of the 6,500,000 pregnancies conceived in the U.S. this year, 2,145,000 will end in miscarriage

---

SOURCES: American College of Obstetricians and Gynecologists; National Center for Health Statistics; medical texts cited in Bibliography.

How to Use This Book

After you read this chapter, I'm sure you will immediately turn to the part of the book that deals with your particular complication. Great! That's exactly what you should do. When you start reading about your complication, you'll find several references to other chapters in the book. I strongly urge you to read these as well. You should allow yourself to become as knowledgeable about your condition as possible. In addition, there are several chapters of this book that I consider MUSTs for you to read. They are:

- *Chapter 2: When Pregnancy Is Perfect.*   This chapter tells you what physical changes a woman's body goes through during pregnancy, under normal circumstances. It's important for you to know which of your symptoms are the result of the normal part of your pregnancy. Most of the bodily sensations and discomforts you will feel while pregnant are the result of these natural and amazing changes. If you don't know what's normal, how will you be able to spot what is not normal?

- *Chapter 14: What to Expect When You Go to the Hospital.* This chapter explains hospital admissions procedures and tests, hospital routine, and how to maneuver your way through the system. A great many complications require that you spend some time in the hospital before you deliver, possibly on very short notice. Knowing what it's going to be like before you get there will help you to feel more in control and therefore less panicky. And it doesn't hurt to know in advance how to work the system so that you are treated as well as you possibly can be.

- *Chapter 15: Bedrest: Keeping Yourself from Going Bonkers.* Many complications are treated in part or in whole with bedrest. If you don't know what to expect, what you can do to make your confinement as pleasant as possible, how to cope, and where to turn for emotional support, bedrest can really drive you nuts. This chapter tells you what to expect both physically and emotionally. It provides an exercise regime (to be done only with permission from your OB) that you can follow and offers practical suggestions on how to get to the other end of bedrest with your sanity intact.

- *Chapter 8: Preterm Labor and Premature Rupture of Membranes.* Unfortunately, many complications put you at risk for preterm labor and delivery. Almost 85 percent of all neonatal deaths and injuries are due to the complications of prematurity. You may think that you have no control over this, but you do! If you know what to look for and how to monitor yourself for contractions, you *will* have control! No one can stop preterm labor from starting. But once it starts, it can be successfully arrested and the pregnancy prolonged in 80 percent of all cases.

• *Chapter 13: Cesarean Section.*   One out of four of *all* pregnant women deliver by cesarean. For those of us with complications, that figure is even higher. You owe it to yourself to be prepared for this possibility. If you know what's going to happen ahead of time, you'll be less frightened, and you may really be able to enjoy the birth of your child. It *is* possible for a cesarean to be a positive birth experience, but usually only if you are well-prepared and have a good attitude! This chapter leads you step by step through preparation for the surgery, the operation itself, the recuperation period, and the road to recovery.

• *Chapter 10: Pregnancy Loss: When the Worst Happens.* There is no way to raise this subject easily: Even though the vast majority have happy endings, some complicated pregnancies end with the death of the baby. Even women with otherwise perfect pregnancies can lose their child to a birth accident. What makes this tragedy even harder for the bereaved parents is that often they receive little support and guidance from their hospitals, clergy, friends, and relations. This chapter will tell you what to expect of yourselves and others during the first painful days after a loss, explain the broad range of options you are likely to have, and inform you of your rights as parents.

In all likelihood your pregnancy will have a happy ending. It's often hard even to consider that it might not. And for that reason, it may be that you just can't bring yourself to read this chapter right now. That's perfectly understandable. In that case, I suggest that you ask your husband or a close friend or family member to read it, so that someone close to you will know what to do and how to help guide you through the terrible first days if the worst does happen.

• *Chapter 16: For the Fathers: What Happens to You When Pregnancy Isn't Perfect?*   This chapter is for your husband. In complicated pregnancies, men are almost always left to cope on their own. In many respects, their job is as hard as yours, yet they will not receive the kind of support and counseling that is available to you. Even if support is offered, most men won't take advantage of it. But most men will do a little reading. Ask your husband to read Chapter 16 and the other chapters that are must reading for you, *plus* the chapter(s) on your condition(s). He cannot be your best advocate and support person if he lacks the basic information he needs to understand your situation and to work with your care providers.

A Note on Repetition and Use of Gender in This Book

I fully expect that most people who read this book will not read it cover to cover. Rather, they will use it as a reference tool, focusing on their own particular complications and the "must reading" chapters. Therefore, certain facets of hospital procedure and suggestions for coping are repeated in a number of chapters, as appropriate. If you hit some of these sections more than once, just skip them the second time around.

For ease of understanding, and for no other reason, when I refer to doctors in this book, I use the pronoun "he." I most often call the male half of a couple the "husband," and I label the woman "wife." I call all babies "she" (except, of course, when the real baby referred to in the text is male). I am well aware that many doctors are women, that many couples are not married, that not all mothers are part of a couple, and that all babies are not females. I apologize if I offend some people with this system of labeling.

Best Wishes

When you finish reading this book, you will know everything I didn't know but wished I did when I was pregnant. My hope is that you can use what you learn here (and from the other good texts recommended in the Other Reading and Resources section) to take control of your situation when you can and to counter your fear and feelings of isolation.

Those who went down this road before you got to the end, and so will you. No matter what happens to you in the next weeks or months, in the long run, you'll be okay. If you work with your doctor, do your part in following treatment, use the support systems offered in the book, and have just a little luck, you'll come out of this pregnancy stronger, happier—and the proud mother of a healthy, normal baby!

2

When Pregnancy Is *Perfect*

Deborah's pregnancy was very difficult for her. She vomited three times a day from her fourth week through her fifth month. Her stomach was so unsettled that it took hours for her to get dressed and ready to leave the house every day for work. As a result, her productivity at her job fell to "half of what it might have been otherwise."

She was exhausted all the time—"a kind of exhausted that I'd never felt before. Sleeping extra didn't even begin to make a dent in it. And because I was so tired, I just didn't care about anything. I was miserable all the time. I was disinterested in life. I hardly went out. I hardly saw anyone. I fell asleep every day sitting up in my office. I was terribly depressed."

On top of that, Deborah had "horrible constipation," severe abdominal cramping, back pain, and shooting pains down one leg.

Yet medically, there was nothing wrong with Deborah—except that She was going to have a baby. Deborah's was a perfect pregnancy. She had no medical complications. She gave birth, at term, to a healthy, lovely baby boy. Deborah's complaints were the normal, natural consequences of regular, uncomplicated pregnancy.

YOU'RE KIDDING! I THOUGHT PERFECT PREGNANCIES WERE JUST THAT—PERFECT.

No. The truth is, for most women, even a perfect pregnancy is no picnic. The majority of normally pregnant women vomit—sometimes a lot. They get constipated. They have hemorrhoids and varicose veins. They have trouble sleeping, and eating, and, toward the end of pregnancy, they even have trouble breathing. Their bellies, backs, and legs ache. Their noses run. They have to pee all the time. They cry easily. They're exhausted. Their breasts are sore.

Now these aren't things that most women who have had babies emphasize when they discuss with newly pregnant women what pregnancy will be like. And such complaints pale in comparison to what it's like to be on contraction-stopping drugs, to name just one example. But I think that knowing these things may help you a lot. When you're in the throes of preterm labor, or lying in bed for the twelfth week in a row, it's easy to idealize other people's pregnancies and feel like you've been cheated out of the blissful, carefree experience that should have been yours.

"Maybe one of the reasons that we all think pregnancy is as easy as falling off a log is because as soon as we have that baby, amnesia sets in," said Theresa, who had two "perfect" pregnancies. "The truth is, until you asked me to think about it, I had blocked out that for me, it was generally, overall, a bad time of life. What I remember most about my pregnancy is that any complaint that I had, the midwives said was normal. I had migraine headaches for the first five months of my second pregnancy. I can remember waking up in the middle of the night and feeling like there was a drum inside my head. I'd walk down to the freezer like Frankenstein and get ice cubes to put on the back of my neck. That was one of the things that I forgot. The farther you get away from the pregnancy, the more amnesia you have."

Yes, pregnancy is a natural part of life. But as Theresa said, "it's not necessarily all it's cracked up to be." It's important that you try to keep the basic realities of pregnancy in perspective as the months roll by in your own complicated pregnancy.

Learning about how "normal" pregnancy affects the body will help you in several other ways: First, it will help you understand which of your symptoms are due to your complication(s) and which are just the usual consequences of pregnancy. And even though you have complications, they will not affect every aspect of your pregnancy. Some of the aches and pains, fears and doubts you will have are the same ones experienced by complication-free women. In other words, a lot of what goes on with you will be *normal.*

Next, knowing what normal physical and emotional changes during pregnancy are may also help you recognize when something might not be quite right with you. After all, how can you know what is *not* normal if you don't know what *is?*

Finally, this chapter is here to remind you that, even though you have complications, you still have a great deal in common with women who have normal pregnancies and that, while things certainly could be going better—maybe much better—for you, almost no pregnancy is without its little problems.

Body Changes During Pregnancy

Virtually every system in a woman's body undergoes changes when she is pregnant, all to support the fetus and accommodate its presence in the uterus. It's amazing, really, that the human body can alter itself so much for such a relatively short period of time. Equally incredible is that within hours of the baby's birth, the mother's body undergoes further changes to convert some of its energy to producing milk for breastfeeding; then, within days of the delivery, most of the mother's other body systems begin to return to their prepregnant state.

Some of these processes are internal only; you will not see them. But you will feel their effects. Others manifest themselves in visible bodily changes. Many of these adaptations by the body produce uncomfortable side effects for a majority of women.

CHANGES IN THE UTERUS

The first thing most of us think about when we contemplate the physical changes that pregnancy brings is our belly. We know that the uterus will enlarge to accommodate the baby. We've all heard that we'll lose our waists along with sight of our toes. And changes in our size are certainly the most visible of all aspects of pregnancy.

Before a woman becomes pregnant, her uterus is a fist-sized, pear-shaped, almost solid organ. It weighs only about two and a half ounces and has a space—or cavity—inside it that holds only about one-third of an ounce of liquid. But do those numbers ever change by the end of a pregnancy! By the end of pregnancy, the average uterus weighs a little under two and a half pounds and has a capacity of about five and one-quarter quarts!

In order to accommodate such an incredible expansion, a number of changes occur: The uterine muscle cells stretch. Fibrous and elastic tissue forms in the external muscle layer of the uterus. The size and number of blood vessels, as well as the lymphatic system in the pelvis, increase tremendously. And the shape of the uterus changes from pear to round to oval as the fetus grows and the contents of the womb stretch it out.

In the first three months of pregnancy, this process is caused by hormonal changes. After that, changes are stimulated by pressure on the uterus from within, as the growing fetus and its support systems—

the placenta, amnion, amniotic fluid, and so on—press outward. Perhaps in anticipation of the vast stretching, during the first trimester the walls of the uterus thicken. Then, as pregnancy progresses and the baby grows rapidly, the uterine walls stretch and thin until they are less than three-quarters of an inch thick.

During early pregnancy, these changes may cause a dull ache in the pelvis or a feeling of fullness in the lower belly. You may feel swollen. As pregnancy advances, other physical symptoms may crop up, but these arise more from the other changes the body must go through to make room for the growing uterus than from the uterine changes themselves.

STRUCTURAL CHANGES: BONES AND CONNECTIVE TISSUE

As the womb enlarges, other structures inside the body also move and change to accommodate the growth and prepare the body for the delivery. The ligaments of the pubic symphysis (the place where the pubic bones come together in the mid-front of the body under the pubic hair) and sacroiliac joints (connections between the sacrum, or the base of the spine, and the broad bones of the pelvis in the back) loosen and stretch, which helps create enough room for the fetus to pass through the pelvis during birth.

For some women, this relaxation and stretching can be quite painful at times. Some women experience aching, others sharp but brief pains when they change position. Almost all women experience some degree of discomfort from the process, especially later in pregnancy.

As the uterus bulges up and outward, it also tends to pull one's normal center of gravity off-balance. You compensate for this by arching your lower back and leaning somewhat backward. Your gait changes to a shuffle or swagger as you work to maintain balance when you walk. Almost all women experience back pain because of this shift of posture and positioning. The pain may be steady, or intermittent, but is usually relieved with rest, changes of position, or a heating pad. Often, the aching interrupts normal sleep at night.

LUNGS AND BREATHING CHANGES

The enlarging uterus also affects breathing. As the womb grows, it pushes up the diaphragm—the muscular membrane that separates the abdominal cavity from the chest cavity. The diaphragm's contractions and expansions are what make us breathe. The rib cage also expands during pregnancy. This pressing up of the diaphragm and expansion of the rib cage allow you to inhale and exhale about 30 to 40 percent more air. But your reserves of air—that is, the amount you retain in your lungs after exhaling completely—drops about 20 percent. With these and other changes, your total lung capacity falls about 5 percent. You may experience this small decrease in capacity as shortness of breath, which increases in the late second trimester, is worst during the eighth month, and is relieved somewhat in the ninth month by the "dropping" of the baby deeper into the pelvis. This lessens pressure on the diaphragm, allowing the lungs to retain more air.

In addition to shortness of breath, many women also feel like they have a cold all the time. During pregnancy, all mucus membranes in the body produce more mucus and swell. The nasal passages are no exception, and this leads to the sensation of having a permanently stuffed nose.

How the Digestive System Changes

The hormonal changes and the enlargement of the uterus also create alterations in the digestive tract. As the womb gets bigger, it pushes up against and compresses the stomach, actually changing its shape. The stomach can no longer hold as much food as it did before pregnancy. Thus, it is easy to eat what feels like too much food, because the stomach literally doesn't have the room to accommodate it.

At the other end of the system, in the rectum, the pressure from the enlarging uterus elevates pressure on certain blood vessels, called the hemorrhoidal veins. Combined with the hormonally caused dilation and swelling of all blood vessels in the body, this pressure causes the hemorrhoidal veins to bulge into the rectum (the lower portion of the large intestine; it connects to the anal canal). The bulges are called hemorrhoids, and they can hurt, burn, or itch, especially when stool passes over them during defecation. And hard stools can make the veins bleed, sometimes quite profusely.

Hard stools and constipation—that is, infrequent bowel movements—are two other common changes in the digestive system brought on by the size of the uterus and hormonal changes during the pregnancy. In the early months of gestation, the body produces massive amounts of hormones to sustain the fetus. These hormones work throughout the body, not just in the uterus.

These substances slow down peristalsis, the rhythmic, wavelike contractions of the smooth muscles surrounding the intestines and the rest of the digestive tract. Thus, food travels through the system more slowly and loses more fluid along the way, making stools harder than normal. Also, the uterus may actually press on the large intestine and make it more difficult for the waste products to pass through. The result: feelings of constipation and difficulty in elimination.

Then there's heartburn. The esophagus is the tube that connects the mouth with the stomach. A band of tissue at the bottom of the esophagus (the esophageal sphincter) closes once food reaches the stomach. During pregnancy, the esophogeal sphincter tends to relax. It is this relaxation, combined with the upward pressure of the enlarging uterus on the stomach and other internal organs, that often allows gastric juices to escape up into the esophagus. When that happens, the tissue in the lower esophagus can become irritated and sometimes painful. This causes the hot, burning sensation called *heartburn.*

Couple this feeling of fullness with the slowdown of peristalsis and the sensation of heartburn in the lower esophagus, and add the extra hormones of pregnancy. The result: 60 percent of all pregnant women experience nausea and/or vomiting in their first trimester. Although it's called "morning sickness," nausea of pregnancy can occur at any time of the day or night. Vomiting up to several times a day is considered normal. These symptoms set in as early as the second week of pregnancy and usually disappear by the sixteenth week, although some women say that they are nauseated from the very beginning of their pregnancy and well into the fifth or sixth month.

Hormonal changes also affect the condition of most women's gums. The gums swell, turn redder than usual, and are likely to bleed when the teeth are brushed. Sometimes small cysts form on the gums, only to recede completely after the delivery.

URINARY TRACT CHANGES

Virtually every woman notices changes in urination when she is pregnant. That is, we all need to pee more. Once again, this is due in part to that growing uterus. During pregnancy, the kidneys enlarge somewhat to accommodate the greater amount of waste products that pass through them, as you take in more liquids and pass waste from the fetus through your own blood system. Also, pressure on the ureters—the tubes leading from the kidneys to the bladder—increases because of the development of extra blood vessels in the pelvis, increased blood volume, and the enlargement of the uterus.

As the fetus grows and the uterus and soft tissues in the pelvis stretch and swell, the bladder is pushed up and flattened somewhat. In late pregnancy, as the fetus settles into the pelvis, the part of the baby that is lowest in the womb puts pressure on the base of the bladder, which hampers the drainage of blood and lymph. Another consequence of increased pressure is that some urine stays in the ureters and bladder at most times.

The bladder, in its compressed state, simply cannot hold as much urine as it normally does. And since more urine is being produced by the kidneys, the result is the urge and need to pass more urine. For some women, the extra peeing becomes quite bothersome, waking them up in the middle of the night and creating the necessity of numerous extra ''pit stops'' on long trips.

In addition, the extra pressure on the bladder, combined with poor muscle tone in the pelvic floor—the muscles encircling the urethra, vagina, and anus—can cause a small, uncontrolled leakage of urine at unpredictable times. Urine may leak out upon sneezing, coughing, or laughing, or, less frequently, in a fairly constant drip.

CHANGES IN THE CERVIX, VAGINA, VULVA, AND PERINEUM

All women experience extra secretions of vaginal mucus during pregnancy. The amount of extra mucus and fluid flowing from the vagina varies from woman to woman. Some women find the secretions quite annoying, but for most women, this is not an inconvenience.

The increase in secretions is a result of the body's preparation of the vagina, cervix, vulva, and perineum (the tissue between the vagina and the anus) for the delivery. In the cervix, the tissue becomes soft and swollen. Mucus production increases, the mucous membranes thicken, and a thick mucus plug stops up the cervical canal, which prevents bacteria and other contaminants from reaching the fetus.

The perineum and vulva become more vascular, and their tissues soften in preparation for the stretching during birth. The vagina's connective tissue also softens. Because of the added veins and blood in the pelvic region, the vulva and vagina become an almost purple color. This is called ''Chadwick's sign.''

CHANGES IN THE CIRCULATORY SYSTEM

Pregnancy also makes the body produce more blood and lymph. When you become pregnant, your blood system undergoes major changes. Your heart has to work harder and pump more blood—about 40 percent more blood during a normal pregnancy—and the heart rate accelerates up to 15 percent. Your blood supply increases between 20 and 100 percent—mostly because of an increase in plasma. This increase in plasma volume alters the balance of fluids in your body. Even though your kidneys filter your blood up to 50 percent faster, you tend to retain more sodium in your tissues, which makes you retain water. Your veins and arteries usually become more elastic, and your vascular capacity expands to handle the additional blood volume and heart work. Blood pressure throughout a normal pregnancy is usually below what is normal for you in your prepregnant state.

In later pregnancy, the uterus becomes so large and heavy that it can completely compress the major vessels that underlie it when you lie down. These changes mean that lightheadedness is common when rising from lying to sitting or sitting to standing. You may find it harder to exercise, and when you do work out, you can't do it for as long. You may feel tired, and your ankles may swell.

CHANGES IN THE BREASTS

The breasts begin to change early in pregnancy. By the fourth week of gestation, they usually become tender and heavy, and you may feel like your breasts or nipples are tingling.

During the first trimester, the breasts enlarge quickly and continue to grow larger throughout the pregnancy. This is due in part to the engorgement of the vessels in the breasts. Milk ducts and glands that will produce milk after birth also enlarge.

The nipples enlarge, too, becoming darker and bumpier. During the latter half of pregnancy, the nipples often leak a yellow fluid, called colostrum, the forerunner of milk.

Every woman experiences different levels of sensation and discomfort in her breasts during her pregnancy. Some women find that these changes cause only temporary, mild discomfort; others can barely stand to have clothing touch their breasts because the nipples feel so sore. Sometimes the enlargement of the breasts causes backache because the additional weight and bulk of the breasts puts a strain on upper back muscles. Most women find that a maternity bra with good support provides relief.

ABDOMINAL CHANGES

As the internal organs shift inside, and as the uterus and baby grow, the muscles and skin of the abdomen must expand, too. Every woman "shows"—that is, her stomach becomes larger, her waist starts to thicken—at a different time. Most often, you'll first notice a change in your figure at the waist. By the fifth month of pregnancy, most women have had to switch to a maternity wardrobe.

In the last few months of pregnancy, your navel will pop up like a button or knob. Some women—first-time mothers especially—feel like their skin is "tight as a drum," or as if they will burst. They don't. The skin, fat, and muscle always stretch to accommodate the baby.

However, for about half of all women, the accommodation includes stretch marks (straie gravidarum). These are red or purple irregular lines that form on the underside and/or sides of the belly, thighs, buttocks, and breasts, as the connective tissue in the skin is overstretched. Rubbing oils into the skin does not prevent stretch marks, nor does keeping weight gain low; either you are genetically predisposed to them or you're not. Within two years after birth, the redness fades to a silvery white, but the lines themselves never fully disappear.

OTHER SKIN CHANGES

Many women also undergo other skin changes. About seven in ten white women get red raised patches with spidery veins running out of them—called *spider veins*—on their upper body; 10 percent of black women get them. After delivery, the spiders disappear.

Most women also get dark patches somewhere on their bodies. This is due to elevated levels of the hormones that stimulate the production of pigment. The darkening of the skin turns the nipples and areolae a darker brown, the belly button and the line from the navel to the pubic hair in the center of the stomach may also become brown (*linea negra*), and the perineum may turn brown as well. But all these changes reverse themselves in the early months after pregnancy.

Some other skin changes do not. One example: Elevated levels of sex steroids in the body can create blotchy dark spots on the face—called the "mask of pregnancy." These spots can fade after delivery, but may never go away completely.

The Stages of a Normal Labor

When the fetus begins to reach maturity, thirty-seven or thirty-eight weeks after fertilization, the shape of the uterus changes and the baby descends lower into the pelvis. Until now, the lowest part of the uterus—called the lower uterine segment—has not developed to the point where it can stretch enough to accommodate the baby for the birth process. Now the lower uterine segment is larger and more elastic, and the baby moves downward into it. You may have heard this referred to as the baby "dropping."

Braxton Hicks contractions—tightenings of the uterus that do not shorten or efface the cervix—increase in these last few weeks as well. The cervix begins to *ripen*—that is, to soften more and thin out or efface. Before actual labor begins, it is common for a woman's cervix to open partially, or dilate, a centimeter or two. It is also normal for the cervix to remain firm and high right up until the start of labor.

Usually, within hours to days of the onset of labor, the mucus plug that has stopped up the opening in the cervix is expelled through the vagina. This is called the *bloody show* because it is often tinged with a small amount of blood. At the same time, or soon thereafter, it is common for the amniotic sac to rupture—called *breaking the waters*—

releasing the amniotic fluid, which will drip or gush out of the vagina. But it's also normal for a woman to labor for hours before her waters break. Some doctors call this "prelabor."

Then, either before or after these two events, the uterus begins the contractions that will end in the birth of the baby. For almost everyone, giving birth is hard work. As any childbirth instructor will tell you, that's why they call it *labor.*

Generally, doctors and childbirth instructors separate the phases of labor into three distinct stages:

Stage One. The first stage of labor is the contractions that bring on the full effacement and dilation of the cervix. Normally the cervix is about two centimeters in length and has thick walls. The cervix is considered completely effaced and dilated when it is flat, with almost paper-thin edges, and is open approximately ten centimeters. The length of time that this process takes varies from one woman to another. Average length of time for this stage is twelve hours for first-time mothers; eight hours for women who have already had one or more babies. During stage one contractions, you may have diarrhea, a backache, and discomfort that ranges from mild to strong pain.

Stage Two. The second stage of labor is the expulsion of the baby from the womb. It starts when the cervix is completely dilated and ends when the fetus is expelled through the vagina. For first-time mothers, this phase takes nearly one hour; for women who've had other pregnancies, the second stage averages about twenty minutes. Labor pains—that is, pains from the contractions—are intense.

When the cervix is completely dilated, you usually have what feels like an uncontrollable urge to push or bear down and force the baby out. Up until now, your uterus has been doing all the work. Now you will feel as though you want to help by using all your stomach and back muscles to make the contractions more effective. When the baby's head can be seen through the opening of the vagina, it is called *crowning*—because it is almost always the crown of the baby's head that emerges first. Frequently, the doctor makes a small incision called an *episiotomy* to enlarge the vaginal opening so that the baby's passage does not rip the tissue. The second stage ends when the baby is delivered.

Stage Three. The third stage of labor begins right after delivery of the baby and ends with the delivery of the placenta—or afterbirth—and the membranes that surrounded the baby while you were pregnant. Compared to the rest of the labor, this stage is short. The placenta and the rest of the contents of the uterus usually come out within a few minutes after the baby is born, with one or two pushes on your part, and perhaps some pressure on your abdomen by the doctor.

Now that the baby and the placenta are outside your body, your uterus will quickly start to resume its old size and shape. Although this process will continue for some weeks, the majority of the shrinkage occurs within the first few hours following birth. It is normal for the uterus to continue to contract and for you to have some pain—called *afterpains*—for about four hours after the birth. These hours are sometimes called the *fourth stage* of labor. It is also at this time that the doctor will repair any tear in the perineum, or an episiotomy.

A TIME OF HEIGHTENED EMOTIONS FOR ALL WOMEN.

While all these physical changes—from conception to after the birth—are going on inside you, you will experience a wide range of emotions. In psychological terms, pregnancy is a life crisis, a milestone event that heralds the beginning of a new phase in your and your partner's lives. It is a time of excitement, of fear, of anticipation, and of ambivalence for all women.

"Each time I was pregnant, I worried, how will this affect my life?" said Genie, who had two "perfect" pregnancies and now has two healthy teenage daughters. "I very much wanted a second child, but I began to really worry. How was I going to do it all? I was filled with self-doubt. And I worried each time, was it a healthy child?"

Genie's experience is typical: Any number of different thoughts and concerns occupy new mothers-to-be. It is natural to wonder how the new member of the family will enhance or alter your relationships with your spouse and others who are close, such as parents. At some point in the pregnancy, you can expect to worry about whether you're ready to give up the freedom that just being a couple has given you. You may worry about your ability to be a good mother. You may be concerned about finances, about getting the baby's room ready, about whether the baby will inherit your husband's big ears. And, like Genie, all women worry at various points in the pregnancy about whether their baby will be "normal."

In other words, there's a great deal to consider and have feelings about when a woman is pregnant, under any circumstances.

Added to these event-generated feelings is the heightened emotionality that the physical changes of pregnancy bring on in most women. During pregnancy, the body produces tremendous amounts of hormones to sustain the fetus and help it grow and to assist your many tissues and organ systems in accommodating the extra life inside you. These hormones can affect your mood. You'll cry more easily, become agitated or upset more readily, and may be more excitable than you are normally.

Plus, as the pregnancy advances, especially in the last trimester, most women are physically uncomfortable. Everyone knows that when they aren't feeling their best, their mood is likely to reflect that. It's common to feel cranky and restless.

Many women are actively unhappy with the way pregnancy makes them look. You may feel ungainly, unattractive, and self-conscious, and your self-confidence may falter. "After one particular remark, I forbade my husband to make any comments about my size," Diane, who had a "perfect" pregnancy, told me. "One morning, around my eighth month, I was trying to help him make the bed. But I was so exhausted and miserable that I just lay down on it instead. So he says, 'Gee, honey, you look like a beached whale.' He didn't mean to be unkind, but I just got hysterical. And I *did* look like a beached whale. But I just couldn't hear it from him or anybody else without it making me very very upset."

Once pregnancy is over and the baby is born, it is normal and usual for this heightened emotional state to continue or even become temporarily more extreme. Post-partum depression, or the *baby blues*—feeling sad or depressed, with wide swings in mood—in the days and first weeks following the birth, is quite common. At this time, a woman's hormonal levels are again changing rapidly; at this time the uterus returns to its prepregnant state and the breasts begin to produce milk for the newborn. Some women find that they cannot shake their dark thoughts and must seek professional counseling in order to cope.

These are all universal feelings, true both when pregnancy *is* perfect, and when it isn't. Having a complicated pregnancy is likely, if anything, to intensify one's already sensitive emotions. It will help, as you read this book, and as you go through *your* complicated pregnancy, to remember that whatever you feel during this special time is normal, natural, and *completely* understandable under the circumstances. All pregnant women suffer from the blues and blahs now and then. And even the most complicated pregnancy has its normal parts, too. What you are feeling may just be a consequence of the normal part of your pregnancy!

3

Hyperemesis Gravidarum

I was nauseous practically from the first day of my pregnancy. I never did throw up, but I felt constantly on the verge. Only cereal, plain noodles, and, sometimes, cottage cheese sat well with me. By the beginning of my fourth month, though, the nausea started to subside. I remember feeling particularly brave one night and asking my husband to make fish for dinner. He spent hours in the kitchen preparing an elaborate meal of fresh vegetables, rice pilaf, and sole almondine. Just before he was ready to serve, I got the faintest whiff of fish cooking. My stomach reeled.

My husband looked so proud—and the meal looked so perfect—when he brought in my plate, that I didn't have the heart to tell him how awful I felt. I took a deep breath and reminded myself how hard he had worked on this meal, just for me. Yes, I would eat this meal, smiling. But my stomach didn't share my mental fortitude. I just couldn't do it. I took one bite, burst into tears, and had to ask him to take the dishes away. I ate dry toast and tea for dinner instead.

For most women, mine is a familiar story. By the time we get pregnant, the majority of us know that a little nausea, a little queasiness, and perhaps even some vomiting come as part of the territory during the first trimester. We call it "morning sickness." Actually, the term is misleading, as nausea and vomiting in pregnancy can happen at any time of the day or night. The pattern of each woman's morning sickness is different. Some only feel queasy and never vomit. Some women are only nauseated at night; others, only in the morning. Six out of ten of us will have some degree of nausea during our first sixteen weeks of pregnancy.

But for one to three in one thousand women this unpleasant side effect of pregnancy turns into a harrowing complication so debilitating that it requires hospitalization. For these few, the vomiting and nausea become constant and relentless. They sometimes vomit more than a dozen times a day, for days on end. Repeated loss of food and fluid creates a danger of dehydration, which in turn exacerbates the nausea.

Amy was one of these unlucky ones. She began to have indigestion and nausea immediately upon getting pregnant. She didn't know anybody else who vomited from morning sickness so often, only people who said they felt very queasy. But Amy had days when she just kept running to the bathroom and vomiting. She couldn't care for herself. Once she was so weak she blacked out in the shower.

"I remember one time," she told me, "during my second pregnancy, my husband was opening a can of salmon in the kitchen, and I was in the living room, two rooms over. Just the sound of the can opener was enough to make me start vomiting."

Amy had the complication called *hyperemesis gravidarum*. If left untreated, the effects of excessive vomiting can damage the kidneys and liver and ultimately threaten the life of both mother and child.

Duration and Prognosis

The key words to remember about hyperemesis are "if left untreated." Serious organ damage, or worse, happens only when vomiting and dehydration are left untreated—that is, when you don't consult your obstetrician and/or do not follow his advice and allow him to treat your condition. There is no reason, in this day and age, for a woman to die from hyperemesis. In other words, if you have this problem, your prognosis is excellent.

And so is your baby's. Possibly the best news about having this complication is that it will not result in your baby's being deformed, retarded, jaundiced, or small for gestational age. Hyperemesis will not make you develop hypertension or toxemia, and it will not make you miscarry or have preterm labor. With proper medical care, you and your baby should both fare well.

Carol vomited up to ten times a day for her entire pregnancy. She told me that as miserable as she felt, she tried to keep a positive attitude. After all, she said, she was "getting a baby out of the deal." Besides, she recalled, "some of my friends told me that the vomiting was a good sign—it meant the baby was taking hold."

In fact, pregnancies in which nausea and vomiting occur are more likely to have a favorable outcome than those without this problem. Another comforting thought: No matter how bad your vomiting problem is, it *will* end. Within three days of delivery, if your hyperemesis lasts until then, your appetite and ability to keep food down will be back to normal.

How long will your hyperemesis last? That depends on the individual. Although hyperemesis tends to lessen by the sixth month of pregnancy, some women report throwing up until the day they deliver. Even those women say that the nausea is not as bad during the last trimester.

But don't let the good statistics lull you into complacency. A good outcome for you and your baby depends upon your being responsible in the way you deal with the problem. You must discuss your vomiting with your obstetrician, and do exactly what he or she tells you to do. Following treatment instructions and, if your doctor thinks it is necessary, spending some time in the hospital are the two ways you can minimize the risk of serious complications that hyperemesis gravidarum can cause.

Why Are Women More Prone to Nausea During Pregnancy?

Some of the physical changes that the body goes through during pregnancy affect the digestive system and predispose you to vomiting. During the early months of pregnancy, the body produces massive amounts of hormones to sustain the fetus. These hormones work throughout the system, not just in the uterus. In the digestive tract, they also slow down peristalsis, the wavelike rhythmic contractions of the smooth muscles surrounding the intestines that move food through the system. Food travels through your system more slowly.

The hormones also relax a band of tissue at the bottom of the esophagus—the esophageal sphincter. This relaxation, combined with the upward pressure of the enlarging uterus on the stomach and other internal organs, often allows gastric juices to escape up into the esophagus. This causes the hot, burning sensation called *heartburn.*

As the uterus enlarges, it pushes up against and compresses the stomach, actually changing its shape. The stomach can no longer hold as much food as it did before pregnancy; it literally doesn't have the room. Couple this feeling of fullness with the slowdown of peristalsis and the sensation of heartburn in the lower esophagus, and add those extra hormones. The result: For 60 percent of women, nausea and vomiting. Women with hyperemesis have a heightened physical predisposition to vomit.

What Causes Hyperemesis?

The answer to this question, unfortunately, is that nobody knows for sure. There are some good guesses, however. The most-often-advanced medical theory is that severe vomiting occurs in women who have a particularly elevated level of human chorionic gonadatropin (hCG) in their bloodstream. HCG is essential for sustaining the fetus during early pregnancy. Doctors think hCG may be a factor in hyperemesis because its levels are normally rather high during the first trimester, the same time that nausea and vomiting are most common.

Another hormonal theory is that women who experience hyperemesis in pregnancy have higher levels of estradiol, the most powerful form of estrogen, in their bodies than women who do not suffer from excessive vomiting. The estradiol theory is relatively new, has not been proven conclusively, and is causing some controversy within the medical community. A third theory is that women with severe hyperemesis have an elevated thyroid function—hyperthyroidism—which causes the thyroid gland to produce too much thyroid hormone. There are more medical hypotheses that remain unproven.

The Emotional Factors

Almost every authority cites psychological factors as a key contributor to abnormal vomiting in pregnancy. According to these experts, as many as 80 percent of women with severe hyperemesis in pregnancy (those requiring hospitalization, intravenous feeding, and drug therapy) suffer definitive psychological problems that contribute to the vomiting problem. For example, the mother-to-be may be unusually fearful and uncertain about her ability to be a good mother to her unborn child. Or she may subconsciously resent her baby, and the vomiting could be a figurative rejection of the pregnancy. Another key psychological factor can be stress, either from the woman's job or at home.

Carol attributed her vomiting to her job's being stressful. She was a lawyer, and at the time she was pregnant, she was doing divorces—something she stopped after giving birth. She had cases to present in court all over her city, and she said that they made her tense. She even worked out a routine of vomiting into a paper bag outside the courthouse before she went to argue a case in front of a judge. She told me that she is much less "stressed out" now that she has stopped handling divorce cases. But, at the time, it was her job and she was obligated to her clients to keep going. She concluded that the stress of her job was a key factor in her vomiting.

Of course it is also natural, especially for a first-time mother, to worry a little about whether she is up to the job of motherhood. Certain fears about the pregnancy, its outcome, and the changes in the relationship between partners that a new life will bring are also quite normal. Ambivalence about the pregnancy is common as well. Thoughts such as "Do I really want this baby now?" and "I don't know if I'm ready to give up my freedom" are natural, understandable, and to be expected from time to time.

The problems arise when such natural questioning becomes overwhelming, and you find no outlet for dealing with the fears or expressing them to others. Perhaps you are worried that your partner might not understand your concerns or might make fun of them. Or perhaps you never knew anyone else who admitted to having such feelings, and so you feel abnormal, embarrassed, or ashamed about expressing yourself. Maybe you have spoken to someone you know and, not receiving the response you hoped for and needed, are afraid to talk about it again.

Whatever the reasons for her reticence, it is important for the woman with hyperemesis, and for her family, to be aware that there may be more than just physiological factors at work. However, don't make the mistake of assuming that if a psychological component is involved it means that the problem is "all in your head." Far from it. Hyperemesis is a real and potentially dangerous condition that requires close medical supervision. Resolving emotional difficulties, if they exist, usually provides some relief from the constant vomiting, but even if such psychic problems are dealt with, some degree of hyperemesis may remain.

How Do I Know I Have Hyperemesis and Not Just Morning Sickness?

Hyperemesis and morning sickness begin at the same time during pregnancy, usually around the fifth or sixth week of gestation. During pregnancy some vomiting is normal. Women who experience morning sickness may vomit several times a day during the first trimester. Hyperemesis is defined as severe, persistent vomiting that results in fluid and electrolyte disturbances and nutritional deficiencies.

The general symptoms that various medical textbooks advise doctors to look for to distinguish hyperemesis from morning sickness will help you make the distinction. You're suffering from hyperemesis if:

- Nausea and vomiting are severe and persistent—that is, you are vomiting repeatedly and cannot keep any food or liquid down.
- You become dehydrated (signs include skin losing elasticity, and a noticeable lowering of the volume of urine output).
- You have fainting spells that you associate with lack of food retention.
- You develop a fever but do not have other symptoms of illness other than the vomiting.
- You lose more than 5 percent of your body weight (if, for example, you began pregnancy at one hundred and twenty pounds and lose six pounds after the onset of vomiting).

In other words, if you are vomiting numerous times a day, feel that you aren't holding down any of the food you are trying to eat, and cannot keep liquids down either, you should call your obstetrician. Together you can figure out what the problem is.

You and your doctor may find it helpful if, before you call, you keep track of exactly how often you have vomited during the past twenty-four to forty-eight hours, how soon after a meal or a snack you vomit, and how much you think is coming up. Also, note any other symptoms you may have, such as faintness, fever, or a lower-than-normal urine output. If you haven't been keeping "score," try to recall these items and write them down, so you have something to refer to as you talk. That way you won't forget any information you meant to offer.

By giving your doctor complete information about your problem, you will also combat the tendency some physicians may have to discount your concern as overdramatization. Some medical texts to which doctors refer, or with which they received training, state that pregnant women tend to exaggerate descriptions of vomiting in terms of frequency and severity. Describing your subjective experience of nausea and vomiting is just that—subjective. Your obstetrician has nothing to go on but your account of the problem, so be as accurate as you can.

Treatment for Hyperemesis

STANDARD TREATMENTS

How aggressively your obstetrician treats your problem depends on how severe your symptoms are. The standard advice that doctors give their pregnant patients who suffer from slight to moderate nausea is:

- Eat light, dry foods (toast, crackers, broth). Have six small meals a day rather than three large ones.
- Increase fluid intake, but take fluids one hour after eating rather than with the meal.
- Rest.
- Try to eliminate sources of stress and conflict.
- If necessary, see a psychotherapist to identify and resolve conflicts.
- Take a mild sedative if your doctor prescribes one.
- Alter household routines so that you don't do the things that make you feel more nauseated.

For instance, if you are usually the cook, try to switch household routines with your mate. Have him cook, so you don't have to be near food when it's prepared. Or have friends and neighbors help out. During her second pregnancy, one woman I spoke to even had the neighbors come in and change her toddler's diaper because the smell made her too nauseated.

Another woman who talked to me offered this advice for fellow hyperemesis sufferers: "You have to realize that you are the one who knows when you can keep foods down. My advice is, avoid any possible situation that's going to start things off. I couldn't even look at prepared foods at the supermarket. You have to go with what your body's telling you."

If vomiting and nausea are severe, and you have been unable to keep anything down, or if you have developed a fever, are in pain, or are dehydrated, your obstetrician may admit you to the hospital for treatment. Most likely, the treatment will consist of:

- Complete bedrest until there is improvement. This may include an order for no bathroom privileges (on the theory that the less you move around, the less likely you are to throw up).
- No food by mouth for forty-eight hours.
- An intravenous drip of fluids that include all the nutrients your body needs for full nutrition and hydration (this is called parenteral feeding).

If you improve after forty-eight hours, you'll graduate to a dry diet of six small meals a day, with clear liquids, but you may still need the

IV until your doctor is sure you're out of any danger. If you don't improve, you may simply continue the intravenous feeding or be fed a well-balanced baby formula or other pureed food through a nasogastric tube (a tube placed into your stomach through your nose).

In addition, after discussing the probable sources of stress in your life that could be exacerbating your problem, your doctor may recommend psychotherapy. If he determines that the stress is caused by your living situation, your doctor may order no family visiting hours for you until you can hold down food again. He may also place you in a private room to help reduce your tension further.

In some instances, vomiting may continue despite this regimen. In those cases, one option is to continue on total parenteral feeding; this can be sustained, if necessary, for months. If you have to go this route, once you stabilize, your doctor may release you from the hospital and allow you to continue the feeding at home—under close medical supervision, of course.

Amy tried the IV-at-home routine, with good results. Her husband was a physician, which undoubtedly helped. Amy said she wanted to come home because her three-year-old daughter was quite traumatized by Amy's vomiting, and she worried that her little girl would become more upset if Mommy had to stay in the hospital.

"Being at home with the IV was difficult," Amy said. "But at least I was home. In the long run, I may have been better off being in the hospital, because I think I would have been more relaxed." But she said, the IV calmed down her stomach and ended the cycle of vomiting. And, most important, her daughter was reassured that Amy was home.

HOSPITAL TESTS AND PROCEDURES

Whenever you are admitted to the hospital during your pregnancy, there are certain tests and procedures that are routine. These are explained in Chapter 14, What to Expect When You Go to the Hospital. Besides that standard drill, there will most likely also be laboratory workups that are specific to your hyperemesis condition. Your doctor will want to rule out any physical cause of your vomiting other than pregnancy. He will want to monitor your body's fluids, so that he can order the correct intravenous regimen. He will also want to check out your mineral levels and electrolytes to make sure you have not sustained any organ damage.

What this means is that nurses, residents, or interns will probably take blood samples at least several times during your stay, and you'll be asked for urine samples on a regular basis. In some instances, your doctor may order the nurses to monitor closely your fluid output and intake. Your urine will be collected; so will your vomit. The staff will also carefully monitor the liquid you're taking in through intravenous feeding.

And you will have to have an intravenous line put in, so that you can take nourishment (remember, nothing by mouth for forty-eight hours in many cases) and stay hydrated. Properly installed, an IV is not painful, and after a short while, you will often forget that it is there. It does hurt or sting going in, but not a lot, and the pain will disappear after five or ten minutes at the most. All this may be bothersome, but it is necessary for the proper treatment of your condition.

WHAT ABOUT ANTI-NAUSEA DRUGS?

Your doctor may also prescribe one of a number of anti-nausea drugs (called antiemetics) to stop your vomiting if the total bedrest, no-food-by-mouth, intravenous treatment seems not to be working and you continue to lose weight and/or you have kidney or liver complications. In general, the obstetrical community has moved away from drug therapy for hyperemesis, as none of the drugs on the market has conclusively been proven safe for use during pregnancy.

When you are thinking about the safety of anti-nausea drugs, or any drug during pregnancy for that matter, it is important to understand that in medicine, as in the rest of science, there are very few absolutes. No good doctor will promise you that there are no risks in a given course of treatment, no matter how good its safety record. That's because there is always the slightest chance—the one-in-a-million odds—that something may go wrong. When risk is that small, it is often better to accept that remote possibility and to go ahead than to be scared away by a statistic and refuse a treatment that could help you or even save your life.

Rather than panic if your physician wants to prescribe drug therapy for your vomiting problem, you will do better to ask him, in a nonconfrontational way, for the information you feel you need to make a reasoned decision about whether to take the medicine. You may want to ask him to tell you specifically why he wants you to take this medication and what risk you run if you do not. You could ask what alternative courses of action are open to you, what the side effects of the medication are, if any, and whether there are conclusive studies showing effects on the fetus. If there are no conclusive study results, you could also ask what the preliminary results have been so far. You would also want to know if there are likely to be long-term effects for you or your baby.

Most of the drugs that can be prescribed to relieve hyperemesis fall into three categories, in terms of their demonstrated safety:

- Those drugs about which studies have demonstrated no fetal risk in animals and there have been no studies in women;
- Those drugs about which studies have shown some adverse effect on animal fetuses, and there are no confirmed problems in women during the first trimester; and
- Those drugs about which studies have found adverse effects on animal fetuses, and no controlled risk studies have been done in humans.

These may be the categories your doctor uses in explaining the potential risks of the drug he chooses for your treatment. Your doctor will not administer drugs from the third category unless the potential benefit of taking them justifies the risk to your baby.

Since every case of hyperemesis, like every pregnancy, is different, your doctor will be working with the objective laboratory data he gets on your condition, as well as his subjective feeling about your unique circumstances. Most medical texts warn doctors to shy away from drug treatment for hyperemesis unless absolutely necessary. If you trust your doctor, you may assume that he would not ask you to take an anti-nausea medication unless he really thinks it is required in your particular case.

Oral Hygiene: An Ounce of Prevention . . .

There is another kind of physical damage caused by hyperemesis, one that you might not normally be inclined to think about—damage to the teeth and gums. When you vomit frequently, the acid from the stomach can eat away the tooth enamel, cause gum tenderness and swelling, and, if not treated, can lead to gum loss and tooth decay. The amount of tooth erosion from stomach acids relates directly to how often you are throwing up and for how many months.

Every time you vomit, the backs of the teeth, especially the upper teeth, are bathed with strong acid. Over a nine-month period, if you do not engage in vigorous preventive measures, the loss of tooth enamel can be extensive.

All women are more prone to certain dental problems during pregnancy. Hormonal levels make the gums and soft tissues of the mouth more susceptible to swelling, erosion, and inflammation. During a normal pregnancy, the American Dental Association recommends that you see your dentist at least once every three months for tooth cleaning, instead of the usual semi-annual visit. Brushing more frequently and avoiding sugary foods that promote tooth decay are also recommended.

But if you have vomiting problems during your pregnancy, seeing a dentist three times in nine months is not enough. At the very least, each time you throw up you should immediately clear any debris from your mouth and rinse your mouth thoroughly with cool water.

If you can tolerate the taste (that is, if it doesn't make you nauseated all over again), and if you have no other complications that might make extra salt intake dangerous (such as a hypertensive disorder), instead of rinsing with plain water, try rinsing with a mixture of one teaspoon of baking soda dissolved in a glass of water. This will actually neutralize the acids remaining in the mouth, further reducing the possibility of damage to the teeth and gums. Before you start rinsing with it, you should consult your obstetrician about whether you can safely use bicarbonate of soda.

In addition, it would be wise—again, if you can tolerate the tastes—to brush your teeth with toothpaste. Follow up with a fluoride rinse. Fluoride speeds the remineralization process in your teeth.

In the most severe hyperemesis cases, you can even have your dentist construct a physical barrier for you, much like the dental retainers fitted for people who have just had their braces taken off. The device should be inexpensive and could be quite effective. However, for the few months that you will be vomiting, such a barrier is usually not medically necessary.

Your best bet is to go with the simple measures. Rinse with water or, better yet, with baking soda and water each and every time you vomit. Follow by brushing your teeth and rinsing with a fluoride rinse. And when you are up and around, make sure you get to the dentist for a consultation, just to make sure that what you're doing is working for you.

Finally, try to remember that no matter how bad the vomiting gets, it will end. You will go back to eating food and liking it. You are not sick, you are pregnant! As my friend Carol reminded herself: ''You're getting a baby out of the deal.''

4

Placenta Previa

Jennifer was thirty-one weeks' pregnant when the bleeding started. "I was sitting in a chair on my front lawn, watching my daughter ride her bike. And I felt a gush. I thought it was just the usual discharge I'd had through my pregnancy. But then there was a second gush, and a third. My best friend was sitting next to me, and I told her, 'There's something wrong.' We got me to the house and into the bathroom. It was blood, lots of blood and clots. My husband works the night shift, so I woke him up and he drove me to the hospital." Jennifer was given drugs to prevent contractions and was transferred to a metropolitan hospital by helicopter. She stayed in the city hospital for five weeks. "I never did bleed again," she said. Her six-pound boy was born by cesarean section at thirty-six and a half weeks, with mature lungs and no complications. When she told me her story, little Jesse was seven weeks old and weighed over twelve pounds. Mother and son were doing just fine.

Jennifer's was a classic case of *placenta previa*. It happens when the placenta—the spongy mass of blood vessels and tissue that forms within the uterus to supply the baby with nutrition via the umbilical cord—forms unusually low in the uterus and covers part or all of the cervix. The first symptom is usually bright red, painless bleeding that comes between the twenty-eighth and thirty-eighth weeks of pregnancy. The initial episode of bleeding may or may not be followed by others. The mother is invariably placed on bedrest, under strict medical supervision, and is delivered as close to term as possible, almost always by cesarean section. And, in the vast majority of cases, both mother and child do quite well.

A GREAT PROGNOSIS—NINE OUT OF TEN PREVIAS
SELF-CORRECT.

Up to 43 percent of all pregnancies start with the placenta lying close to, or even over, the cervical opening (called the cervical os— the opening from the uterus to the vagina). But by the end of the second trimester, almost all placentas have migrated higher up inside the uterus, safely away from the cervix. Only one in two hundred to two hundred fifty pregnancies that result in a live birth go into the third trimester with a placenta previa. And even in nine out of ten of these, by the time the woman is ready to deliver, the placenta has moved up out of the way.

So that's the good news. If you've been diagnosed as having a placenta previa, you have a 90 percent chance that the condition will correct itself by the time your baby is ready to be born. Even if you've had terrible bleeding problems. Even though you're hospitalized for this complication, or you've been sent home on strict bedrest. That means that you've got an excellent shot at a normal, uncomplicated, vaginal birth. It's highly likely that your unborn child will be just fine, as will you. In fact, even if your placenta is one of those that doesn't get out of the way, your chances of having a great outcome for both you and the baby are remarkably high.

That's not to say that placenta previa is a minor problem. It's potentially a very serious complication. But with proper medical attention, the worst possibility—fatal hemorrhage, for both mother and child—never comes to pass. Less than one-half of 1 percent of women with previas suffer fatal complications; nine out of ten babies survive.

Still, there are certain problems associated with placenta previa. For the mother, repeated or severe bleeding can result in anemia (low red blood cell count) and low blood volume, both of which can be countered through transfusions. There is also the possibility of hemorrhage before or after delivery, because of the failure of the uterus to contract tightly enough to shut off blood vessels opened when the low-lying placenta detaches from the uterine wall. This can result in shock, which is treated by infusion with intravenous fluids and blood products, and may require drug therapy to assist the uterus in contracting well. Also, a woman with placenta previa may get a uterine infection after delivery. This is treated with oral or intravenous antibiotics.

Women who have had one or more previous cesarean section(s) and a subsequent placenta previa may have a condition called *placenta accreta,* in which the placenta forms an unusually firm attachment to the uterine wall. This leads to severe bleeding when the doctor tries to deliver the placenta and may require hysterectomy as the only workable treatment.

For the baby, the gravest danger after birth is respiratory distress syndrome (inability to breathe properly and take in enough oxygen) due to premature delivery. With modern neonatal intensive care facilities and topflight medical care, babies born with respiratory distress do better now than ever before, although some suffer visual and hearing loss and learning problems, even with the best of care. And some babies do still die.

Placenta previa can also cause the baby to be small for gestational age (called "intrauterine growth retardation"—see Chapter 5). Babies of mothers with placenta previa seem too to have a higher incidence of jaundice at birth (readily treated by exposure to special lights in the neonatal intensive care nursery). And about 10 percent of babies of mothers with placenta previa lose some blood along with the mother when bleeding occurs in the uterus. Sometimes the bleeding is severe enough that the baby needs a transfusion shortly after birth.

Despite this list of possible complications and side effects, the vast majority of women with placenta previa and their babies have an excellent outcome from the pregnancy. Remember, nine out of ten previas self-correct. Those are great odds to hold onto while you wait for your child to be born.

The Placenta: Form, Function, Formation

The placenta (Latin for a circular or flat cake) is a disc-shaped spongy organ that forms during pregnancy and is expelled from the body by the uterus shortly after the fetus is born. By passing nutrients and oxygen from the mother to the fetus, the placenta acts as the growing baby's lungs, liver, and kidneys. It also produces several of the hormones necessary to sustain the pregnancy.

The development of the placenta is a complex process that actually begins just after conception, when the cells start to divide and multiply and begin taking on the different functions that will eventually become the fetus, the placenta, the umbilical cord, and so on. Within six to seven days after conception, the fertilized egg has divided into many cells and formed a hollow ball—called the blastocyst—and has traveled out of the fallopian tube into the uterus. The hollow ball then implants itself in the uterine lining (the endometrium), where it begins to produce the hormones to sustain the pregnancy.

After a series of cellular changes, the blastocyst cells connect with the mother's capillaries and begin to form areas that will later serve as the spaces in the uterine lining through which oxygen and nutrients pass from her blood to the baby's.

By the time twenty-one days have elapsed, the fetus has established its own blood supply, which is filtered through what is rapidly becoming a dense forest of fingerlike projections called *chorionic villi*. Within forty to fifty days of conception, the villi have branched, like upside-down trees, into masses called cotyledons. Eventually there will be ten to twelve main cotyledons, forty to fifty medium-sized, and about one hundred fifty rudimentary ones. The cotyledons lie in the spaces in the uterine lining. The mother's blood and lymph flow around the cotyledons, delivering oxygen, nutrition, and antibodies that are then carried to the baby. The mother's blood also picks up waste products passed by the baby's blood in the cotyledons. The baby's blood and the mother's blood do not actually mix.

At first, the placenta is quite small. By the beginning of the second trimester, it is the same size as the fetus. When the baby is born, the placenta is usually about one-sixth her weight, or one pound, and about six inches in diameter and around three-quarters of an inch thick. The body expels the placenta after the baby is born (hence the term *afterbirth)*, and its condition is a useful diagnostic tool for the obstetrician, who can tell from looking at it whether certain neonatal complications are likely.

Under normal circumstances, the placenta tends to form in that portion of the uterus that has the best blood supply—the front, back, or top of the upper two-thirds of the womb—in the same place that the fertilized egg implants after it travels down the fallopian tube into the uterus. Sometimes, however, implantation and then growth of the placenta are in the bottom third of the uterus, where the walls are thinner and the mother's blood supply is not as great. When the placenta develops here, it often covers some or all of the cervical os—or opening—and is called a placenta previa.

Possible Causes of Placenta Previa

No one is really certain why the placenta forms too low in some women and not in others, although the medical community has identified some factors that seem to increase the likelihood of placenta previa: if the woman has had one or more cesarean sections or other surgery that left a uterine scar; if she has had five or more pregnancies (in which case she is called a *grand multipara);* or if she is over the age of thirty-five. Placenta previa is also more common in women who have had previous pregnancies than in those who have never been pregnant before. Women who have had one previa in a previous pregnancy are significantly more likely to have another than a woman who has never had a previa.

The common thread here seems to be damage to the uterine lining, or endometrium. With the grand multipara, the theory is that each pregnancy damages that part of the uterine lining that lies underneath the placenta—that is, makes it less well-supplied by blood than other areas. As implantation tends to occur in the area of the uterus best supplied by blood, a woman who has had many pregnancies is more likely to have an implant where no damage has been done before— lower in the uterus.

But a woman who has had one or more c-sections—usually performed on the lower part of the uterus—and thus has damage to the uterine lining there, also has an increased chance of a previa. One theory here is that the scar may alter the blood supply to the area or alter the uterine lining in some way. It may also change the shape of the uterus. Another theory suggests that the scarring may require the placenta to grow to a larger-than-normal size, to compensate for the reduced blood supply of the lining. And the larger the placenta, the more likely it is to encroach on the cervical opening.

Are All Previas the Same?

No. There are degrees of placenta previa, each named for the amount of the cervical opening covered by the placenta. A *total* placenta previa (placenta previa "centralis") covers the entire cervical os. A *partial* placenta previa (placenta previa "partialis") extends over part to most of the cervical opening. A *marginal* placenta previa (placenta previa "marginalis") can range from barely encroaching upon the opening to within six centimeters (or about two and a half inches) of the cervical os. This last category is also called *low-lying placenta* or a *low implantation*.

The total previa is the least likely to migrate up and out of the way as the pregnancy progresses. The marginal or low-lying previa is the most likely to move up to a better position. All three types of previa can cause severe bleeding problems.

Why Does the Placenta Bleed When It's a Previa?

As the pregnancy progresses, both the baby and the placenta grow larger, requiring the uterus to stretch to accommodate them. Especially during the last trimester, the lower third of the uterus (called the *lower uterine segment*) stretches and thins somewhat, both to make room for the developing fetus and in preparation for the birth. This stretching and thinning often cause a low-lying placenta to tear somewhat at its margins, causing bleeding.

If the placenta is lying partially or totally over the cervical opening, bleeding is virtually assured at some point. As every woman comes closer to term, the cervix begins to soften and change shape in preparation for the birth. It shortens (effaces) and begins to open up (dilates). Many women have some degree of these cervical changes weeks before labor begins. These cervical movements create a problem for the placenta in a previa position. As the cervix starts to open up, it shears off the blood-filled placental attachments on top of it, causing the mother to bleed, sometimes dangerously.

If the woman is at term and begins to labor, or goes into labor prematurely, the shearing becomes worse, and bleeding increases. Since the lower part of the uterus does not contain strong muscle tissue that contracts well, the blood vessels that open up from the shearing of the placenta tend not to be clamped off well, even during contractions. Unattended to, the bleeding can be catastrophic for both the mother and the child.

Fortunately, the vast majority of previas are discovered before disastrous bleeding occurs. First bleeding episodes are rarely life-threatening. Rather, they are a serious warning sign. Properly treated, the mother's condition can be stabilized, and an uneventful birth by cesarean takes place at or close to term.

How Will I Know I've Got Placenta Previa?

There are two ways you are likely to find out that your placenta is too low. Either you'll start to bleed one day out of the blue, or your doctor will discover your condition during an ultrasound exam that he's ordered for another reason.

For example, Colleen's previa was diagnosed by an ultrasound that her doctor had ordered because he felt that she was carrying much too large for the amount of time she had been pregnant, which might have meant she was carrying twins or had another complication that causes too much amniotic fluid to form. With an ultrasound scan, he found that at thirty weeks, she had a total placenta previa. After eight weeks of complete bedrest, Colleen gave birth, via c-section at thirty-eight weeks, to a healthy baby boy. And although her placenta never migrated away from her cervix, she never bled once during the entire pregnancy.

While more and more previas are being discovered earlier in pregnancy, most of us with placenta previa still find out we have it in the old-fashioned way: One day, unexpectedly, we simply begin to bleed.

Sometimes the flow is heavy; for others it's just a little spotting. My placenta previa showed up unusually early (very early second trimester). I had gone to the bathroom and happened to look down and was astounded to find the bowl bright red with what I thought had to be a tremendous amount of blood. I never even felt it happen—no pain, nothing. I continued to bleed for about an hour—a panic call to the doctor told me to lie down and not get out of bed except to pee until forty-eight hours after the bleeding stopped—and then gradually the bleeding slowed down and turned darker, until it finally turned brown.

In my case, one of my twins was a low implantation, and the leading edge (closest to the cervical opening) had torn. I had a number of other "bleeds" before the placenta grew upward away from my cervix and the problem resolved itself.

Except for the timing, mine were classic symptoms: bright red blood that shows up with no pain or cramping.

What to Do if You Start to Bleed

[Note: If you have already read Chapter 9, Bleeding, Hemorrhage, and Placental Abruption, the following four sections will be repetitive for you. However, placenta previa is a serious complication, which almost always results in bleeding. Therefore the information bears repeating here.]

If you experience these or similar symptoms, or any kind of bleeding during your pregnancy, call your doctor immediately, *no matter what time it is.* Call him even if it's just a tiny spot of blood. Any time during pregnancy, except when you expel the mucus plug just prior to a full-term labor, bleeding is a sign that something is wrong. Don't stand on ceremony or worry about waking the doctor up. Getting calls in the middle of the night comes with the territory of being an obstetrician.

If you are not bleeding heavily, your doctor can tell you whether he wants to see you immediately, whether you can wait to see him, and whether he'll see you at his office or in the hospital. He will explain to you that bleeding during pregnancy can be caused by many conditions, most of which are benign.

A Word About Describing the Bleeding

Your doctor is going to want to know whether you are bleeding only slightly, moderately, or heavily. You are probably going to be a little upset (to say the least) at the sight of bright red blood coming out of your body, and you are likely to overestimate how much blood has passed. Nonetheless, try to be as objective as you can in describing your problem to the doctor. Are you just spotting, like you would at the beginning or end of a period? Is it every time you go to the bath-room? Are you soaking through pads every few hours, every hour? (If it's every few minutes, go to the hospital right away. . . . Is the blood bright red, like from a cut? Or is it darker? Try to estimate amounts and to decide whether you feel that it's subsiding or not. Your OB is going to make his judgment based on what you tell him. So try as hard as you can not to minimize or to dramatize.

If you are bleeding heavily (a cup or more at a time, or persistently soaking through pads at a rapid rate), or if you wake up in the middle of the night in a pool of blood, call the doctor's office or service and tell them you are on the way to the hospital and very briefly why. Don't wait for the doctor to get back to you; just get to the hospital as quickly as you can. His explanations about potential causes can wait. His answering service will tell him to meet you there.

If you haven't been instructed earlier to go directly to the labor and delivery or maternity section of the hospital, go to the emergency room. Don't wait for your husband or neighbor to park the car. He'll find you. If the ER is crowded, for heaven's sake, don't stand on line or wait around for others to take their turn. Get yourself attended to *right away*. Prompt, excellent care is key to a good outcome. Usually, and especially at night, there is a guard or attendant right at the door who will quickly get you a wheelchair or put you on a guerney (table with wheels) and make sure that someone comes to your aid.

It will help you stay calmer if you know these facts:

- The bleeding is not necessarily from a placental problem. There are many other reasons for bleeding of this sort, such as blood vessels in the outside of the cervix or vagina rupturing or lesions in the vaginal walls.
- It is extremely rare for a first bleed from a placenta previa of any kind to be fatal to either the mother or the baby.
- With modern diagnostic tests, you will find out quickly what is causing the bleeding.

How Will the Hospital Treat My Placenta Previa?

If you rush to the hospital with profuse, bright red, vaginal bleeding, you should be prepared for some drastic intervention on the part of your doctor and the hospital staff. Exactly how they will treat you will depend on how many weeks along you are, whether you have also started having contractions or are in active labor, just how badly you are bleeding, and whether your baby is in distress.

Essentially, there are two standard courses of treatment: immediate delivery by cesarean; or what doctors call "expectant management"— that is, strict, in-hospital bedrest and frequent monitoring until the baby is mature enough to live without a respirator outside the womb. Either way, you can expect some rapid initial testing and procedures:

- The doctor will examine your abdomen to determine whether the uterus is soft (meaning you're not having contractions) and to assess the position of the baby.
- He will listen to your heart and check your blood pressure (which can help to tell him how much blood you've lost).
- He will place a fetal monitor on you to find your baby's heartbeat and assess the baby's condition. This is a noninvasive microphone that is strapped to your belly along with some jelly to conduct the sound waves. A second monitor will check to see whether you are having contractions, and if so, their intensity and how far apart they are.
- The doctor will insert an intravenous line into your arm and start infusing you with fluids to replace the blood you've lost and prevent shock and to ready a vein in case you need a transfusion or drugs to stop contractions.
- The nurse will draw several blood samples from you to type your blood and check it for infection and composition (another way to tell how severe the blood loss is).
- You will have an ultrasound scan of your uterus to assess the exact position of the placenta and the baby and determine whether the placenta is really the cause of the bleeding. (Some hospitals now use magnetic resonance imaging [MRI] for the scan instead of ultrasound. This is a noninvasive test that uses magnetic waves to create images of your tissues.)
- If you are in labor, the doctor may start you on tocolytic drugs to stop the contractions, because contractions can worsen the bleeding.
- The doctor may also perform an amniocentesis to assess the lung maturity of your baby.

All of these procedures and tests will probably happen in rapid succession if you come in bleeding heavily. More time can be taken if the bleeding is slowing down or has stopped. You'll probably be asked to use a bedpan if you need to urinate, on the theory that the more you move around, the more likely you are to provoke more bleeding.

Or the doctor may order the insertion of a catheter (a plastic or rubber tube) into your bladder to drain urine, so that you don't have to move at all. Having a tube stuck up your urethra (the natural tube through which you pass urine from the bladder to the outside of the body) is a bit painful, especially when you are tense. But the pain lasts only as long as it takes to insert the tube—usually less than thirty seconds. Once the catheter is in place, you won't feel a thing.

A Note About Your Feelings

If you go to the hospital with a bleeding emergency, it will be absolutely normal for you to feel overwhelmed and frightened. The rapid change of scene, the frenetic pace of the treatment you'll be receiving, and your concerns about the well-being of the baby are likely to scare and disorient you. You will also feel grateful for the intervention and efficiency of the staff and safer knowing that you're in the hands of people who can help you.

Remember that the staff will be working fast to give you and your baby the best chance of making it to term, and the urgent nature of your problem may make staff dispense with the niceties.

This doesn't mean that you should give up all your say in the matter. If you have questions, ask them. If you have concerns about some procedure, say so. Don't assume that, just because you are in the hospital, everybody who enters your room is going to know completely about your condition. You must take responsibility for informing people about what's going on with you, for your own sake.

One story—repeated to me in other versions by other women with previas—is especially apt. Ann was hospitalized for placenta previa for ten weeks before giving birth by cesarean to her seven-pound, thirteen-ounce son. One day, after she had been in the hospital several weeks, she had another bleeding episode and was rushed downstairs to the labor and delivery suite. A medical student who was unaware of her real condition came in and told Ann that he was going to give her a pelvic exam (routine and frequent with women who are at term and in normal labor, to check the amount of dilation of the cervix). Ann refused, because she knew that with placenta previa, even gentle probing with a finger in the late second trimester or third trimester can provoke uncontrollable bleeding. Had she allowed the student to proceed, it could have been a disaster.

For a woman with placenta previa, pelvic or rectal exams are *never* supposed to be done unless she has been taken to a delivery room or operating room set up and completely ready for an emergency c-section (called a *double set-up*). That means a full team of nurses, her doctor, a pediatrician on hand for the baby, and an anesthesiologist standing by. It also means preparing her abdomen for surgery (shaving, disinfecting) and having several units of blood on hand to replace lost blood.

IF YOU ARE THIRTY-SIX WEEKS OR MORE ALONG . . .

If you have reached your eighth month of pregnancy, and the baby's lungs are mature, and your previa has started bleeding, it is common to deliver the baby immediately, rather than risk full labor and more severe blood loss. That means that the hospital staff will prepare you for a cesarean. Chapter 13 will tell you everything you need to know about the procedure. The one twist with placenta previa is that if it is a true emergency operation, you will probably have general anesthesia instead of regional anesthesia, and so you may be asleep for the birth.

IF YOU ARE LESS THAN THIRTY-SIX WEEKS PREGNANT . . .

If you are less than thirty-six weeks pregnant, it is likely that your baby's lungs have not matured sufficiently to allow her to breathe on her own outside the womb. In that case, unless your situation is critical, your doctor is going to do his utmost to keep you pregnant until the baby can breathe without assistance.

What does that mean for you? Well, complete bedrest, most likely in the hospital, for as long as it takes (or as long as you can hold out before going into labor—up to 25 percent of women with bleeding previas go into labor spontaneously when they bleed). However, staying in the hospital long-term is extremely expensive, not to mention disruptive of your lifestyle. If you are financially unable to handle weeks in the hospital, or if you have other small children at home, your doctor may allow you to rest at home once your condition has stabilized, if you can meet certain restrictions.

Most physicians will allow you to rest at home only if you live no farther than fifteen to twenty minutes from the hospital and have reliable transportation and if another adult can be with you at all times in case you start to hemorrhage. If you do go home, you will have to follow your doctor's instructions to the letter, for your own safety as well as for the well-being of your child. You will be on bedrest either until the baby's lungs are mature or the previa self-corrects and moves up out of the way (remember, this happens in 90 percent of all cases).

If you must spend more than a few days on bedrest in the hospital, it may help you to read chapters 14 and 15. Chapter 14 discusses long-term hospital stays; Chapter 15 will answer your questions about what to expect from prolonged bedrest and how to cope with it.

New Developments in the Treatment of Placenta Previa

Recent Advances in Ultrasonography

Ultrasound testing involves extremely high-frequency sound waves that are inaudible. In ultrasonography, these sound waves are directed at a hidden part of the anatomy, and their reflected echoes are then translated into a picture of that organ or cavity.

The procedure is completely painless and noninvasive: The woman lies on a table with her abdomen bared. A technician puts a conductive gel on the abdomen and presses an electronic "microphone" in a circular motion on the gel until she is able to get a clear image of the uterus and baby inside. This image is projected on a monitor, like a picture on a television. The technician working the ultrasound equipment can even take photographs of the image and then develop them, like X rays, on film.

Ultrasound has been used for diagnostic purposes in pregnancy for some years and is presumed completely safe for both fetus and mother, although no long-term follow-up studies have been completed to confirm this. The reigning consensus among the medical community is that ultrasound is much safer for the unborn child than X rays, which are known to pose a health risk and are not as accurate.

Until recently, ultrasound of the uterus was done only through the mother's abdomen (transabdominally). Images taken through abdominal tissues are 95 to 98 percent accurate. But sometimes, especially for images of the cervix and lower third of the uterus, the density of the mother's overlying tissues (bladder, muscles, fat) obscures the images or makes them cloudy.

Since 1987, advances in ultrasound technology have made it possible to image the cervix and lower portion of the uterus with almost 100 percent accuracy. The images are taken transvaginally—with sound waves directed up the vaginal cavity directly at the cervix. Since no other tissue is in the way, the cervix, and the placenta above it, are clearly visible on the screen, making it easy to see exactly what degree of placenta previa is present.

If the woman's condition is so unstable that it is unwise to place the transducer (the *microphone*) into the vagina at all, clear images can also be obtained by using the ultrasound machine against the perineum (the skin between the vaginal opening and the anus).

Not all physicians have training in the use of these new methods, nor do all hospitals and clinics have the equipment to perform transvaginal and transperineal ultrasound. But it is worthwhile asking your obstetrician about the possibility of its use, since the new procedures reduce the margin of error significantly.

New Use for an Old Technique: Cerclage

Cerclage (French for "hooping" or "circling") is a minor surgical procedure, done with anesthesia in the hospital, in which a suture or stitch (one to several) is placed around or through the cervix to keep it tightly closed. Doctors usually prescribe cerclage when the woman has a weak or "incompetent" cervix—that is, one that prematurely opens (dilates) or shortens (effaces), leading to premature labor and birth. Cerclage has long been a proven aid in prolonging pregnancy under such conditions.

Now, some obstetricians are successfully using cerclage to prolong the pregnancies of women with placenta previa. By keeping the cervix closed with a suture, less shearing—and therefore less bleeding—seems to occur. Recent studies indicate that cerclage, combined with bedrest and, in some cases, drugs to prevent contractions, helps women with previas maintain their pregnancies long enough to allow the baby to develop mature lungs.

Many doctors still consider cerclage an experimental treatment for placenta previa, so there is not yet consensus within the medical community on its benefits. However, it is reasonable to discuss this development with your obstetrician to see whether cerclage is an avenue open to you under your unique circumstances.

Banking Your Own Blood

If your doctor discovers your condition early enough in your pregnancy, you may be able to take advantage of a recent advance in treatment: storage of your own blood for later transfusion. Many women with placenta previa require transfusions before or at delivery.

As recently as 1987, using your own blood was not even an option in most parts of the United States. But with spreading fear of contamination of the U.S. blood supply by the AIDS virus and hepatitis, doctors have started to rethink the position that a pregnant woman should not bank her own blood.

The technology also exists to recapture blood lost through vaginal bleeding, clean it and replace it intravenously in the woman's body. This is called *autotransfusion.* The American Medical Association's Council on Scientific Affairs endorses autotransfusion as a practice, stating that "the safest blood a patient can receive is his own." And, according to the council, autotransfusion is as economic or less expensive than giving a woman blood from a blood bank.

Autotransfusion is still limited in obstetrics and gynecology practice—principally due to lack of training in its use for obstetric purposes and unfamiliarity with or lack of the proper equipment. But a growing number of physicians are beginning to view the practice as the wave of the future.

However, autotransfusion does have its limitations: It isn't recommended for women with blood contaminated with bacteria, or for women with cancer (because blood-carried cancer cells could cause cancer to develop in other areas of the body).

As there is no safer blood supply than one's own, these are options that you should definitely discuss with your obstetrician.

5

Intrauterine Growth Retardation (IUGR)

I was lying in my OB's examining room waiting for the results of a sonogram I'd had to assess any changes in the placenta previa affecting one of my twins. I was about twenty weeks along and hadn't had a bleeding episode for sixteen days. When my doctor came into the room, she looked a little subdued, but her tone was upbeat: "Laurie, I've got some good news and some bad news for you." The good news was that the previa had corrected itself, so I wouldn't be bleeding anymore.

The bad news, she said, "is you have to stay on bedrest. Your upper twin is showing signs of having intrauterine growth retardation."

I didn't like the sound of that. What the hell was intrauterine growth retardation? My doctor explained that one of the babies was now smaller than it should be for the length of time I'd been pregnant. It didn't mean the baby would be mentally handicapped, just that she'd be born smaller than normal, with a lot of catching up to do.

What it did mean, she told me, was that I'd have to be on total bedrest to allow the smaller baby to take as much nutrition and oxygen from my body as possible. I'd probably deliver a couple of weeks early (common anyway with twins). I should go home and try not to worry. Both babies were likely to be all right at birth. In fact, the little one might just be genetically predisposed to petiteness and not be growth-retarded at all. I should consider the prescription of bedrest at this point a necessary precaution. If the baby really turned out to have growth retardation, I'd be doing everything possible to assist her proper growth. We scheduled another sonogram for three weeks later. The doctor would know better then how the smaller baby was growing.

What Exactly Is Intrauterine Growth Retardation?

Intrauterine growth retardation—IUGR, for short—is a term that describes a complication that principally affects the fetus rather than the mother. Doctors define a child with IUGR as one who at birth falls below the tenth percentile of normal for height and weight. In general, this means that any child born weighing less than five pounds and shorter than eighteen inches is considered growth retarded.

This definition (the "one who at birth" part) stems from the time when growth retardation of the fetus could only be found out after the fact—that is, after the baby was born. Until ultrasound testing became available in the early 1970s, no accurate diagnostic tests existed to detect slow growth inside the uterus.

Today, ultrasonography can detect abnormally slow fetal growth quite early in the pregnancy. Since IUGR is now frequently diagnosed before birth, another, more descriptive term is often used to label the condition: The baby is referred to as being "small for gestational age"—SGA for short. Such a baby is smaller than it should be for the length of time it has been growing (gestating) in the womb. Doctors also call these babies growth-retarded or "small-for-dates."

Between 3 and 10 percent of all babies born in the United States each year—that's 117,000 to 390,000—have some degree of intrauterine growth retardation. No one is perfectly clear on the exact numbers, and the range changes depending upon which expert or medical text one consults for the data.

Is every child born at or below 10 percent of the norm growth retarded? No. There are several instances in which unusually small babies are not considered growth-retarded. For instance, women who are small themselves tend to have smaller infants. That doesn't mean that these children are growth-retarded. Genetically, it may be normal for a very petite woman to bear a very petite child.

Another category of babies born underweight and short, but not necessarily SGA, is preemies. Infants born prematurely are usually much lighter and smaller than their full-term counterparts. Most preemies are born at a weight and length that are normal for their degree of development; they are just born too early, and, had the pregnancy gone to term, would have been at a normal weight and height. Growth-retarded babies born prematurely are normally even smaller than preemies.

My twins are a good example. They were born six and a half weeks early. My son weighed four pounds, fourteen ounces at birth—hearty for thirty-four weeks' gestation. My doctors estimate that had he gone to term, he would have been a healthy seven pounder. My daughter, born one minute later, weighed only two pounds, twelve ounces. She was SGA. Even if she had been born at forty weeks' gestation, it's likely she would have been under five pounds.

The Prognosis: Generally Good

If your baby has been diagnosed as SGA or "small-for-dates" during your pregnancy, and the doctor has found no major complications, he should already have told you this good news: Your baby is likely to do well after birth. She is likely to be of normal intelligence, although she'll probably never be the tallest in her class. Provided she receives excellent medical attention during delivery, good intensive care after birth, and excellent nutrition in her first year, she is likely to catch up in both weight and height (that is, move above the tenth percentile in the normal range) by the time she is between two and eight years of age.

How each SGA baby fares is a function of how extreme the growth lag is, what month it sets in, and whether it is accompanied by birth defects or disease. Growth retardation is often caused by other underlying problems in the pregnancy that tend to reduce the amount of oxygen and nutrition the fetus receives from the mother—such as hypertension, placenta previa, or uncontrolled or longstanding diabetes.

Babies who suffer IUGR later in pregnancy have the best chances of catching up in growth and the least chance of serious complications due to their petiteness. That's because late-onset IUGR is usually of the "brain-sparing," or asymmetric, type. That means that the head and brain continue to develop normally, while the body falls behind in growth.

Eight of every ten growth-retarded babies have asymmetric IUGR. After birth, they grow quickly. While there is some chance of minor learning disabilities and other minor residual ailments, most asymmetrically growth-retarded babies develop without any lingering problems.

But 20 percent of SGA fetuses lag behind in both head and body size. This is called symmetrical IUGR and is usually linked to chemical or drug exposure, chromosomal abnormalities, birth defects, or poorly controlled insulin-dependent diabetes. In these instances, the baby continues to develop, but at an abnormally slow pace, with the head remaining proportional to the body. If this slowed growth pattern sets in very early in the pregnancy, brain capacity and other body organs can be permanently affected. Symmetrical SGA babies tend not to do as well as asymmetrical IUGR infants in terms of catching up outside the womb or avoiding post-pregnancy complications.

Each case of IUGR is different and depends upon the unique circumstances of the mother and the overall health of the baby. Still, there are some rules of thumb with IUGR. In general, barring major birth defects (most of which can be detected well before birth), the later the onset of IUGR in the pregnancy, and the longer the baby can be safely kept inside the mother, the better the baby does after birth. Thus, IUGR babies born after thirty-six weeks' gestation tend to have excellent outcomes (assuming a nontraumatic delivery); infants born at thirty-four to thirty-six weeks also do quite well. Very premature infants—that is, earlier than thirty-four weeks—can still do well. But all very preterm babies are at high risk for post-birth complications caused by their prematurity, and IUGR babies are no exception.

A bit of good news: Even though they are often born prematurely, SGA babies usually avoid the most serious potential post-birth problem—respiratory distress syndrome. When a fetus undergoes the severe stress of IUGR, the experience helps the lungs mature more quickly than had it been a normal pregnancy. The result is that SGA babies, even quite premature ones, often breathe on their own right from the start.

How Do Babies Grow During a Normal Pregnancy?

In a normal pregnancy, the placenta—the flat, cakelike organ that delivers oxygen and nutrients from the mother to the baby and takes away the baby's waste products—is large. Blood flow in the uterus, the placenta, and the fetus's umbilical cord is high. The baby receives and takes in plenty of nutrition and oxygen. With adequate nutrition and the proper hormonal balance, the baby gains weight during most of the pregnancy, as it grows and changes and readies itself for birth. At fourteen to fifteen weeks of gestation, the fetus gains about five grams (one-sixth of an ounce) each day. By the twentieth week, that rate has doubled to ten grams/day (one-third of an ounce). At thirty-two to thirty-six weeks, the baby is adding nearly an ounce or more a day (thirty to thirty-five grams). After thirty-six weeks, the baby's weight gain slows down as the placenta matures. Growth stops completely at forty weeks and the baby is born.

What Causes the Baby to Grow Too Slowly?

A number of factors can keep the baby from receiving and/or taking in enough nutrition. These factors can be divided into three categories: medical problems of the mother; medical problems of the baby; and problems due to environment. Some of these impediments to growth can be removed by altering one's behavior; others are completely out of the mother's control.

The factors directly linked to the mother's behavior during pregnancy include smoking, drinking, and drug use. By smoking cigarettes during her pregnancy, a woman is likely to decrease the birth weight of her child by two hundred to three hundred grams (a little less than one-half to three-quarters of a pound). Those precious ounces can spell the difference between growth retardation and normalcy. Similarly, a woman who has a drinking problem can severely affect the growth of her unborn child by her alcohol intake. In fact, some physicians feel that even "social" drinking can cause IUGR.

Drug abuse—including the only occasional use of marijuana or cocaine—can have a devastating effect on the growth of the fetus. And inadequate nutrition—that is, if the mother doesn't eat well enough to gain at least twenty-five pounds while she is pregnant—can also cause the baby to be SGA.

The mother's medical condition when she enters pregnancy, or as pregnancy advances, can also stunt fetal growth. Whether she begins pregnancy with them or catches them while she is carrying, infections such as herpes, cytomegalovirus (a specific type of herpes virus), rubella (German measles), or toxoplasmosis (an organism transmitted principally through contact with animal feces—such as contaminated cat litter) can affect the fetus and cause IUGR. (See Chapter 11, Other Fairly Common Medical Complications During Pregnancy, for information on these problems.)

Women who have certain chronic illnesses that affect the blood flow or its nutrient-bearing ability, such as diabetes or kidney or heart disease, are more prone to have SGA babies. Anemia can also cause growth retardation, as can hypertension, whether it is pregnancy-induced or chronic.

Cecilia told me that she had "a perfectly wonderful pregnancy until about the sixth month." She had had mild hypertension before she became pregnant—so mild it was controllable through good attention to diet. But at a routine checkup close to the end of the sixth month, her blood pressure had shot up to 165 over 120 (normal range during pregnancy should not exceed 140 over 90. See Chapter 7, Hypertensive Disorders of Pregnancy). Her doctor hospitalized her immediately. A sonogram done that day showed Cecilia's daughter was healthy and growing. But in a follow-up ultrasound the next week, the baby's growth had nearly ceased. Little Ellen was born by cesarean during Cecilia's thirty-fourth week, weighing only three and a half pounds. When I spoke to Cecilia, her daughter was just turning two. Ellen was still a bit small, but was talking in short sentences and had just about "caught up" in her physical ability.

Certain pregnancy-induced problems also cause IUGR. Placental abnormalities like placenta previa (see Chapter 4) or placental abruption (see Chapter 9) can deprive the baby of nutrition and oxygen and stunt her growth. Gestational diabetes that is poorly controlled can also cause IUGR (see Chapter 6).

Genetic disorders such as birth defects and chromosomal abnormalities can cause growth retardation as well. Between 10 and 30 percent of all IUGR babies have some sort of physical problem that causes them to grow unusually slowly. Most of these defects are detectable early in pregnancy through diagnostic testing (amniocentesis, chorionic villus sampling, ultrasonography, or blood tests). Parents then have advance warning and can choose how or whether to progress with the pregnancy.

Then there are environmental and situational factors. Women who live at altitudes greater than ten thousand feet above sea level may have decreased blood flow to the placenta caused by the thinner atmosphere. This can lessen nutrient exchange and affect the baby's ability to grow. Women who become pregnant very soon after giving birth may have an SGA child. And it is not unusual in multiple pregnancies for one or more of the babies to have IUGR. In 15 to 20 percent of all twin pregnancies, one fetus takes the majority of the nutrition the mother has to offer, which leaves the other growth-retarded. With triplets or more, the probability of IUGR is even higher.

How Will I Know That My Baby Has IUGR?

In all likelihood, you won't be the one who figures it out. Your obstetrician either will discover the condition during an ultrasound scan or will suspect it based on your medical history and routine office visit results.

Until the advent of ultrasound, even doctors had a hard time discerning who among their patients might bear an SGA child. Part of the problem stems from the fact that it's usually quite difficult to pinpoint exactly when the woman became pregnant.

Despite the inexactness of dating the pregnancy, it is crucial for the fetus that IUGR be detected early and treated aggressively. The best outcome for an SGA baby is obtained when the doctor knows ahead of time that the child is unusually small.

So how does the doctor know? His first hint may come from your medical history. If you've had a previous IUGR pregnancy, it's more likely that the current baby will be SGA. If your sister or mother or her mother had an SGA child, it increases your chances of having one. If you smoke, drink, or take drugs, you are also at risk for IUGR.

If you have any long-standing medical condition, such as diabetes, kidney disease, heart disease, or hypertension, you are at risk for IUGR. At your very first obstetrical visit, you will be asked whether you suffer from any of these maladies. Always volunteer the information if you are not asked.

The doctor or his staff can also measure your belly to chart the growth of your uterus. This is done with a tape measure from the pubis (the pubic bone) up over the belly to the fundus (the top of the uterus). Your belly should grow a certain amount between each visit to the doctor. When the same person measures you each time you are at his office, tape measurement is 70 to 80 percent accurate for spotting potential growth problems.

The most reliable method of spotting an IUGR fetus is to measure the baby's head, abdomen, and leg bones for sustained growth. This is done through ultrasound examinations repeated at two- to three-week intervals during the latter half of the pregnancy. (See Chapter 4 for an explanation of ultrasonography.) The technician takes pictures of the baby's head and body, then measures their circumference. She also measures the length of the femur (thigh bone). The radiologist uses standardized ratios and mathematical equations to chart the size of the baby against a curve for normal growth. Although not 100 percent accurate, these measurements—especially if initially taken early in pregnancy—create a baseline against which future growth can be mapped.

How Will My Doctor Treat IUGR?

The first thing he'll tell you is not to worry unduly. Most IUGR babies survive quite nicely once they're born. There is no drug treatment yet to combat IUGR. But, there are things that you can do to help your baby. Your most important job is going to be following the doctor's instructions faithfully. Your OB will ask you to take certain measures over which only you can exercise control. These include immediately ceasing smoking, drinking, and drug taking.

The doctor may want you to eat more and/or alter the content of your diet so that you can provide the most nutrition possible for your baby. Once my OB diagnosed my daughter's IUGR, he asked me to increase my caloric intake to thirty-five hundred calories/day. (Remember, I was carrying twins. Unless you're pregnant with multiples, you won't have to eat *that* much.)

You will also have to rest more. You may even be placed on total bedrest, lying on your left side (the best position to increase blood flow to the uterus) until you deliver. If this is the case, I suggest that you read Chapter 15, Bedrest. The idea behind the bedrest is that the less oxygen and nutrition you use to fuel your own activity, the more there is for the baby to absorb.

If early labor or contractions are a problem—and they often are—your doctor may prescribe oral or intravenous (if you are in the hospital) contraction-inhibiting drugs (tocolytics). Contractions temporarily rob oxygen from the baby, a situation to be avoided at all costs with an IUGR pregnancy. Chapter 8 contains a list of tocolytic drugs, how they work, and their side effects.

Your doctor will also order a series of ultrasound exams to chart the baby's growth and determine the ideal time to deliver her. There comes a point in most IUGR pregnancies when the baby will definitely do better in the external environment of a neonatal intensive care unit (NICU) than inside the uterus. That point usually comes before you are at term.

"That's why I was delivered early," said Kim. She was pregnant with triplets, and the smallest of the three babies—all boys—just was not getting his fair share of the nutrition in the womb. "The doctor told me," Kim recalled, "that if Kevin stopped growing completely, they'd take all of them right away." That happened when Kim was thirty-two weeks pregnant. True to form for SGA babies, Kevin, who weighed only one pound, fourteen ounces at birth, had mature lungs and never had to be placed on a respirator. It was the biggest of the bunch—normally grown but very premature—who spent weeks on mechanical ventilation. All three boys are now healthy toddlers.

One of the ways your obstetrician will decide whether the baby is better off inside or outside of you is through a series of what are called fetal nonstress tests (NST). A monitor is placed on your belly and tracks the baby's heartbeats over a period of about thirty minutes to one hour. Your doctor will order NSTs at least twice each week. If your doctor or the technician spots trouble, and it's close enough to term, you can expect to be promptly delivered (after confirmation by retesting).

Later in the pregnancy, you may also take a contraction stress test (CST)—or oxytocin challenge test. This test also monitors the baby's heartbeats, just like in the NST. But the CST technician analyzes the baby's reaction to contractions. If the chart indicates fetal distress, the doctor will have to decide whether it's time to deliver your baby. Many physicians feel that the CST is a more accurate indicator of fetal well-being than the NST.

The test is done one of two ways. You will be asked to stimulate your own nipples (which releases a natural hormone, oxytocin, that causes uterine contractions) until you have had three contractions within a ten-minute period. Or the technician will administer just enough oxytocin into your bloodstream to induce several small contractions (not enough to throw you into premature labor . . .).

You will also be asked to keep a twice-daily record of your baby's movements. To do this, your doctor will tell you to recline comfortably after a meal and count the number of kicks that the baby makes over a ten-minute period. Babies tend to be most active right after the mother eats.

The normal range of movements or kicks over that time span is between five and twenty. After a few days, you'll get to know your baby's "range." If, over the course of a day or two, the activity drops suddenly, or stops altogether, call the doctor immediately. He'll want to confirm by NST and ultrasound that the baby is not in trouble.

Most likely you will deliver early. And, for the baby's sake, you will probably have a cesarean section. IUGR babies are fragile, and most do not react well to the pressures of vaginal delivery.

Another reason that OBs prefer c-sections for IUGR babies is that because of the stress many have passed meconium (the first stool) prior to delivery; and often the babies have drawn some of this thick, tarry liquid into their throats. It's crucial for the obstetrician and then the neonatologist to remove the meconium before the baby breathes it into the lungs, causing respiratory distress and possibly infection. Cesarean sections limit these possibilities because they avoid the contractions that can force fluid into and out of the baby's lungs. A full discussion of what to expect if you have a cesarean is in Chapter 13.

If you insist upon vaginal birth, or if the doctor allows it, your baby's vital signs will be continuously monitored. You can expect the doctor to insert an in-scalp fetal electrode that picks up the baby's heartbeat and allows for fetal scalp blood sampling to assess oxygen uptake through the umbilical cord. If the baby shows any sign of distress during labor, an emergency c-section may have to be performed to prevent suffocation and brain damage.

No matter whether you deliver by cesarean or have a vaginal birth, you can expect the delivery room to be crowded with medical personnel. The delivery room will be set up for surgery, with everything necessary to give your baby the best possible care. At the very least, your doctor, an anesthesiologist, a nurse to assist in the surgery, one to attend to you, and another neonatal or pediatric nurse will be present. So will a neonatal specialist or pediatrician for the baby.

A Note About the Level of Care Your Hospital
Can Provide for the Baby

If you have received a diagnosis of IUGR for your pregnancy, most medical authorities urge you to deliver in a medical center equipped with the highest level of neonatal intensive care possible—a level-3 NICU. Such hospitals are prepared to administer the most complicated treatment to newborns, including chest surgery if needed. At a facility with a level-3 NICU, you can be assured of the best care for your baby.

This is crucial, as experts agree that immediate excellent neonatal care is necessary for the best outcome. SGA babies have particular problems that are optimally handled only in the NICU. For instance, abnormally small infants do not have the fatty deposits that full-term, normal babies do. Therefore they become cold easily and must be kept in incubators to maintain a proper body temperature. SGA infants may have respiratory distress from inhalation of meconium. And they'll be in the NICU for as long as it takes to bring them up to a weight of at least five pounds.

If you are planning to deliver in a facility that does not have a level-3 NICU, many authorities suggest that you change where you are going to have the baby, even if it means changing doctors—for the baby's sake. Changing hospitals is possible even if you are already hospitalized. You can be transported by ambulance, or by helicopter in some regions.

Should you wish to consider such a change, you should discuss your thoughts and reservations about your current facility with your doctor. Every case of IUGR is unique, and you should make your decisions based upon as much information and input from your OB as possible.

6

Gestational Diabetes

Hazel's was a great pregnancy. She didn't have a single complaint—no morning sickness, no swollen ankles, nothing out of the ordinary in any way. In fact, she felt that she'd never been healthier than while she was pregnant. She ate the right foods. She exercised daily. So it came as a big shock when, in her seventh month, she was diagnosed as diabetic. "I had no indication that this was happening," she told me.

Hazel's doctor immediately sent her to a nutritionist, who placed her on a special diabetic's diet that required her to weigh every morsel of food she ate and count every calorie. She had to make extra visits to her obstetrician, where a blood-sugar test was given at each appointment. There were also several extra sonograms to measure the baby's growth inside her, and, as her due date approached, other tests to see how the baby would react to the stress of delivery. At home, she now tested her blood for evidence of sugar at least four times a day. "It was a drag," Hazel remembers.

But all the bothersome testing and the special diet paid off. Hazel never had to be on insulin therapy. And she delivered a healthy, nine-pound baby boy without surgery. As soon as the doctor delivered the placenta, Hazel's blood tested normal, and for the first time in two months, she could eat what she wanted. "I'd been dreaming about Reuben sandwiches and strawberry shortcake," she told me, "something I couldn't have on the diet. As soon as my son was born, we had it right there in the delivery room!"

Every year in the United States, there are 117,000 to 468,000 Hazels—women who develop diabetes during pregnancy. Like Hazel, the majority of these women are unaware that they have this condition until their obstetrician tells them. And, in the vast majority of women, gestational diabetes can be controlled through diet alone.

This type of diabetes, the kind that manifests itself during pregnancy, is the complication called *gestational diabetes*. It is the most frequently occurring metabolic disorder in pregnancy. Three to twelve in one hundred women develop gestational diabetes, usually after their twenty-fourth week—that is, in the second half of pregnancy. In more than 95 percent of all cases, gestational diabetes is controllable through diet alone. The remaining small percentage of women must inject insulin one or more times per day to control their condition.

I was in this latter category. From the twenty-sixth week of my pregnancy, I injected myself with insulin twice a day, every day, until the day I gave birth. I have not had to take insulin since.

Duration and Prognosis

That's the good news, if you have gestational diabetes. In almost every case, as it was in my own, within hours to days of delivery, your pancreas will be able to make sufficient insulin for your body, your blood sugar levels will then return to normal, and you will no longer be clinically diabetic.

Provided that your condition was diagnosed early, and that your blood sugar is strictly monitored and controlled from then on—through supervised diet and, possibly, insulin therapy—it is extremely likely that you will suffer no permanent damage from this complication. And your baby, too, has an excellent chance of being normal and healthy.

However, even though the vast majority of gestational diabetics and their babies have an excellent outcome when the diabetes is well controlled, they still have a higher-than-normal chance for certain complications. That does not mean that *you* will have complications, simply that it's a possibility of which you should be aware. For instance, gestational diabetics have a higher rate of premature labor and delivery, and so they receive close monitoring to detect and stop early labor. Sometimes this means having to stop working and going on bedrest in the latter half of their pregnancy to avoid triggering premature labor. Statistically, gestational diabetics also have a higher rate of cesarean sections than their nondiabetic pregnant counterparts. These are due in part to the baby growing to an excessive size or growing too slowly.

These possibilities make it imperative that you work hard at keeping your blood sugar levels in check. That means doing whatever your doctor tells you is necessary, whether it is altering your diet, taking insulin, or otherwise changing your routine. This is one complication where your active participation in your care is crucial. Don't let the fact that you most likely will not be on medication for the problem trick you into thinking gestational diabetes is nothing to be concerned about.

If a woman allows her diabetes to progress uncontrolled or ill-controlled, there is a dramatic increase of the chances that she or her baby will have one of a host of problems. The mother risks a 50 percent chance of developing a hypertensive disorder, such as hypertension, preeclampsia, or eclampsia—which can lead to seizures, swelling of tissues, and, if not caught in time, respiratory and heart failure. Severe water retention can occur with twenty times the frequency of normal pregnancies. In the worst cases, the woman can die of such complications.

For the baby, the mother's untreated or poorly controlled gestational diabetes creates a strong possibility of stillbirth. Death shortly after birth is also likely, frequently caused by respiratory distress syndrome—a condition in which the baby's lungs cannot properly use the oxygen in the air she takes in.

Babies of uncontrolled diabetic mothers can grow to an excessive size—defined as over nine pounds at birth. The condition, called *macrosomia,* almost always results in a cesarean section for the mother. Macrosomatic infants who are delivered vaginally can suffer traumatic birth injuries to the head and limbs; the mother's pelvis, cervix, and vaginal tissues can also be injured by the baby's passage.

Conversely, in severe cases, the mother's condition can also prevent the baby from taking enough nutrition through the umbilical cord, making it small for gestational age—a condition called *Intrauterine Growth Retardation* (IUGR). (See Chapter 5, Intrauterine Growth Retardation, for a full explanation of this complication and its treatment.)

How can you avoid these problems? I can't stress it enough: *strict* adherence to the diet, insulin requirements, self-testing procedures, and doctor's orders. If you have gestational diabetes, you can return your chances of having a good outcome to your pregnancy almost to normal by doing everything that's required of you to keep your condition in check.

Why Are Women Prone to
Develop Diabetes During Pregnancy?

It begins with insulin. Insulin is the hormone that helps the body to break down carbohydrates into the glucose (sugar) that the body needs for energy. In a normal, nonpregnant woman, the pancreas produces just enough insulin to keep muscles, the kidneys, and fat tissue running properly. When the body does not manufacture enough insulin, or when its ability to use insulin is impaired, diabetes ensues. Excess sugar, fats, and protein build up in the bloodstream, which the body then tries to flush out through the kidneys.

When this happens, a series of uncomfortable symptoms arise, as well as some effects that cannot be detected without medical testing. Urine output increases to as many as two to three liters/day. Hunger and thirst also increase, but, because the body cannot utilize extra food, weight is lost and the person my feel weak or debilitated and appear emaciated. The skin itches, particularly around the genitals, and skin eruptions are common.

The worst complication—heart disease, permanent eye damage and kidney damage—are not likely to afflict the gestational diabetic. Her diabetes lasts only twelve to sixteen weeks in most cases, and if she submits to the routine blood tests all OBs administer to their pregnant patients, her obstetrician will catch the problem and intervene before any damage can be done. Your doctor should be fully aware of the possibility of diabetes in his patients, because pregnancy itself is a "diabetogenic state"—that is, it tends to bring on diabetes in a certain percentage of individuals. The American Diabetes Association (ADA) has recommended to all doctors that their pregnant patients be tested for gestational diabetes between the twenty-fourth and twenty-eighth weeks of pregnancy.

During a normal pregnancy, the body and the fetus demand an increased production of insulin from the mother's pancreas, as her body adjusts to provide enough nutrition for itself and the baby. During the first half of pregnancy, the fetus continuously removes glucose and amino acids from the mother's circulation. The mother meets this demand by eating more, which creates the need for additional insulin to break down this extra food into usable glucose.

To compensate for the baby's needs, the mother's body stores up fat in early pregnancy. As pregnancy progresses, her body uses this fat increasingly to fuel her energy needs, thus reducing her own need for glucose and amino acids from the food she eats. The burning of the fatty—or adipose—tissue is stimulated by human placental lactogen (hPL), a hormone produced by the placenta.

But hPL tends to block the body's ability to use insulin, even as the body creates the need for more of it. Other hormones of pregnancy—estrogens and progesterone and cortisol—may also contribute to this blocking process. In the normal pregnant woman, the pancreas counteracts the effect of this hormonal cocktail by producing and releasing extra insulin—as much as 30 percent more than her prepregnant state—to maintain the correct balance of glucose.

The actions and interactions of hPL, the other hormones, and the fetus's need for nourishment prove too much for some women's pancreases, and they either cannot make enough insulin to keep up or are blocked by the hPL from using efficiently the insulin that they do make. The result is gestational diabetes.

Once the pregnant woman develops gestational diabetes, the disease manifests itself just as diabetes does in nonpregnant people, but with the added dangers for the mother and the fetus. Nutrients cross the placenta as nourishment for the fetus. If the mother's blood nutrient levels are elevated, the baby's will be, too, which means the baby gets too much to "eat." This can prompt the fetus's pancreas to produce too much insulin, causing excessive fetal growth. This condition is thought to play a significant part in fostering stillbirths, respiratory distress syndrome, low blood sugar, and other neonatal problems.

A NOTE ABOUT CLASSIFICATION OF DIABETES

Doctors have a number of ways of classifying non-pregnancy-related diabetes. These depend upon the severity of the diabetes, the complications it has caused, and the patient's age at the onset of the disease. So you may hear any one or more of a number of different descriptions of your condition. You can ignore most of them. All you have to remember is that you have gestational diabetes. But so you won't be confused when the numbers and letters start flying, or if you do further reading on diabetes (for suggestions see the Other Reading and Resources section at the back of the book), here is a brief explanation:

In general, diabetics are grouped into two main categories. One is non-insulin-dependent diabetes mellitus (NIDDM). These are the 85 to 95 percent of diabetics whose condition is controlled through diet alone (exact statistics on percentage vary). Then there is the insulin-dependent diabetes mellitus (IDDM) group—the other 5 to 15 percent—who *must* take insulin by injection to normalize blood sugar.

In pregnancy, classifications can become confusing, because there are two different systems that are used to describe diabetics. One is numeric; the other, alphabetical. The alphabetical system is called the White criteria. The system runs from Class A diabetics—those who test abnormally for glucose tolerance, but whose diabetes can be controlled through diet alone; to Class T—diabetics of long standing who still have kidney impairment even after a transplant. Between Class A and Class T are the various other stages of the disease. Every class after A requires insulin. Gestational diabetes is no longer part of the White Class's alphabet soup.

The other classification system uses the ADA (American Diabetes

Association) criteria, which assigns numbers instead of letters and calls the classes "types." Type I is IDDM, usually with onset of the disease before the age of twenty. Type I diabetics are usually thin. Type IIs have NIDDM, are often obese or have a history of obesity, and usually develop the disease after age thirty. The ADA lumps all other diabetics (a tiny percentage) into "Other types."

Now, a class all by itself: It's the GDM category—gestational diabetes mellitus, known as gestational diabetes, for short.

There is no way to tell, until pregnancy is over, whether a woman is a "true" or "frank" diabetic. If her diabetes continues past pregnancy, then a woman with gestational diabetes will be reclassified as a true Type I or Type II.

How Do I Know if I Am at Risk for Gestational Diabetes?

Although developing gestational diabetes is not necessarily linked to a family history of diabetes, previous illness, weight, or diet, medical texts state that certain factors, if present, indicate that a woman may be at risk for the problem during pregnancy. These factors are:

- a strong family history of diabetes
- a previous stillbirth
- a previous birth in which the baby weighed nine pounds or more
- obesity
- hypertension
- a history of skin, genital, or urinary tract infections
- age over twenty-five years

There is also some indication that a woman pregnant with multiples—twins, triplets, and so on—may be more prone than other pregnant women to developing gestational diabetes. However, there is no conclusive study that proves or disproves this contention.

Which factors have the most bearing on whether you will develop gestational diabetes? That is a matter of some dispute within the medical community. Many physicians believe that obesity is the single greatest contributing component to the disease. Others feel that age and genetic propensity to develop the disease are the most significant factors.

Even if you are diagnosed as having gestational diabetes, you probably won't get a solid answer on why you developed it, although you may clearly have several of the risk factors working against you. Mine is a good example.

I became pregnant at the age of thirty-two (strike one, I was over twenty-five). I was considerably overweight (strike two, and I'm not telling how much . . .). And I was carrying twins (strike three). But did I develop diabetes because of these things? Nobody could tell me for sure. The bottom line is, medical science just does not know the exact whys of this disorder.

How Will I Know if I Have Gestational Diabetes?

Most likely, you won't know until your doctor tests your blood-sugar levels. Some of the more readily observable symptoms of diabetes, such as frequent urination, thirst, and weight loss are easy for a woman to mistake for the regular discomforts of normal pregnancy. All women urinate more when they are pregnant because the growing fetus puts pressure on the bladder, leaving less room for urine and creating a feeling of fullness.

Pregnant women tend to be thirsty because their body's fluid volume increases during pregnancy, and they need to take in more liquids to accomplish the task. With this in mind, doctors urge their pregnant patients to drink extra milk and water, and a woman may not notice that she is taking in even more fluids than her caregiver has recommended.

Finally, 60 percent of all pregnant women suffer from some degree of nausea during their first sixteen weeks of pregnancy, and the nausea can extend far into the second half of the pregnancy in some cases. Dehydration caused by the vomiting can seem as likely a culprit as blood-sugar problems.

For these and other reasons, your doctor is not going to leave diagnosing gestational diabetes up to you. He will test you for it.

The Test: How It Works and What It's Like

There are several ways in which your doctor will determine whether you need a glucose tolerance test (GTT), the test that definitively determines whether you have gestational diabetes. You may have noticed that as part of your monthly prenatal visits to your obstetrician you must routinely give a urine specimen. One of the reasons for this sample is to test the urine for excess sugar and protein.

If you consistently come into the office with excess sugar in your urine, your doctor will probably ask you to come in the next time without having ingested anything but water for the previous twelve to fourteen hours—called "fasting." He'll draw a blood sample, for a "fasting blood sugar"—to see whether the amount of glucose in your bloodstream is in the normal range (in pregnant women, it should be less than 105 milligrams per deciliter of blood—105 mg/dl). If this test result is abnormal, no further tests are needed: An elevated fasting blood-sugar result makes the diagnosis.

If your fasting blood work came back in the normal range, many doctors do a one-hour glucose tolerance test as a routine screening procedure at your twenty-four-week checkup, as recommended by the ADA.

The idea behind the test is to get a reading on the way you metabolize carbohydrates. If your body is unable to properly utilize them, there should be an excess of glucose in your bloodstream within an hour after eating. If you have gestational diabetes, there may even be excess glucose in your blood after you wake up, but before you've eaten.

So you will be asked to go to the office early in the morning while fasting. The nurse or the doctor will draw one vial of blood (that's your fasting blood sugar). It's just like a regular blood test, no worse. Then, you'll be asked to drink fifty grams of glucola—a thickish sugar syrup. It comes in orange and cola flavors, and it tastes like you've just drunk the contents of your sugar bowl (but you'll be able to get it down without wanting to die).

Then, if you have no restrictions on walking around because of other complications, you'll probably be told to go out for an hour, without eating anything else. When the hour is up, the staff will draw another blood sample. That may be it, or your doctor may ask you for one further sample after another hour goes by, again with no eating in between. And that's that until the results come back.

If your test results show a fasting blood sugar below 105 mg/dl, and a one-hour level above 140 mg/dl, then you may have a problem, and you will probably be asked to come back for a full-blown GTT.

This is not the time to panic. You may have eaten more carbohydrates and sugars than normal the day before, or the lab could have misread the results. So if the mini-GTT shows high levels for you, the doctor does the GTT to confirm *or rule out* the possibility of gestational diabetes.

For the GTT, it's basically the same drill, only longer. Again, you'll go to the office early, on a fast, and have one vial of blood drawn. This time you get to drink one hundred grams of glucola (lucky you . . .). Then the staff will take three more samples of blood, at one, two, and three hours after you've drunk the glucola. You will be diagnosed as having gestational diabetes if two or more of the samples come back above the norm—105 for fasting, 190 at one hour, 165 at two hours, and 145 at three hours.

You Have Gestational Diabetes. Now What?

That depends largely on how far along you were when you were diagnosed and how out of balance your blood sugar is. It also is somewhat dependent on how aggressively your doctor treats gestational diabetes. There is a school of thought that says all gestational diabetics should be put on prophylactic insulin therapy—that is, insulin therapy to prevent excessive growth of the fetus no matter how slight the woman's glucose intolerance is. This is a matter that is not universally agreed upon within the medical community, and you should discuss your doctor's reasoning with him if he wants you to go on insulin right away, without trying diet control first.

You may also want to ask your obstetrician how often he treats gestational diabetic patients. If his experience is limited, some authorities suggest that you consider changing to a caregiver who specializes in this complication, or one who at least has strong experience in the area, and has access to specialists who could consult on your case.

Another reason some experts give for considering changing caregivers is if the hospital at which your doctor practices does not have a neonatal intensive care unit equipped to handle respiratory distress and other problems in newborns. Since the leading causes of fetal death due to complications from gestational diabetes are congenital anomalies, stillbirth, and respiratory distress syndrome, having at hand the appropriate facilities to deal with the problem can be crucial. Also, infants of diabetic mothers need close monitoring in the first days of life to make sure, among other things, that they have no blood sugar problems of their own.

Don't let these ideas panic you. There is no rule that says you *must* change doctors to deal with gestational diabetes. I didn't. But I did ask the questions and satisfied myself that my obstetricians had strong experience with gestational diabetics. I also inquired and found out that the hospital where I would be delivering had a neonatal intensive care unit well skilled in respiratory distress cases. Your doctor should not be offended by your questions and should understand that your concern is to get the best care for your baby, not to disparage his abilities. If you decide to change physicians, your own doctor should be able to recommend a specialist to you.

No matter what you decide, as long as you take this problem seriously, work with the doctor, and follow the regimens he prescribes, you have an excellent chance of a happy ending to your pregnancy.

Amy's pregnancy turned out just fine. Her gestational diabetes was discovered in her twenty-fourth week. She says she wasn't really surprised by the diagnosis, since she was thirty pounds overweight, was over thirty, and had diabetes in her family's history. She took her condition very seriously. "Even though the diet was difficult for me," she says, "I was able to stick to it—first time in my life that I could—because I knew my baby's life depended on it." Amy went to a dietitian at the hospital in which she worked, who geared the ADA diet to her body weight, height, and level of physical activity. After sixteen weeks on the diet, she delivered a healthy, normal, seven-and-a-half pound girl by cesarean. "How did I deal with it? I looked at it like, okay, here's another hurdle. It was nothing in comparison with all the surgery I'd had to get pregnant in the first place!"

Since at least 90 percent of gestational diabetics do control their condition through diet alone, there is a high probability that your doctor will want to try a diet first, before recommending insulin. Like Amy, you will go to a nutritionist or other diet specialist who puts you on the diet and who acts as your diet counselor until you deliver—at term!

Note: This is not a weight-loss diet. Pregnancy is no time to try to lose weight. The diabetic's diet is designed to provide balanced nutrition to both mother and child, with enough calories to maintain a weight *gain* that is normal for pregnancy. However, you also need to know: It's a lot of food to eat.

Lea didn't gain any weight during her pregnancy, because, she told me, she couldn't eat all the food she was asked to take in. "It was too much," she said. In fact, a number of women I spoke with said that they gained very little weight once they were on the diet. The reason may be that on the diabetic diet, a woman eats from five to seven times a day. In late pregnancy, when most women are diagnosed, it is difficult to eat large amounts of food, because of the baby's pressure on and compression of the stomach. One tends to feel full after only a small portion.

Once your diet is in place for a week or so, you'll be retested after a fast and after having eaten, to see whether your condition has stabilized in the normal range. If it has, you will simply continue on the diet. From then on you will be closely monitored to make sure that the baby is growing at the right speed and that your blood-sugar levels stay where they should.

Taking Control

With gestational diabetes, as with any major complication of pregnancy, it is easy to let yourself slip into helplessness, give up all control, and feel powerless against the problem. *Don't!* You must take an active part in working on your care, and the diet is a great place to start. A diabetic diet is complicated, and you'll need guidance and support to carry it out properly.

Let people know about your condition. You needn't keep your gestational diabetes secret, nor should you. First, assuming you have no other complications, you will still be visiting friends and going out for meals. You cannot expect your family and friends, let alone strangers, to divine your dietary needs. You'll have to tell them. Don't be shy about it. Your loved ones will feel better knowing that there is something they can do to help. You will feel supported in your hard task if you let them help you stick to your diet.

Second, if you can get around normally, and you are on insulin, you *must* wear a Medic Alert® bracelet or necklace identifying you as a diabetic, in case you are in an accident or have a sudden mishap. Without the tag, if you are in an accident, paramedics or hospital emergency personnel might give you treatment that could jeopardize both you and the baby. Remember, your diabetes is unrecognizable unless blood tests or urine samples are taken. You may not be lucky enough to be accompanied by one of the few people who can explain your condition to a doctor before any emergency procedures are performed. Medic Alert® tags are routinely carried by many pharmacies. If you cannot find one there, ask your doctor where to get one. And if you cannot bear the idea of wearing a bracelet, wear the tag on a neck chain that you can hide under your shirt.

To help you do your part in addressing your diabetes, your doctor should be recommending a nutritionist, dietitian, or diabetologist for you to consult. If he doesn't, ask him for a referral. The dietary program that you go on to control your diabetes must be tailored to your individual needs—your height, weight, activity level, and whether you are carrying a singleton or more than one fetus. Being ''careful'' about what you eat won't suffice. Work with your caregiver to establish the proper diet for you; have it explained to you in detail and then have it monitored to make sure you're doing it right. In most cases, it is *your hard work* that is going to keep you off insulin and protect the health of both you and your baby.

If you must control your diabetes with insulin, the going is tougher. Not only will you be on a diabetic diet, doing all the weighing and measuring and counting that diet-controlled gestational diabetics must do, you will also have to learn how to inject yourself with insulin once or twice a day, until the day you deliver.

Here's what will probably happen. Your doctor will tell you that the diet alone is not working; you'll have to start on insulin. He will most likely ask you to enter the hospital for a three- to five-day stay. (A few doctors begin insulin therapy on an out-patient basis, but most prefer to begin treatment on an in-patient basis, because they can better monitor your condition that way.)

After you check in at the hospital, and after the initial usual ritual of urine and blood work, there's not going to be much for you to do except try to accustom yourself to the routine. If you haven't already, please read Chapter 14, What to Expect When You Go to the Hospital. It will give you the information you need so that you won't be more upset than you have to be about making an unplanned hospital stay.

There are, naturally, some tests and routines for diabetes control that you should expect on top of the usual pregnant-lady-in-the-hospital drill. One you can be certain of is that you will be asked to give blood samples four times a day for the whole time you're there. These samples are used to monitor your blood-sugar levels and adjust insulin intake.

THE TWO-STICK RULE

It will seldom be your own obstetrician who draws your blood, or, for other complications, places the intravenous line (IV), and medical personnel come to you equipped with varying degrees of expertise in the needle department. The more relaxed you can be about getting your blood drawn or putting the IV in, the easier it will be for all concerned. I happen to have what nurses and doctors call *bad veins*— that is, they aren't big, tend not to sit in one place for the needle, and collapse when I get upset.

So, when I was in the hospital to bring my gestational diabetes under control, I learned to adhere to what the residents called the "two-stick rule." If whoever is trying to take a blood sample does not hit the mark after two tries, refuse to let them go for a third. Ask for someone else to do it. You can ask in such a way that you won't offend the person trying to do the blood work. I often found that whoever was trying seemed tremendously relieved to be asked to quit. They didn't like hurting me, and it was embarrassing for them to try over and over to "hit paydirt."

If your doctor anticipates having to order a lot of blood work on you over a period of days—as is always the case for gestational diabetes analysis—he may order the insertion of something called a *heparin lock,* also known as a *hep lock.* This is like an IV, but has no line attached to it. Its function is to keep a pathway to your vein open, so that each time you have to have blood drawn, the needle goes into the gizmo, not into you. It decreases your discomfort and makes it easier for the staff to do their work.

However, sometimes the hep lock doesn't work well (gets plugged up, or shifts out of the vein), and then it may be back to sticking you each time a blood sample is needed. (I was in this category.) If the hep lock isn't used, over a period of days, your arms might get fairly sore. In that case, you could ask the resident or nurse doing the drawing to use a "butterfly" needle. A butterfly is a smaller gauge needle. It's usually used on children or elderly people with delicate skin. Because it's smaller, I found it hurt less than the regular, larger needle. Not all hospital personnel have a lot of experience with the butterfly, so it may be hard to find someone who can work with it on you.

Sometimes there's no avoiding repeated pokes, but the two-stick rule should help you keep from feeling like a pincushion and your arms from looking like a battle zone.

Injecting Insulin

The other diabetes-control routine you will learn is how to inject yourself with insulin. At first, the nurses will administer these shots. But you'll be taking over that job soon: The whole idea is to make you self-sufficient so that you can continue the therapy at home.

Nobody, especially you, should be surprised if it upsets you even to consider the idea of pushing a needle into your own body twice a day, never mind actually *doing* it. Who do you know who *likes* to get shots? Feeling apprehensive and squeamish is perfectly natural. Self-injection is even daunting to the professionals who inject others as part of their job.

"It was weird to inject myself, after I found out the diet didn't work," said Lea, who happens to be a nurse. Because of Lea's nursing experience, her obstetrician started her on insulin therapy on an outpatient basis. Even though she had experience injecting others, Lea told me, she had to give herself pep talks when it came to using the needle on herself. "I figured out just how many shots I would have to take, and each day I would say 'I can handle this. For just this much longer I can handle this.' "

I also counted the number of injections I had to give myself—144 in all by the time I delivered. Tallying up how many doses I had to take helped make the problem finite. I always had an end in sight, and that end got closer every day. Other women have told me that the counting helped them to make a manageable concept out of the condition that at first seemed overwhelming and totally foreign.

But how do you do it . . . how do you inject yourself? It's really not so hard. You'll be injecting into fat tissue, probably in your legs, and not into a vein. And the syringes you'll be using will have extremely small gauge needles—nothing like the ones used to take your blood. The nurses on the floor will show you how. Sometimes they demonstrate on an orange (just as you may have seen it done on a TV medical show . . .); or, if you're like Willa, the nurse who taught me, you'll be your own target practice. "Honey," she said, "never mind wasting your time on that piece of fruit. You're gonna have to do it to yourself sometime, and today is that day."

I was terrified. I cried. I said I couldn't, I wouldn't, I wasn't ready. But I did exactly what she showed me, and it worked! It didn't even hurt, really—it was more like a pinch, and not much of one at that. Once I got the hang of it, I went on to learn how to fill the syringe, flick out the air bubbles, and care for my supply of insulin. I got so used to the routine that when I was readmitted to the hospital with premature labor, I insisted on giving my insulin injections to myself. It made me feel more in control.

A Note About Insulin

There are several types of insulin available for injection, some from animal sources, the others synthesized human insulin. It is most probable that your doctor will prescribe one of the brands of human insulin for you to inject, rather than the animal forms. If he does not, ask him to. Gestational diabetics have the least possibility of allergic reaction or antibody formation to human insulin. If animal insulin is used, the woman may show a sensitivity to it if she redevelops diabetes when she is older.

Both human and animal insulin are manufactured in three different varieties according to how quickly they act and how long they work inside the body. There is fast-acting insulin, which takes effect within one-half hour of injection and lasts for twelve to sixteen hours in the body. Intermediate-acting insulin takes effect within two to three hours after injection and lasts eighteen to twenty-four hours. And there is long-acting insulin, which takes effect between six and eight hours after injection and lasts for twenty-four to thirty-six hours. Your doctor will require that you use a combination of these categories, with the aim of keeping your blood sugar stable throughout the day and while you sleep. You will not have to refrigerate your insulin. But, take care that you never leave it sitting out so long that it becomes overheated or allow it to become frozen.

On top of the extra blood work that you will have and in addition to learning how to inject insulin, you can expect at least one visit from the hospital dietitian, who will explain the diet you will be on while you're there, and what you must do dietarily once you check out and return home. Even if you feel that you've got the diabetic diet down pat, this talk is worth a serious listen. This is your opportunity to ask any nagging questions you might have about your diet and to begin to understand how the diet interacts with the insulin you will now start to inject.

You will also learn how to perform self-monitoring—that is, testing your own blood for glucose. At first you do this procedure from four to six times each and every day to measure your blood glucose levels and make sure your diabetes is strictly controlled. The measuring can be done by several different types of machines or, if your doctor allows it, by sight—using specially treated strips of paper. This latter method is less accurate and will probably require you to go to the obstetrician more often to give a sample of your blood for checking there.

Although the automatic machine readers vary by brand, they all require essentially the same procedure: You prick your finger with a handy automatic device that looks like a large fountain pen; take a drop of blood, put it on special blotter paper, and then run it through the scanning device that gives you a digital readout of your glucose level. These devices can be purchased or rented from medical supply houses. Or your doctor or hospital may lend the machine to you if there is one available.*

An important part of the self-monitoring process is reporting what you find to your doctor. He will tell you how often he needs to hear from you, the times of day to do the monitoring, and what the levels mean. Be prepared to have him adjust your insulin intake upward as your pregnancy progresses. Gestational diabetes tends to become more severe as your baby grows, and it is likely that you will need more of both long-acting and fast-acting insulin to maintain stable blood levels.

---

*Both of the rentals (the finger sticker and the automatic reader) as well as the blotter paper are tax-deductible medical expenses, as are the syringes and insulin you will use. Since the scanners cost up to several hundred dollars (they do range in price), you can also consider donating the machine, and any unused, leftover trimmings, to your local hospital, a nursing home, or similar facility that might need one. This might be an alternative tax deduction for you if the institution is not-for-profit and your medical expenses aren't high enough to reach the 7.5 percent threshold of adjusted gross income on your return.

The Importance of Being Scrupulous About Your Care

All diabetics are more susceptible to infection than people with normal metabolism. Yeast and fungal infections are possible, and urinary tract infections are common. This is especially true in gestational diabetics, as all pregnant women are prone to urinary infections. Bacterial infection is also a risk if you don't properly care for cuts or abrasions. Ditto for gum infections if you don't brush regularly.

Your best defense against these problems is excellent personal hygiene. Make sure you dry your feet, underarms, and crotch thoroughly when you bathe, to prevent fungus infections (which like warm and moist places). When you urinate, wipe only from front to back, even if your belly makes it awkward to do so. And take good care of your teeth and gums; make extra visits to the dentist. Finally, and most important, always wash your hands carefully before injecting yourself or doing a finger stick for self-monitoring.

What Are My Chances of Getting Diabetes Again, Later On?

Unfortunately, your chances are high. If you have had gestational diabetes once, you are likely to suffer a recurrence with any subsequent pregnancy. What's worse, you also have between a 30 and 60 percent chance of developing full-blown, permanent diabetes within ten to twenty years after your bout with gestational diabetes.

Many doctors believe that the reason so many gestational diabetics go on to develop permanent diabetes later in life is that they are genetically predestined to do so. These women show up with gestational diabetes because pregnancy puts such a strain on the body that their pancreas temporarily cannot cope, in the same way that it will falter later in life. It's just a matter of time for these individuals before they have a permanent case of the disease. But that doesn't mean that *you* are going to be one of those four to six out of ten women.

What Can I Do to Prevent the Later Onset of Diabetes?

There are steps that you can, *and should,* take to minimize your chances of a return engagement, both in subsequent pregnancies and later in life.

First, if you were overweight when you became pregnant, or have had your baby and are overweight now, lose the weight. I know from long personal experience that this is easier said than done. And, as the experience of your pregnancy fades with time, you may remember your temporary sojourn into diabetes as somewhat less unpleasant than it is right now. It becomes easy to avoid dealing with your weight problem, especially as you denied yourself so many of the foods you like while you were pregnant. But as much as you probably don't want to think about it right now, you really should. The Expert Committee on Diabetes of the World Health Organization has singled out obesity as the most powerful risk factor in prompting diabetes.

Do whatever you have to, but lose those pounds. Your obstetrician may not make a big deal out of your weight. It's not his job. Once he's delivered your baby and both you and your child are up and around and doing fine and you've had your six-week postpartum checkup, you won't even see him until your next yearly exam. It's up to you.

And, if you were a sedentary person up until your pregnancy, try to become more active. At the very least, take up walking a mile or two several times a week. Regular exercise is a key to keeping weight off and helping to maintain a steady metabolism.

These are things you owe not only to yourself but to your child. Keep in mind that bringing a healthy baby into the world is just the beginning. Within two years, you're going to have a rambunctious, active toddler on your hands. It will be easier for you to keep up with her if you are the proper weight for your height, and if you have built up your stamina through exercise. She's going to want a mommy who is well, and later on, one who sticks around long enough to enjoy the grandchildren she's going to give you.

With early detection, prompt treatment, and careful control of your blood sugar, the worst that having gestational diabetes is likely to be is an annoying disruption of your routine. Women whose gestational diabetes is strictly controlled have nearly identical chances as nondiabetic pregnant women of delivering a healthy, normal child.

7

Hypertensive Disorders of Pregnancy, A/K/A Toxemia

The first half of Marilyn's pregnancy went easily. She felt terrific. It came as quite a surprise to her when, at the five-month checkup, her doctor became concerned that Marilyn's blood pressure was slightly higher than it should be. Marilyn had been completely unaware that anything was wrong.

The doctor wanted Marilyn to stop working, but Marilyn felt it was necessary for her to continue at her job for as long as she could. So the doctor recommended that Marilyn take medication to lower her blood pressure. But the medicine made her drowsy, and it didn't bring her blood pressure under control. A second drug worked better, but not well enough. Finally, Marilyn had to stop working and rest in bed, on her left side, for the majority of each day.

With rest and drug therapy, Marilyn's blood pressure was brought under control. Her doctor checked her blood pressure three to four times each week at his office; he also looked for signs of swelling and tested her urine for protein—indications that her condition would be worsening. She had several ultrasound exams and weekly tests to monitor the baby's movements and heart rate. In all, Marilyn was on bedrest and blood-pressure medication for three and a half months. Marilyn's compliance with her doctor's orders paid off: Her blood pressure remained under control, and she delivered a healthy, eight-pound, ten-ounce baby boy.

The following August, Marilyn became pregnant for a second time. "I had no blood pressure problems at all in that pregnancy," she told me. Her daughter was born in May 1989, weighing in at a hearty eight pounds, two ounces. "I was so relieved," she said. "I consider myself very lucky."

Marilyn *was* lucky—and smart. Lucky, because her high blood pressure, called "pregnancy-induced hypertension," or PIH, was spotted quickly and treated promptly by her physician. Smart, for two reasons: Marilyn kept all her prenatal appointments with her doctor, which gave him the opportunity to discover the problem; and, once the condition was diagnosed, Marilyn complied exactly with the regime her doctor recommended.

Had she failed to keep her appointments, and/or had the doctor failed to note the rise in Marilyn's blood pressure, her PIH would likely have grown worse and progressed to the more severe and dangerous condition called *preeclampsia.* Among other symptoms, her kidneys could have stopped functioning properly; she could have retained tremendous amounts of fluid, so that her feet, legs, hands, and face would swell badly; there could have been protein in her urine; and her blood volume could have dropped.

Left untreated, the preeclampsia could have escalated, becoming severe. Her vision could have become blurry, or she might have become blind. Her liver and kidneys might have sustained permanent damage. She could have come down with unremitting, violent headaches. Finally, she could have gone into seizures—whole body convulsions—called *eclampsia,* that would put her into a coma and, untreated, could possibly have killed her, or the baby. Even under treatment, eclampsia can kill or seriously injure the fetus.

These three conditions—PIH, preeclampsia, and eclampsia—are collectively called the *hypertensive disorders of pregnancy.* They are a progression of the same disease, and all include abnormally high blood pressure. Hypertensive disorders are among the most serious complications a woman can suffer during pregnancy because untreated, the symptoms tend to progress and can permanently harm or even kill both mother and child. However, when they are treated, most cases turn out like Marilyn's—with a healthy baby and a mother who is not permanently damaged by the disease. And, better yet, good prenatal care often prevents hypertension from turning into preeclampsia or eclampsia.

But I Thought This Complication Was Called Toxemia . . .

It used to be. Several different, and therefore confusing, systems of names are used to define the various stages of hypertensive disorders in pregnancy. Your regular obstetrician might use one set of terms to describe your condition to you. Then, when you get to the hospital, the staff may call the same problem by its other terms. If this happens, ask for clarification so that you won't stay confused.

One of the most common labels for hypertensive disorders of pregnancy used to be *toxemias of pregnancy*, or just plain old *toxemia*. This term referred to the erroneous belief that the condition was brought on by toxins circulating in the bloodstream. Although this is now understood to be untrue, the term is still around.

These days, hypertensive disorders are considered a progression of a disease and are labeled according to their intensity and date of onset. Hypertension diagnosed before pregnancy or that persists after three months postpartum is called *chronic hypertension* and may have many causes unrelated to pregnancy in any way. Hypertensive disorders brought on by pregnancy are called *pregnancy-induced*. The remainder of this chapter addresses only pregnancy-induced hyptertensive disorders.

Prognosis

If you have PIH, preeclampsia, or eclampsia, you have a lot of company. Hypertension is one of the most common complications of pregnancy. As many as 25 percent of all women who give birth in the United States each year (that's 975,000 women) have abnormally high blood pressure by the end of their pregnancies. And, between 6 and 7 percent of all women who give birth in the United States each year (that's 234,000 to 273,000) have pregnancies complicated by preeclampsia. Around 5 percent of this latter group (about 13,650) go on to develop full-blown eclampsia. And, of these, an unfortunate six hundred or so die from the complications. That's far less, by the way, than 1 percent of all women who develop hypertensive disorders of pregnancy. But for women carrying multiples, all of these rates are at least doubled.

PIH and the other hypertensive disorders rarely set in before the twentieth week of pregnancy, unless the hypertension is a condition that the woman brings into the pregnancy. Almost 95 percent of all cases of PIH and preeclampsia/eclampsia occur after the thirty-second week of pregnancy.

Who gets PIH and/or the other disorders? Almost 75 percent of the time, PIH happens to women who are pregnant for the first time (*primagravidas* or *nulliparous*). Hypertensive disorders of pregnancy are ten times more prevalent in first pregnancies than in later ones. Unfortunately you have an increased chance of having hypertension or preeclampsia/eclampsia in subsequent pregnancies if you have one pregnancy with such disorders.

The conditions tend to occur either early or late in a woman's reproductive life: Teens and women over thirty-five are most susceptible.

For some reason, PIH is more common in blacks than in whites, possibly because of the poor diet and inadequate medical care common among poor women. The bad diet/poor prenatal care theory for black women remains unproven but popular, since as a percentage there are many more impoverished blacks in the United States than whites. Hypertension in the general population (men, women, children) is more prevalent among blacks than among whites, possibly because of similar factors.

Whatever a woman's race, the tendency to develop preeclampsia seems to be inherited, passed on from mother to daughter. So, if your mom had preeclampsia (probably called *toxemia* in her day), you may have a higher probability of coming down with the disease when you become pregnant.

Certain medical conditions that a woman brings to her pregnancy or that may develop during pregnancy also can predispose her to preeclampsia or eclampsia. These include diabetes, whether chronic or pregnancy-induced (gestational), kidney disease, and heart disease. Just because you have one or more of these factors does not guarantee that you'll get PIH. If you do get it, no one will be able to tell you exactly why you and not another woman with a similar medical history contracted it.

No matter why you come down with PIH and/or preeclampsia or eclampsia, once you've got the condition(s), both you and your baby are at risk for further complications. PIH and eclampsia can cause the deterioration of function in many organs and systems.

PIH affects the heart, making it work harder. It constricts the blood vessels, which lowers the amount of blood and nutrients carried to the placenta for the baby. As PIH worsens (as is usual without treatment . . .) it also can cause a woman to develop less blood volume than normal for pregnancy, either because of constriction of the blood vessels or because of loss of fluid from the circulation into tissue outside blood vessels (which causes the woman's legs, feet, hands, and face to swell up, a condition called *edema*).

Lowered blood volume makes a woman less tolerant to the normal amount of blood loss pregnant women have during birth. She may also experience an abnormal decrease in the number of blood platelets in her blood—the part of the blood that is essential for normal clotting when a vessel or tissue is injured. Both of these problems may mean that she'll require a transfusion before, during, or after giving birth if blood loss is significant.

Most women retain some water during pregnancy. But if PIH progresses to preeclampsia, water retention goes up dramatically. The kidneys stop functioning properly and can become enlarged (although most often, permanent kidney damage does not occur).

If preeclampsia becomes severe, cellular changes occur in the liver, and its functioning deteriorates. If the condition worsens, the liver can become enlarged, and there may be pain in the upper right side of her body. Most but not all of these symptoms tend to reverse themselves after delivery. In severe preeclampsia, visual disturbances are common. These include shimmering of the vision, blurred vision, and, rarely, detachment of the retinas and blindness.

Untreated, the woman's condition deteriorates further. She can develop violent headaches, changes in temperament, and nausea. Finally, if the condition remains untreated and/or gets out of control, the woman's condition turns into eclampsia: She goes into whole-body seizures, which are typically followed by coma. Convulsions can be so violent that the woman literally flings herself out of bed or into furniture or walls, causing bruising and even broken bones. She may bite her own tongue or lips, bruising or tearing them. The woman may also suffer bleeding in the brain—that is, a stroke. Such damage from eclamptic seizures can be permanent. And last, you can die from it.

For the baby, PIH and preeclampsia or eclampsia dramatically increase the chances of premature birth. And although the stress of the pregnancy speeds development of the fetus's lungs, severe prematurity can still place the baby in grave danger of death or severe, permanent disabilities. Before birth, the baby may develop *intrauterine growth retardation* (IUGR)—the condition in which the fetus grows too slowly inside the womb (see Chapter 5)—because PIH and preeclampsia lower the amount of blood and nourishment flowing to the placenta.

Up to one-third of all women who have placental abruptions— premature separation of the placenta from the uterine wall—have been suffering from one of the hypertensive disorders (almost always, it is either severe preeclampsia or eclampsia). If the placenta abrupts or if seizures take place, the baby may lose too much oxygen and suffocate or suffer brain damage.

These are frightening prospects, I know. But with proper prenatal care, attention to early signs and symptoms, and prompt treatment, your PIH should not end up as eclampsia, and your baby has a good chance of being born close to or at term and healthy. And for all three hypertensive disorders, delivery of the baby is the guaranteed cure. Unless you have underlying chronic hypertension, after you deliver, your hypertension and other symptoms should disappear fairly rapidly. If you still have symptoms after three months, it usually means that you carried the hypertension into the pregnancy—that is, you had undiagnosed chronic, or permanent, hypertension, which can be caused by many factors. And because chronic hypertension can be controlled through medication, you stand an excellent chance of resuming a normal life.

What Exactly Is Hypertension?

Sometimes blood pressure becomes too high, causing too much pressure—or tension—on the walls of blood vessels, making the heart work overtime pumping against this heavy pressure. The term *hypertension* refers to this condition—*hyper,* from Greek, means *excessive; tension,* from the Latin *tensio,* meaning *a stretching.*

That's how the term is derived. But in order to understand what hypertension is, you must be familiar with the concept of blood pressure. Blood pressure is the force that blood places on the walls of the arteries and is a function of a number of variable factors. High blood pressure can result if the walls of the arteries are tense, stiff, and contracted, or the volume of blood is too great. Blood pressure is low when the walls of the arteries are elastic, relaxed, and the energy with which the heart pumps the blood through the system is low.

How Is Blood Pressure Measured?

You may recall that when the doctor tells you your blood pressure, he gives you two numbers: for instance, 100 over 80. The first number is always greater than the second. This is because blood pressure readings measure pressure at two different points in the heart's beat. The first number represents the *systolic blood pressure*—the greatest force caused by the contraction of the left ventricle of the heart. The second number represents the blood pressure during the relaxation phase between heartbeats—called the *diastolic blood pressure.*

The doctor takes these two measurements with a blood pressure cuff—the cloth and Velcro wrap that the nurse puts around your upper arm and pumps up until it's very tight. A hose connects the cuff to a glass-encased column of mercury, which looks much like a thermometer. Numbers expressed in millimeters (mm) are printed along the column. As the cuff exerts pressure, the column of mercury rises.

(Newer, more state-of-the-art blood pressure cuffs have a digital readout.)

How the numbers come out can change from reading to reading depending upon such factors as whether you are nervous, have just been exercising, are lying down or standing up. And everyone's blood pressure is different, because of their unique mix of other variables, including their age, size, physical condition, sex, and the amount of stress they are under. Thus, "normal" blood pressure is expressed in a range that allows for these differences. Generally, normal blood pressure ranges from 100 to 140 mm of mercury for the systolic pressure and 60 to 90 mm of mercury for diastolic—or 100/60 to 140/90.

The American College of Obstetricians and Gynecologists (ACOG) defines hypertension as a systolic blood pressure of at least 140 mm of mercury and a diastolic blood pressure of at least 90 mm of mercury. But even if your blood pressure doesn't reach the 140/90 level, you could still be hypertensive. ACOG also defines hypertension as a rise in systolic blood pressure of 30 mm of mercury over normal *for the individual,* and 15 mm of mercury in diastolic pressure over normal. That means that if your normal pressure is, say, 105/60, you'd become hypertensive at 135/75.

Why Does Pregnancy Tend to Bring on Hypertensive Disorders?

No one really knows. There are so many hypotheses as to why this progressive syndrome occurs that hypertensive disorders of pregnancy are called *diseases of theories.* A few of these are:

- Somehow the mother and the fetus are incompatible, and the mother is "allergic" to the fetus.
- The mother is "allergic" to the chorionic villi that become the placenta.
- The mother has a calcium deficiency.
- Extra pressure on the lower body created by the growing baby and uterus combined with a mother's being on her feet might initiate hypertension in susceptible women.

What doctors do know is that when a woman becomes pregnant, her blood system undergoes major changes. (See Chapter 2, When Pregnancy *Is* Perfect, for a description of these changes.) But sometimes the woman's circulatory system fails to accommodate to these changes. Blood vessels and arteries become more tense, rather than more elastic. Blood pressure rises. When it rises above 140/90, the condition is considered severe diastolic hypertension—that is, abnormally high blood pressure.

How Will I Know I've Got PIH?

You probably won't. The initial symptoms are painless and can be detected only by blood pressure and urine checks. This is why prenatal care and keeping every appointment for a checkup is so important. Every pregnant woman should have her blood pressure checked every two weeks during her seventh and eighth months and once a week during the ninth month. This is especially critical if you have one or more of the factors that predispose you to PIH.

One of the major problems with having hypertension in pregnancy is that at first, you'll feel just fine. So when the doctor tells you that you have become hypertensive, it may be hard to believe. And so it may also be hard to comply with the treatment he recommends.

That's what happened to Cecelia. She went to her doctor for a routine checkup when she was six months along. Her doctor measured her blood pressure and, without saying much about it, recommended that she see an obstetrician who specialized in hypertensive disorders. "I didn't know anything was wrong," she told me. "It was real hot out and my legs were kind of swollen, but I figured it was the weather. I felt just great. When I went to see the specialist that Saturday, he told me that my blood pressure was really high. I asked what to do about it, and he said that he'd like to check me into the hospital. He said it was the best place for me. That was the first inkling I had that anything was wrong."

Cecelia said that once she was admitted to the hospital, she "pulled a couple of no-nos," like walking the halls and visiting with other patients. She didn't understand that bedrest was essential in bringing her blood pressure under control. When she saw her doctor the next day, she asked him why the nurses had been so upset with her for walking around. "I asked him what to do. He said just lie there on your left side. You can take a shower and that's it. But I didn't feel sick, and I had trouble complying."

Once Cecelia better understood the seriousness of her condition, she stayed put in bed. Her blood pressure continued to escalate, but was brought under control with medication. She delivered her daughter prematurely, at thirty-four weeks. And although the baby weighed only three pounds, five ounces at birth, the little girl was healthy and is now a normal, active toddler.

How Can My Doctor Tell I Have PIH?

For one thing, he'll know whether you are predisposed to high blood pressure based on the medical history and assessment he takes at the beginning of your pregnancy. Physically, the doctor will be looking for a significant rise in your blood pressure. Every time you go in for a prenatal visit, your doctor or the nurse takes your blood pressure. If your blood pressure has risen more than 30 mm of mercury over what is normal for you, and the diastolic pressure is up 15 mm or more, the doctor will be concerned.

He will want to recheck your pressure soon. Hypertension is diagnosed if two readings taken six hours apart are 140/90 or higher, or 30/15 greater than your usual pressure. The idea here is to let enough time go by that the doctor can discount transitory rises in blood pressure that can be caused by external factors, like nervousness or recent physical activity. Letting a little time go by and rechecking your pressure tends to cancel out these momentary rises in pressure—if that's what's causing the abnormally high reading.

Will I Be Able to Tell if I'm Developing Preeclampsia?

You may not be able to know for sure, but there are several signs that you can watch for. If these develop, you should call your doctor and ask to come in and have your blood pressure and urine checked. The signs are:

- *Swelling of the hands, face, feet, and legs.* Most women have some degree of water retention during pregnancy. For that reason, doctors no longer rely just on swollen feet and ankles to diagnose preeclampsia. But if the swelling progresses to the upper half of the body—if your rings become too tight to wear or get off or if your eyes swell up or your face puffs up markedly, it may be a sign of preeclampsia.
- *A sudden increase in weight.* If you start gaining more than two pounds per week or six pounds in a month, something is wrong. Average weight gain during the last trimester of pregnancy is one pound per week. Keep an eye on the scale. But also remember, if you pig out over a holiday weekend or spend a week indulging a craving for a pint of ice cream with fudge sauce every night, you could gain two real pounds in a fairly short time.

- *A headache that won't go away.* This isn't a headache that lasts just a few hours. It must linger no matter what you do to relieve it. With preeclampsia, such headaches are very serious; severe headache almost always precedes the first convulsion of eclampsia. If this happens to you, call your doctor, explain the symptom, and ask to come in right away.
- *Visual disturbances.* These can range from slight blurring of the vision to partial or complete blindness. In extreme cases, the retinas can even detach (but tend to reattach spontaneously after birth). Again, these are very serious symptoms and need prompt medical scrutiny.
- *Pain in your upper right side and shoulder.* In preeclampsia, this is caused by enlargement of the liver and is a sign that preeclampsia is headed for eclampsia.

If you have one or more of these symptoms, you should call the doctor promptly. The last three—headache, visual disturbances, and upper right side and shoulder pain—are very serious signs that something is wrong. Although preeclampsia tends to set in gradually and slowly worsen over a period of weeks, the condition sometimes strikes suddenly—in a matter of hours or a few days. This is called *fulminating preeclampsia* and is quite dangerous to you and your baby.

So call the doctor. Ask him to check your blood pressure and look at your other physical symptoms. It's possible that it's a false alarm—but as with any complication of pregnancy, you are better safe than sorry. Your doctor would rather have you be embarrassed than have you self-diagnose away a serious problem.

How Can the Doctor Tell I've Got Preeclampsia?

From your blood pressure readings and the same symptoms that you will be on the lookout for. Plus, he'll also be checking your urine to see whether your kidneys are excreting protein. High levels of protein in the urine are a dead giveaway for preeclampsia.

If you come in complaining of persistent headaches, right shoulder pain, and/or visual changes, your doctor should be very concerned. These are usually treated as red flags that you and the baby are in danger.

Preeclampsia almost always precedes the convulsions of eclampsia. So both you and your physician will have some warning that your condition is turning grave. It is extremely rare that convulsions just "come on" without these other signs and symptoms.

What's an Eclamptic Seizure Like?

Marcia's recollection of her experience is typical. In her thirtieth week she developed such severe preeclampsia that her doctor felt that despite the prematurity of her baby, delivery was crucial. Her son was delivered at thirty weeks' gestation. In the three days following the delivery, instead of getting better, Marcia's condition grew worse. Her blood pressure continued to climb, and her weight shot up. On the fourth day after the birth, Marcia's doctor sent her for an X ray to check for pneumonia.

As far as Marcia is concerned, what happened next is anybody's guess. "I was in the X-ray room, and that's the last thing I remember. I was in a coma. It was all such a strange experience. I was so in and out of consciousness so much. When I finally woke up, I had a respirator down my throat. I had been on life support. I had no idea what had happened to me. I would wake up periodically, when they were sticking a tube down my nose. I remember a nurse asking the doctor questions. Then I passed out again for a day and a half. I woke up on a Tuesday. I had had the convulsion on the previous Sunday. I couldn't walk for days after the seizure. To this day I really still don't know what happened to me."

Like Marcia, few women actually remember the convulsion itself once it has started. It often begins with facial twitching, but soon the whole body has involuntary muscle contractions that make it rigid. This phase lasts from fifteen to twenty seconds. Then the muscles of the face, including the eyelids and then the rest of the body, alternately relax and contract, so forcefully that she may bite her own tongue, or throw herself out of bed or into other objects. She foams at the mouth. She stops breathing. This phase lasts about one minute. Gradually the spasms decrease in intensity until she becomes motionless. She lapses into a coma and does not remember the events immediately before, during, or after the seizure. The length of the coma varies from individual to individual and can last as long as a week or more.

This is a description of a *grand mal* convulsion. The eclamptic woman usually has more than one and may, in severe, untreated cases, have up to one hundred seizures or more. In between convulsions, the woman usually regains some consciousness, although it's likely she won't remember these brief periods of wakefulness.

Eclamptic convulsions can occur after the birth as well as before or during labor. If, as in Marcia's case, the seizures set in after the birth, they usually occur within forty-eight hours after delivery. However, they can take place up to ten days to two weeks after birth.

Still, even with eclampsia, within two weeks of the delivery, the blood pressure usually returns to normal. But other systems of the woman's body may not fare as well. In Marcia's case, she sustained permanent kidney damage. Although uncommon, permanent visual changes, brain function disorders, and damage to other organs may occur.

When I spoke with her, Marcia wanted other women to know that even though she suffered permanent effects from her condition, her baby turned out to be okay. Although he had a difficult first few months in intensive care, when I spoke with Marcia, the baby was two and a half and healthy. "You'd never know by looking at him that he was a high-risk baby," she told me. "He seems to be just fine. Now that I do know what happened to me, I feel very lucky."

How Am I Likely to Feel Emotionally if I Have One of These Disorders?

If all you have is PIH, you probably won't feel anything but terrific—that is, until you hear the diagnosis. Then it will be perfectly normal for you to feel nervous, anxious, or downright terrified. You may be worried about yourself as well as your baby.

It may be difficult for you to believe at first that anything is really wrong. And that may make it hard for you to comply with doctor's orders. This is one of those times that you really just have to take it on faith that what the doctor is asking you to do is good for you.

Of course, that doesn't mean that you should be a Pollyanna about it. It is natural and normal for you to feel angry at having your life so abruptly disrupted. It's also okay to be sad that your pregnancy will no longer be the experience you had come to expect. Any woman who has had major pregnancy complications, who has had to go on bedrest, or face the possibility of premature birth will tell you that she's felt that way. It comes with the territory.

"When I was going through it," Kate told me, "I actually found myself wishing sometimes that I'd have a miscarriage. It was so bad. And I felt terrible to have such feelings, but I was so depressed. The second time I was pregnant and had preeclampsia, I saw a psychiatrist, who told me that what I was feeling was perfectly normal."

You can also expect that your condition itself—if you have preeclampsia—and the drugs used to treat it will affect your mood (see discussion of drug use to combat hypertension and preeclampsia, below). You may feel depressed, disoriented, sleepy, jittery, anxious, or combative. "All I did was lie there and cry," said Sue. "I couldn't focus on conversation. Things became garbled. I couldn't talk. The nurses tried to calm me down. But I blamed myself. Did I do something wrong? The nurses kept telling me no, that with preeclampsia, they really don't know why it happens.''

Sue's nurses were right. You must remember that you did not bring your condition on yourself. It's a physiological process related to pregnancy that the best minds in science have yet to figure out. Remember, you're already under enough stress with all you're going through. Don't add to it by beating yourself up mentally. You did nothing wrong.

And if you find your feelings overwhelming you, seek help. Talk to your loved ones about what you're experiencing. Or reach outside your usual circle of support and make contact and use the services of volunteer and professional groups that specialize in high-risk-pregnancy support. Chapter 15 on bedrest, provides suggestions on how to cope with prolonged bedrest and offers information on support organizations that can help you stay sane while you wait for the baby to be born. You don't have to go through this alone!

How Will My Doctor Treat My Condition?

Essentially there are two ways to treat the hypertensive disorders of pregnancy: immediate delivery of the baby, if the mother is close to term or is in grave danger of developing seizures; or expectant management, which is the treatment of hypertension with bedrest, drugs if necessary, and close observation for changes in the woman's condition. The definitive treatment for preeclampsia and eclampsia is delivery. As soon as the placenta is expelled, the woman's system begins to get back to normal (unless there is underlying chronic hypertension). Within three months after the birth, all symptoms should have disappeared.

The goal with expectant management is to get the mother as close to term as possible without unduly jeopardizing her or her baby, so that the baby has a reasonable chance of breathing on her own once she's born.

What You Can Expect with Expectant Management

If you develop PIH or the other disorders before your baby has matured enough to breathe on her own outside the womb, your doctor will work to prolong your pregnancy until the baby is viable. That will mean bedrest, and plenty of it, with or without antihypertensive drugs. Sometimes, if your case is very mild, or moderate, your OB will allow you to rest at home. If so, you can count on being asked to stay prone, on your left side, for at least the greater part of every day. If abnormal blood pressure is minimal, just going on bedrest may bring it back under control.

If you are allowed to rest at home, you will also be more involved in monitoring your condition. You may have to learn to take your own blood pressure several times each day and check your urine by dipping specially treated paper strips into a sample to see if your body is excreting too much protein. The doctor will expect you to come to his office for a checkup at least once a week, probably more, and will send you for an ultrasound scan to check the baby's growth at least once every three weeks.

Another alternative to in-hospital care for mild hypertension or preeclampsia is to get your physician to order in-home nursing care (which more and more insurance companies are paying for as part of their maternity coverage). Your doctor should be able to recommend a service to you. (See Chapter 8 on preterm labor, for a list of national home-monitoring companies.) Home health-care nurses or technicians can monitor your blood pressure, test your urine, and assess your condition in other ways. Some in-home nursing or health-care services even provide nurses aides or homemakers to assist in preparing meals, caring for children, and doing light housekeeping—all with the goal of keeping you in bed and complying with doctor's orders.

However, this is not always an option—either because such services do not exist in your area or because your doctor feels that the best outcome for you and your baby lies in having *you* lie in at the hospital. In fact, most doctors will admit the woman to the hospital and keep her there—usually through delivery. If you do have to spend time in the hospital for PIH or preeclampsia/eclampsia treatment, you can count on at least the following tests and procedures:

- You'll be asked for your medical history and be given a general physical.
- Medical staff will question you daily about how you feel. Do you have a headache; have you had any changes in your vision; do you have pain in your upper right side; do you feel like your fingers or face are swelling up?
- Nurses will weigh you daily.
- You will give urine samples for protein testing at least every other day.
- Nurses will take your blood pressure at least every four hours, including through the night.
- Technicians will take blood samples as often as several times each day.

- You will have frequent ultrasound exams to check the baby's growth and amniocentesis to assess your baby's lung maturity.
- The baby's heart will be monitored up to four times a day and her movements and heart rate measured several times a week with a special, noninvasive test called a *nonstress test.*
- When you are close to term, contraction stress tests are performed, which record the baby's reactions to uterine contractions.

If your hypertension or preeclampsia is not severe, you most likely can have a semi-private room and will be allowed to be up and walking at least part of the day. But if you have severe preeclampsia or have had seizures, you might be placed in a private room or even in intensive care, with lights dimmed and no visitors allowed. If that happens, nurses may be provided around the clock to watch you and keep you from hurting yourself if you have convulsions.

You may be given sedatives to help you relax and lower your blood pressure. You may be given an in-dwelling catheter to collect urine, as walking back and forth to the bathroom may be enough to elevate your blood pressure. Also, it's important for the doctor to know exactly how well or poorly your kidneys are functioning. He'll have to measure not only how much fluid goes into you, but what comes out of you as well. You may also have an IV inserted to deliver fluids and/or drugs to your system. Many of the antihypertensive drugs used to treat preeclampsia are administered through an IV, because it is the most precise way to control the amount that you receive—allowing the drug dose to be tailored to your exact condition.

Usually, complete bedrest and strict attention to diet begin to bring PIH and preeclampsia under control. Within twenty-four to forty-eight hours, you should start losing the water weight you've been gaining. You'll be urinating a great deal. However, it is rare for these conditions to reverse themselves entirely and disappear before the baby is born. And if hypertension progresses to preeclampsia, the focus of treatment shifts from watching you closely to actively attempting to prevent the onset of seizures, bleeding in the brain, and permanent damage to other organs.

If I Need Them, What Drug(s) Am I Most Likely to Receive?

Many physicians give pregnant women with PIH antihypertensive drugs in an attempt to normalize blood pressure and prolong the pregnancy. Sometimes these drugs work; sometimes they don't. Most medical experts agree that drug therapy is to be avoided if at all possible, as most of these drugs do cross the placenta and may affect the fetus.

When drugs have to be used, doctors literally have dozens to choose from. The most common of these are described below. Trade names appear in parentheses.

BETA-ADRENERGIC BLOCKING AGENTS

Beta blockers are substances that interfere with the transmission of certain nerve impulses. In the case of hypertensive disorders, they are used to block the impulses that cause the vessels to contract. Use of beta blockers in the United States is still relatively new—but numerous studies are producing evidence that beta blockers can be extremely effective in combating hypertension in pregnancy.

There are a number of different drugs that are beta blockers. Their names are:

- atenolol (Tenormin)
- metoprolol (Lopressor)
- nadolol (Corgard)
- pindolol (Visken)
- propranolol (Inderal)
- timolol (Blocadren)

Beta blockers are designated selective or nonselective. It is usually the nonselective class of the drugs that are prescribed for PIH.

Some beta blockers—propranolol, metoprolol, and timolol—are metabolized by the liver; most of the others are excreted unchanged by the kidneys. The antihypertensive effect of the drugs is felt several hours after administration.

Unfortunately, as with most drugs used in pregnancy, beta blockers can cause numerous side effects. Most of these reactions disappear shortly after you stop using the drug(s). Side effects include:

- bronchospasm (asthmalike constriction of the lungs; so, if you've had asthma, your doctor probably won't use beta blockers)

- slow heart rate (under sixty beats/minute)
- insomnia
- nightmares
- hallucinations
- depression
- dizziness
- poor muscle coordination
- numbness of the limbs
- nausea
- diarrhea
- stomach pain
- constipation
- high blood sugar (hyperglycemia)

METHYLDOPA (ALDOMET)

Methyldopa is the drug of choice for pregnant women with mild to moderate chronic hypertension. Although methyldopa does cross the placenta, it is considered safe for both mother and fetus. It is sometimes used in combination with hydralazine (see below), or a diuretic. But methyldopa should not be used in combination with a diuretic during the second half of pregnancy, because it may disturb uterine blood flow.

It works by depleting the contents of certain nerve endings in the body, while at the same time causing the body to reduce production of some of those agents. It also relaxes vessels in the arms and legs and lowers cardiac output—which means the heart has less of a work load.

Methyldopa can be given orally or intravenously and is relatively slow to reduce blood pressure. When taken by mouth, it takes two or three days before the drug takes full effect; and, whether given by mouth or intravenously, it takes two to four hours for the drug to take effect at all. The body eliminates the drug through urination and defecation.

Like most antihypertensive drugs, methyldopa can cause side effects. These include drowsiness, feeling sedated, and sodium retention. You may feel depressed while on the drug. Your nose may be stuffy. Some people are allergic to the drug (although this is not common) and come down with fevers. Methyldopa can occasionally cause anemia.

HYDRALAZINE (APRESOLINE)

Hydralazine is considered the drug of choice for treatment of moderate to severe hypertension in pregnancy. It is not routinely used for mild hypertension and is rated safe for use during pregnancy. It works by directly relaxing the smooth muscles of the arteries, which causes blood pressure to drop. But this, in turn, stimulates nerve endings in the heart, and that is one of the drawbacks of the drug. The nerve stimulation causes the heart to increase cardiac output, which then counteracts the blood-pressure-lowering effect of the drug. If this counteraction is marked, another drug (such as propranolol—a beta blocker [see above]) can be used with hydralazine to make sure that the heart rate doesn't cancel out hydralazine's effect on the blood vessels.

You can take hydralazine either by mouth or through an IV. It is usually given intravenously, unless used for mild hypertension. The portion of the drug that is not used by the body is eliminated from your system by the liver.

Hydralazine has some common side effects, which are not life threatening and will disappear after you stop taking the drug. These include having heart palpitations, feeling flushed and hot, having the nose and sinuses feel congested, and suffering from headaches, dizziness, and changes in heart rate. Hydralazine may also make you feel nervous.

MAGNESIUM SULFATE

Called *mag sulfate* by most hospital personnel, this is the drug of choice to stabilize severe hypertension, prevent the onset of eclamptic seizures or, once convulsions have begun, repeat seizures. It is also used as a tocolytic (contraction-stopping) drug for premature labor. The wonderful thing about mag sulfate is that treatment of eclampsia with mag sulfate therapy almost eliminates the possibility of death for the mother. For that reason alone, it is a terrific drug.

Mag sulfate works directly on the central nervous system as a depressant and lowers the excitability of muscle fibers, which keeps muscles from contracting. It is also a vasodilator (that is, it causes blood vessels to dilate) and thus increases blood flow throughout the body— including the all-important placenta.

Although the drug can be administered by deep injection into the buttocks (along with some local anesthetic to ease the pain of the poke), it is usually delivered intravenously. First, an amount called a *loading dose*—that is, enough of the drug to bring about quick response to the drug—is administered, which takes effect virtually immediately. Then, continuous, but lesser amounts of the drug are added to the IV drip to keep the body relaxed. The body excretes unused mag sulfate through the kidneys.

Mag sulfate does create side effects in both mother and child. It crosses the placenta and may, in large enough doses, cause the baby to be weak, have depressed respirations, be lethargic, and have poor muscle tone and low apgar scores at birth. But these effects disappear over the first day(s) of life and no long-term problems have been documented from its use.

For the mother, if mag sulfate is given at levels excessively high for her, deep tendon reflexes can disappear and her breathing can become dangerously depressed. She can also, in rare cases, suffer heart failure. Calcium gluconate, which stimulates nerves and muscles, is an antidote for these toxic reactions.

If you have to take mag sulfate, it's more likely that you'll have only the more common reactions to the drug. Unfortunately, it is a most uncomfortable drug to experience, because it makes you feel unbearably hot as it dilates the vessels. Some women describe the drug only as making them feel extremely hot. Others have more potent reactions, feeling as though they are on fire.

The extremes of sensation dissipate after the first twenty to forty-five minutes of administration of the drug, although you will continue to feel feverish. Mag sulfate also makes the muscles feel weak, and you may feel lethargic and woozy. These reactions are mostly reported by women who have taken the drug to stop premature labor. Women who receive the drug to stop seizures are usually unconscious and thus do not remember how it made them feel.

ABOUT THE USE OF DIURETICS—

Diuretics, drugs that make you excrete excess fluids, used to be used commonly for treatment of hypertensive disorders of pregnancy. In recent years it has been found that diuretics, rather than helping the woman, can, under certain circumstances, actually harm her or the baby. They reduce kidney effectiveness and may reduce blood flow to the placenta. They can also deplete key minerals in the fetus and create clotting problems.

Of course, every woman's case is unique. It could be that for you, the dangers of diuretics are outweighed by the potential health benefit to you and your unborn child. Still, if your doctor orders diuretics as part of your treatment regime, it is fair for you to discuss with him whether this is absolutely necessary and what your alternatives are.

What Happens When Drug Therapy and Bedrest Just Don't Work?

It is important to remember that bedrest and drug therapy are not really the decisive methods of treatment for the hypertensive disorders of pregnancy. Delivery of your baby is. Going on bedrest and/or taking the drugs are stopgap measures to get you to the point in your pregnancy at which your child can survive outside the womb—preferably without the use of a respirator.

If you have PIH or preeclampsia, you must be prepared for the possibility that your baby may come into the world prematurely, both for her sake and yours. There may come a time when, because of your condition, it is safer for the baby to live outside your body, in an intensive care nursery if need be, than to go all the way to term inside you. As I've explained, if your condition progresses to eclampsia, it's extraordinarily dangerous to you and the baby.

If you have to deliver well before term, it may help you to know that preemies of mothers with hypertensive disorders fare better—breathe on their own faster—than preemies of women who do not have PIH or preeclampsia/eclampsia. The stress of the pregnancy tends to force early lung maturation.

A Word About Corticosteroid Drugs to Prevent Fetal Respiratory Distress Syndrome

If the doctor expects that you will deliver very prematurely (before thirty-four weeks) and has at least twenty-four hours to play with before you go into labor, labor is induced, or a c-section performed, he may offer you injections of corticosteroid drugs, such as betamethasone, which can speed up the baby's lung maturation process, and may make it possible for the baby to breathe on her own right away, or sooner than she would have without the injections.

Marlene gave birth at thirty-one weeks. She had been in bed with preeclampsia since her twenty-second week. By the end of thirty weeks, her condition had deteriorated so badly that her doctor was afraid for both Marlene's and the baby's survival. So, twenty-four hours before he induced labor, Marlene's OB injected her with corticosteroids. "When he was born," she said, "he only weighed three pounds, five ounces, but he was perfectly fine. He had no problems at all . . . he just needed to put on weight. He didn't need a respirator after the first four hours. Today he's a healthy three-year-old."

Administration of these drugs to women like Marlene is becoming more commonplace, but it still has not been conclusively proven that they are safe for the baby in the long run. Follow-up studies of children whose mothers received corticosteroids are under way, but results will be at least several years off. Still, if the alternative to the drug is a child who may not be able to get enough oxygen even on a respirator, the potential benefits outweigh the risks. You should, for your own peace of mind, discuss these possibilities with your doctor, until he addresses all of your concerns.

It is just as likely that you will not deliver very prematurely, that your condition will be stabilized, and that you will be able to stay pregnant until the baby is mature enough to breathe on her own outside your uterus. In that case, unless there are other factors working against your delivering vaginally, you should be allowed to attempt a vaginal birth. Even women who have eclamptic seizures can deliver vaginally. In fact, many physicians feel it is less dangerous to attempt a vaginal delivery than to do surgery when a woman has had or is likely to have convulsions. If, after a trial of labor—at least six to twelve hours, and sometimes as long as twenty-four or forty-eight hours—you don't deliver, you will probably have to have a cesarean. (For a discussion about what you can expect if you have a cesarean, read Chapter 13 on cesarean section.)

Kate had to have cesareans both times she was pregnant. But each time, her doctor gave her a long trial of labor. "The first one—well, they tried to induce her for two days and she just didn't descend, so finally I had a c-section. With the second one, they waited a week, then had to do a cesarean. Both times I was thirty-six to thirty-seven weeks along when I delivered. Both babies were fine. It was a long nine months, but it was worth it!"

Remember, no matter what happens with your PIH or preeclampsia, compliance with your doctor's treatment regimen is going to be crucial. And knowing what you now do about your condition is going to help you get through it. "I was very ignorant about everything," Marcia, who suffered from eclamptic seizures and coma, told me. "And it was terrifying. If I'd at least known something about what was happening, and the dangers, I would have acted differently in the first place, and could have coped better. I only went in to the doctor once a month, and I never gave them a urine specimen until I was seven months along. I just didn't know. Now that I realize what happened, I feel very lucky."

8

Preterm Labor and
Premature Rupture of Membranes

It was a hot Saturday night in June, and I'd been on bedrest for twenty-six weeks. My husband and I were having a "date." That meant that we'd rented a videotape for the VCR, had a special meal of Chinese take-out, and were eating popcorn (no salt) as we watched the movie in our private "cinema." We were about twenty-five minutes into it when I felt a large gush of warm fluid rush out of my vagina. I remember asking my husband for the Kleenex box and grabbing half the tissues. I pushed them down between my legs. They came up soaked with pink liquid. Then the cramps began. "Oh, my God," I cried, "I'm in labor." It was only my twenty-ninth week.

We called my OB's service and left word to meet us at the hospital. With my husband at the wheel, we careened into Manhattan, me lying in the backseat trying to stay calm and convince myself that if I had the twins that night, they'd be okay. At least they'd be in good hands. But it was so early . . .

The guard at the hospital door put me into a wheelchair, and within minutes I was in the labor and delivery suite, monitors strapped to my belly. I was contracting every three minutes and was one centimeter dilated, and my cervix had effaced 40 percent. My doctor put an IV into my arm and started running fluids, trying to bring the contractions under control. It wasn't working. We had to go to contraction-stopping drugs. My gestational diabetes made me a poor candidate for the most-often-used drugs, terbutaline and ritodrine, so they had to use magnesium sulfate. But I had such an extreme reaction to the drug that it had to be stopped almost as soon as it was started. Luckily, the combination of the fluids and the little mag sulfate that did hit my system brought things under control. At 4:00 A.M. they wheeled me onto the maternity ward.

I would be in the hospital for five and a half weeks. Every two to forty-eight hours, I'd start contracting and gushing all over again. I was in labor and delivery a dozen times. My daughter's growth slowed to a halt, and we made the decision to deliver by cesarean at thirty-four full weeks. But the babies started having distress a few days before the scheduled section date, so they were born by emergency cesarean at thirty-three and a half weeks. My son, who is now three and a half, came out screaming and never had a problem (except that he was scrawny and had to spend time in the NICU to put on weight). My daughter, Jenny, had severe respiratory distress syndrome and fused joints from lack of fluid due to the leak. She died eighteen hours after she was born.

Even though I lost my little girl, I consider myself one of the lucky ones. My children were born so prematurely that I could have lost them both. You see, I never even knew that I was contracting when my water broke that Saturday night. I didn't know that my persistent lower-back ache, the pressure in the backs of my thighs, and the gas pains I was having were all symptoms of preterm labor. I thought it was the normal discomfort of carrying twins and being on bedrest. I never felt the contractions. I had no idea I was in preterm labor, until it was nearly too late.

COMPLICATED PREGNANCIES CREATE A HIGH RISK OF PRETERM LABOR AND BIRTH.

Every year 9 percent (351,000) of the women who give birth in the United States have preterm labor and/or early rupture of their membranes (the amniotic sac), which lead to premature birth of their babies. Those of us whose pregnancies are not perfect—that is, we have one or more complications of pregnancy—are at significantly greater risk for preterm labor and birth than this national statistic suggests. If you have a pregnancy complication such as placenta previa, gestational diabetes, hypertension or preeclampsia, among others, you are, as I was, at high risk for preterm delivery. This doesn't mean your baby will be born early, like my twins were. It means that you run a higher-than-average risk that you will deliver early, and you should do everything you can to learn about preterm labor. You need to be able to identify it if it happens to you and get treatment early, so that the labor has a good chance of being stopped.

Unfortunately, most women who have preterm labor are like me. They recognize their problem after the optimum time for medical intervention has passed—that is, after their cervix has shortened and dilated too much for the doctor to be able to effectively stop the contractions that lead to premature birth. Once the cervix is 80 percent effaced (shortened and flattened—which is a normal part of the labor process) and/or two centimeters dilated, and the uterus is contracting every five to eight minutes, efforts to stop labor often are ineffective. Only 10 to 20 percent of all women in preterm labor call the doctor or go to the hospital before this happens. That's because they simply are not taught about this complication and what to do about it. And that's a shame.

ALTHOUGH THERE IS NO KNOWN METHOD OF PREVENTING PRETERM LABOR FROM STARTING, WHEN A WOMAN KNOWS THE SIGNS AND SYMPTOMS TO LOOK FOR, AND SHE MONITORS HERSELF FOR THEM DAILY, SHE HAS ABOUT AN 80 PERCENT CHANCE OF AVOIDING PREMATURE BIRTH.

And that's the key. Premature birth and its complications account for 85 percent of all perinatal birth-related problems and deaths in the United States. There is a lot of medical help out there for you if you do go into preterm labor, help that most times will keep you pregnant until your baby can survive outside your uterus. The preventive approach works, but it depends heavily on early diagnosis and treatment.

This is one problem in your complicated pregnancy in which you will play a crucial, active role. You've got to know what to look for. You've got to work with a doctor who is experienced in detecting and treating preterm labor and rupture of membranes. And once the problem is diagnosed, you've got to do exactly what the doctor requires of you to keep the contractions under control. This chapter will teach you what you have to look for, what your doctor may do to treat preterm labor, and what you will have to do to give both yourself and your baby the best chance of going to term. Let's begin with the basics.

To Whom Does Preterm Labor Happen?

It can happen to anyone. As I've said, approximately 9 percent of all women who give birth in the United States each year do so prematurely. Blacks are statistically more than twice as likely as whites to suffer from premature labor—due mostly, experts believe, to low socioeconomic status and the poor prenatal care and diet that often go hand in hand with poverty.

As with many complications, preterm birth is more likely to happen to women who are at either end of their reproductive life—that is, those who are in their teens or who are over thirty-five. Any woman currently experiencing certain pregnancy complications is also at high risk—in some cases even higher than the 9 percent national average. These complications include:

- moderate to severe hypertension
- placental disorders (such as placenta previa or placental abruption)
- bleeding
- severe anemia
- physical trauma or burns
- multiple pregnancy
- infections such as pneumonia, or bacterial infection of the uterus and/or cervix
- spontaneous rupture of membranes (see PROM, below)
- distension of the uterus due to hydramnios or multiple pregnancy
- abnormalities of the fetus (which tend to cause intrauterine growth retardation and preterm labor)
- death of the baby in utero

About 50 percent of all cases of preterm labor can be predicted based on the above pregnancy-related complications or from the following physical/medical problems and events in the woman's medical history:

- poor prenatal care and diet
- malnutrition or obesity
- a short interval between pregnancies (less than three months)
- previous laceration or surgery on the cervix
- incompetent cervix
- previous uterine surgery
- abnormalities of the uterus
- excessive cigarette smoking
- stress
- drug taking
- previous preterm labor
- a retained IUD
- previous preterm delivery
- maternal disease (such as kidney or heart disease)

- misdiagnosis of the length of gestation and premature inducement of labor

These are only the *known* possible causes of preterm labor. For the other 50 percent of women with preterm labor, the direct cause is simply never known. It just happens.

Cervical Incompetence

Sometimes premature effacement and dilation of the cervix is not caused by labor at all, but by structural weakness of the cervix itself (called *cervical incompetence*). This weakness can be the result of several conditions or occurrences, mostly to do with previous injury to the cervix or the inherited physical condition of the cervix.

Surgical procedures involving the cervix can make it too weak to hold a growing fetus inside the womb. For instance, a previous D&C (short for *dilation and curettage*—a surgical procedure to empty the contents of the womb) can damage the cervix. Also, cervical cautery (burning with chemicals to remove growths or stop bleeding), cone biopsy (having a cone-shaped piece of tissue removed for study under a microscope where a precancerous condition is suspected), or amputation (removal—usually as a treatment to eliminate cancer) can make the cervix weak. So can physical abnormality of the cervix—usually caused by DES exposure in the womb when the mother herself was a fetus.

When the cervix is damaged in any of these ways, it cannot hold back the weight of the pregnancy. It dilates silently and without contractions or pain, sometimes opening completely. The dilation allows the amniotic membranes to bulge through the opening and eventually rupture, almost always well before the baby can survive outside the womb. This in turn irritates the uterus and brings on preterm labor. In these cases, labor is usually detected when it is far too advanced to stop the process, and the baby is born fated to die from complications caused by her extreme immaturity. Cervical incompetence accounts for 15 to 20 percent of all pregnancy losses during the second trimester.

Sadly, it often takes several of these losses before the woman's problem is properly diagnosed. But once it is pinpointed, the condition is treatable through a surgical procedure called a *cerclage* (French for *hooping* or *circling*). This is considered a minor surgery, although it is done under epidural or general anesthesia in the hospital.

The cerclage is usually performed after the twelfth week of pregnancy, the time after which a woman is least likely to miscarry for other reasons. The doctor places a stitch (one to several) around or through the cervix to keep it tightly closed, the way a purse string holds the edges of a pocketbook together.

After surgery, the doctor monitors the mother closely for development of infection (a risk with any surgery) and contractions, which are sometimes brought on by the procedure. This is usually done on an outpatient basis. After discharge from the hospital, the doctor will often require the woman to remain on bedrest in order to keep pressure off the cervix and increase the chances of retaining the pregnancy until the fetus is viable.

The cerclage can be removed (and usually is) just before the baby is due, so that the woman can give birth vaginally. Or the cerclage can be left in place, and the baby delivered by cesarean. In either case, the mother will often be asked to take tocolytic drugs in the third trimester, to keep contractions from pulling out the cerclage.

Although having a cerclage put in place isn't pleasant, it may be a way of helping the body hold on to a pregnancy when it otherwise could not. Marie's story is typical. She lost several pregnancies, including twins in the twenty-second week, before her weak cervix was revealed as the cause of her premature labor. Once it was discovered, however, Marie became pregnant again, and at fourteen weeks, she had a cerclage inserted through her cervix. With the help of these stitches, which were removed just prior to birth, she was able to hold her next two pregnancies until each baby was viable!

What Exactly Is Preterm Labor?

Preterm labor is contractions of the uterus that start before thirty-seven weeks of pregnancy and result in changes in the cervix that, if uninterrupted, will lead to premature birth of the fetus. Medical authorities choose thirty-seven weeks of gestation as a milestone because by this time the lungs and other organ systems are mature enough for almost all babies to survive outside the womb without mechanical assistance.

But there are surprising exceptions to the thirty-seven-week rule: The lungs of babies under the stress of preterm labor or other maternal complications often mature before thirty-seven weeks' gestation. My son, for example, was born at thirty-three and a half weeks and breathed on his own from his first second of life!

Preterm labor is most often defined as uterine contractions that occur four times in twenty minutes or eight times in one hour, accompanied by effacement and partial opening of the cervix. But preterm labor is actually a progression of symptoms. The trouble is most women experiencing the first stages of preterm labor feel no pain, and they don't associate the abdominal tightenings with labor.

"I had no idea I was having contractions," said Dedi. "I went in to my OB for a regular appointment, and my stomach tightened up. He said, 'Dedi, you feel that, don't you?' I said, 'Yeah, it's the baby moving.' And he said, 'No it's not. You're having contractions.' The next thing I knew, my life as I knew it came to a screeching halt." Dedi was on bedrest and contraction-stopping drugs for twenty-two weeks. When I spoke to her, she had just reached thirty-six weeks' gestation and was about to go off the drugs. Her doctor expected her to deliver a healthy baby vaginally, just in time for Christmas. "And when I do," she told me, "all this will have been worth it!"

How Will I Know That I'm Having Unusual Uterine Activity or That I'm in Preterm Labor?

You're going to learn now. *You* are your baby's first line of defense against preterm birth. Only you can know exactly how your body feels and what is normal for you. It is crucial that you pay attention to how you feel, what your uterus is doing, and whether what you are experiencing is *different* from how you usually feel at any given time of day. You should make yourself take note, on a regular basis, of seven separate feelings and functions:

- your belly hardening—that is, contracting
- cramps in the belly
- low back pain
- pelvic pressure
- bowel function
- vaginal discharge
- your overall sense of well-being

The first order of business is for you to become aware of what feels "normal" for you. Start taking notes early in the pregnancy of what makes your back hurt, how heavy your vaginal discharge is, and so on. Knowing how your body is working before the twentieth week of pregnancy will help you determine if there is something unusual going on for you later in the pregnancy, as the baby grows bigger and your body continues to change. If you are reading this book for the first time during the latter half of your pregnancy, try to recall how your body has been feeling until now. Every woman's physical experience of pregnancy is different, so it is up to you to get to know your body's reactions. Comparing yourself to your friends or relatives won't help you. What is important is *your unique experience of your own pregnancy.*

Once you've started taking stock of your body's normal collection of cranky pregnant habits, you will automatically become more aware of sensations that are outside your usual range of feelings. These are the eight changes you should be looking out for:

- uterine contractions (a hard feeling over the entire surface of the uterus) lasting from twenty seconds up to two minutes each, every fifteen minutes or closer
- menstrual-type cramps, especially if they are rhythmic or wavelike
- dull pain in the lower back, either constant or rhythmic, not relieved by a change of position
- pelvic pressure or a feeling of fullness in the pelvic area or back of the thighs
- persistent diarrhea
- intestinal cramps, with or without diarrhea
- vaginal discharge greater than is normal for you, or whose consistency or color changes (especially if the discharge is pink, greenish, or bloody)
- a general feeling that something is wrong, even if you don't know what it is

If you experience any of these symptoms, lie down for one hour and monitor your uterus for contractions (see How Do I Monitor Myself for Contractions? below); then, call your doctor to discuss your symptoms.

Aren't Some Contractions Normal During Pregnancy?

Yes, in the second and third trimesters, some contractions *are* normal. These are painless uterine tightenings that can occur irregularly from the fourth month on. Some people refer to them as Braxton Hicks contractions.

These normal, irregular contractions usually don't occur more than once in an hour, and they do not bring on changes in the cervix. Preterm labor contractions are contractions that occur in a pattern, and cause changes in the cervix, making the cervix shorter, flatter, and dilated.

If you think you are having contractions, it is *essential* that you monitor yourself for them and then call the doctor or go to the hospital right away.

How Do I Monitor Myself for Contractions?

Once you learn how, the technique is easy to do, and requires only an hour of your time twice a day. It will take some practice for you to get used to the feel of your uterus. Once you learn the technique, ask your doctor or nurse to work with you to confirm that, yes, this is how the belly feels when the uterus is firm, this is how it feels when it's soft.

If the thought of spending two hours a day monitoring your belly makes you roll your eyes and want to complain about the "wasted" time, I empathize, but you are thinking about this exercise with the wrong attitude. This will not be wasted time: You will be actively doing something to prevent the untimely birth of your child. These hours invested will be priceless if they help you keep that baby inside you until term.

The best explanation of how to self-monitor for contractions is stated elegantly in the excellent book: *Preventing Preterm Birth: a Parent's Guide*, by Michael Katz, M.D., Pamela Gill, R.N. and Judith Turiel, Ed.D. Dr. Katz is known throughout the perinatal community as one of the nation's leading experts on preterm labor and its treatment. Here, word for word from his book,* is what you need to do to monitor yourself for preterm labor:

"Monitoring your own uterine activity means lying down and feeling your uterus carefully with your fingertips. We have outlined the method below. We encourage you to ask your health care provider to work with you in practicing these steps until you have learned 'the feel' of your own uterus and its contractions.

It is essential to practice monitoring yourself each day. In this way, you can become familiar with your normal pattern of uterine activity. In addition, you may occasionally have contractions that you will not be aware of unless you have your hands on your uterus.

1. When monitoring, lie down, tilting toward your left side. You may put a small pillow under your hip to support your back. (You should not lie flat on your back during pregnancy for two reasons. First, as the uterus grows, the weight of the baby puts pressure on the VENA CAVA, a large vein that flows underneath the baby. This may cause the circulation to you and the baby to decrease. Second, lying on your back may cause you to have more uterine contractions.)

2. Using your fingertips, gently feel the uterus for tightening.

*Chapter 3, pp. 30–32.

Think of your uterus as divided into four sections, and feel over each of the four sections. When the uterus is relaxed, you will be able to indent it with your fingers. During a contraction, the entire uterine muscle will become firm.

Sometimes you may feel the baby move. The uterus may feel firm on one side while the opposite side remains soft. You may also have localized contractions that cause a bulging on only one side of the uterus. This type of contraction does not cause equal pressure within the uterus and does not cause your cervix to change. You are monitoring especially to detect contractions that feel uniformly firm over all four sections of your uterus.

3. If you feel uterine tightenings, try to determine how often they are coming and how long they last. When timing these contractions, start counting minutes from the time the uterus begins to tighten. The time from the beginning of a tightening until the uterus becomes soft again is the LENGTH, or DURATION, of a single contraction. The number of contractions in any given time period (for example, one hour) is the FREQUENCY of contractions.

4. If you have four or more contractions in an hour, or the time between the beginning of one contraction and the beginning of the next is less than 15 minutes, and this uterine activity persists while you are resting, then you may be in preterm labor and you should contact your health care provider.''

When Should I Monitor for Uterine Activity?

Dr. Katz and his colleagues recommend that you use this technique twice a day, every day, at the times that you feel you normally have the most uterine activity. Some women feel that they have more activity late at night; others, right after they eat lunch. By taking stock of how you feel, you will learn within a day or two what times seem most appropriate for you to monitor. But if you ever feel that you are having unusual activity—that is, an increase in contractions—at another time during the day, lie down for an hour and do the self-monitoring technique. Also, you can and should monitor after any kind of strenuous physical activity, such as swimming, walking briskly (for some women, even a walk to the corner grocery store and back can bring on contractions), or sex (orgasm can bring on uterine muscle contractions, which usually die down within minutes. But if you are at risk for preterm labor, orgasm, in some women, can bring on sustained contracting activity).

As with all other complications of pregnancy: *when in doubt, check it out.* With preterm labor, this means that if you even suspect unusual uterine activity, monitor yourself.

It will help you keep track of your monitoring sessions if you write down the results of each one. This is what you should record:

- the time you began monitoring
- the activity(ies) you were engaged in just before the session began
- the time of each contraction—that is, when it starts, how long it lasts—and how long the interval is between each.
- whether you are having any of the symptoms of preterm labor
- your mood
- the last time you took medication and what the medication is (whether you are on contraction-stopping drugs or other medicines—even over-the-counter remedies, such as hemorrhoid suppositories)
- your pulse rate (if you are on tocolytics)

Keeping a written record serves several purposes: It will help you figure out which activities tend to bring on contractions, so that you can alter your behavior to avoid them. If you do have unusual uterine activity, these items—the length of and interval between contractions, and other symptoms, medication, and so on—are information your doctor will want. This data will help him figure out what's going on with you, and what the next, best course of action will be.

How Should I Alter My Routine if I Am at Risk?

There is no proven way to keep yourself from going into preterm labor. There are, however, certain reasonable measures that you can take to give yourself the best shot at minimizing your chances, even if you already have other complications. If you are bleeding, are hypertensive, or have other complications, you may have to go on bedrest or significantly change your lifestyle to treat them. Being at risk for preterm labor will be an added argument for reexamining your routine. If you do not currently have pregnancy problems that force you to slow down, you may, however, have to come to terms with altering your routine, at least somewhat, to avoid those activities that are most likely to make your uterus contract.

These are decisions that you should not make in a vacuum. Discuss your daily routine with your doctor. Ask his opinion about how much you should curtail your activities, if he thinks you must at all. Some doctors believe that the only place for a pregnant woman at risk for preterm labor is in bed. (And for some, the only good place *is* bed.) Others will work with the woman as an individual and help her tailor activity restrictions to her personal situation.

Preterm Labor and Choosing a Doctor

Management of high-risk pregnancy is a developing field. Not all doctors or other health care professionals have the same level of experience handling pregnancies that may or do result in preterm labor. It is extremely important that your medical care be in the hands of a doctor with experience in handling your type of situation.

This doesn't mean you *must* change doctors if you already have an OB with whom you are comfortable. And even if your OB is not experienced with women in your predicament, you may not have to change to someone else if your doctor can consult with a high-risk specialist as needed. However, if your doctor is inexperienced and cannot or will not (unlikely) consult on your case with someone who is, you may want to think seriously of finding someone who can give you and your baby the best chance of making it to term.

Reprinted below, from *Preventing Preterm Birth: A Parent's Guide,** are ten questions to ask your present OB or prospective doctor. These will help you elicit the information you need to make an informed choice of obstetrician. Also included, from *Preventing Preterm Birth,*** are six other questions to ask yourself when the interview is over. If your answer to any of these six is no, explore the option of choosing another OB.

"**1.** What proportion of pregnant women in his or her practice have been high-risk? (Your provider should either have experience managing high-risk pregnancies or should already have an arrangement for consultation with a high-risk specialist when needed. You may wish to speak with this specialist, too.)

2. How often will you have prenatal visits? Who will you actually see—are there partners involved in your care? Will one person be the primary provider?

3. Will you have any restrictions on your activity prior to the onset of labor? (See whether you and the doctor can work out the best plan for your situation.)

*Chapter 2, pp. 22–23.
**Chapter 2, pp. 23–24.

4. Will she or he help you learn to monitor your own uterine activity? How will you report on your monitoring? Whom can you call if you suspect early signs of preterm labor? What will happen next?

5. How does she or he treat preterm labor? What methods of diagnosis and treatment are most frequently used?

6. What would be the first step if signs of preterm labor are detected? Then what?

7. What kinds of cases does he or she not treat—that is, when is a preterm delivery allowed to occur?

8. What if you feel uncertain or disagree with his or her recommendation?

9. If bedrest seems helpful in your case, will home visits be possible?

10. Where will you deliver if you do have a preterm birth? Will a pediatrician be present at the delivery? Does the hospital have an intensive care nursery?

Things to consider after talking with the physician:

- Do you feel comfortable talking to this person—especially asking questions?
- Does she or he answer questions adequately?
- Does her or his philosophy regarding childbirth and medical intervention agree with yours?
- Do you agree with his or her management of preterm labor?
- Do you think you will be able to participate as you want in the decision-making process?
- Do you feel comfortable about any colleagues or other practitioners involved in your care (such as other physicians or a nurse practitioner)?''

It may feel awkward or go against your nature to question someone so closely. You may feel uncomfortable or embarrassed changing doctors in midstream. It's okay to feel like that, but *don't* let your emotional discomfort get in the way of doing everything you can to assure the best care for you and your child. Remember: Your goal is a healthy, full-term baby.

Pam shopped around for a doctor who would be willing to really work with her. By asking the right questions and choosing carefully, she found a physician who was extremely accommodating. Pam had an incompetent cervix. When she was eighteen weeks along, her doctor inserted a cerclage into Pam's cervix, then put her on tocolytics to keep her uterus from contracting and pulling out the stitches. Pam went on bedrest for two weeks and used terbutaline.

After two weeks, she'd had no cervical changes and wanted to go back to work—a desk job. Pam had learned how to monitor herself, and was also hooked up with a home-monitoring company, which monitored her contractions electronically. Pam said, "I wanted to go back to work. There's a cot in the back of my room. If I had a problem, I knew I could lie down. And I lay on the cot for planned rest periods every day." Her doctor went along with her wishes, on the strict understanding that if there were problems, Pam would go right back on total bedrest at home. She returned to work, and delivered at thirty-six weeks, after having worked full-time until the end.

Most doctors are not as liberal as Pam's. And most women don't have as easy a course once they start preterm labor. But if your body can sustain some level of activity without sending your uterus into contractions, you may be able to avoid total bedrest for at least part of the remainder of your pregnancy. That is, if your doctor allows it.

What Should I Avoid Doing?

Remember, your goal is to avoid doing those things that send you into contractions that may cause cervical changes.

A number of activities tend to cause contractions. These include:

- traveling
- driving
- climbing stairs
- using public transportation
- stimulating your breasts and nipples (as part of preparation for breastfeeding)
- taking prenatal exercise classes

If you do any of these things, you should monitor yourself afterward, to see whether they in fact cause a problem for *you*. Some may; others may not. Each woman's uterus reacts to her activity levels differently. Those activities that cause contractions should be avoided or minimized.

You should avoid rubbing your nipples to "prepare" the breasts for breastfeeding after the birth, as some prenatal books suggest. This always causes the body to release oxytocin, which causes the uterus to contract. Also, if you are at high risk for preterm labor, and you are still allowed to have sex, try not to use nipple stimulation during foreplay and intercourse, for the same reason.

In addition, there are certain physical conditions that tend to cause uterine contractions. Doing what you can to avoid them will help to minimize factors that could lead to preterm labor for you:

- *A full bladder.* A full bladder tends to make the uterus irritable.
- *Constipation.* Eat lots of roughage, and drink plenty of fluids to minimize hard stools and bearing down while you move your bowels.
- *Urinary tract and vaginal infections.* Always wipe from front to back after urinating or defecating. Don't introduce foreign objects, including tampons, into your vagina. Drink plenty of fluids, and empty your bladder regularly during the day.
- *Fatigue.* If you have trouble sleeping, make sure you rest during the day and at night, lying on your left side. This goes for work, too. If you get tired during the day, find a place to lie down, then *lie down.*
- *Improper nutrition.* Avoid sugary foods, don't drink alcohol, don't smoke or take drugs. Eat a well-balanced diet of proteins, carbohydrates, and fats.

Emotional stress is also thought to be a major player in causing uterine contractions. Of course, not all stress is avoidable. Just the news that you are at risk for preterm labor will cause you to feel unhappy and anxious. The idea is for you to try to identify those areas in your life that are stressful, and for you to attempt to minimize or eliminate them. Don't let little annoyances fester. Let go of them, or talk them out. If you feel you can't cope, reach out to those people or organizations that can help you. (Chapter 15, Bedrest, provides a list of groups that offer counseling and assistance to women confined to bed for any reason during pregnancy. Use their service.) Now is not the time for you to take on the world, or new responsibilities at home or at work. Your job is to try and keep yourself on an even keel, to help your uterus stay calm and your baby stay in it.

Premature Rupture of the Membranes (PROM)

PROM is another major cause of uterine contractions. In fact, it causes at least 30 percent of all cases of preterm delivery in the United States. PROM is the rupture of the membranes surrounding the baby—the amniotic sac—prior to the start of labor. When this happens before you've reached term, it is called *preterm PROM*—although most people just say you have premature rupture of the membranes.

When it happens at term, rupture of the membranes is a natural and normal part of labor. But when membranes rupture prematurely, that is, before the baby is mature, there can be problems. The known causes of preterm PROM are numerous:

- infections of the urinary tract, cervix, uterus
- incompetent cervix
- hydramnios (excessive amniotic fluid)
- poor strength of membranes
- family history of premature rupture
- preterm labor

But just as often as not, no one knows why the membranes break too early.

PROM, and especially preterm PROM, can be quite dangerous for the baby. For one thing, after the membranes rupture, delivery, unless it is delayed through the use of drugs, takes place within twenty-four to forty-eight hours. If your membranes rupture very far from term, that could be a disaster for your baby.

When the membranes rupture (also called *breaking the waters*), the umbilical cord can sometimes slip down under the baby and become compressed, shutting off blood flow and oxygen to the fetus. The uterus can become infected (dangerous for both mother and child), and, if the fluid loss is long-term (chronic), the baby may not be able to develop her lungs properly. Fluid loss can also permanently stiffen the baby's joints in some cases.

How do you know when your water breaks? There will be an increase in the amount and change in consistency of discharge from the vagina. The fluid is watery. The increase may come as a sudden, watery gush of clear or pink fluid, as a steady or intermittent trickle, or off-and-on gushing. The size of your belly may shrink afterward.

If you have any reason to suspect your water has broken, especially if you are less than thirty-seven weeks' pregnant, call your doctor immediately! He will want to see you as soon as possible. If you cannot reach him right away, go directly to the hospital. You cannot afford to wait around, because if the umbilical cord slips down (called a *prolapse*), your baby may suffocate inside you.

When you get to his office or the hospital, the doctor will immediately test the fluid coming from the vagina to see whether it is from the amniotic sac. He'll also test the fluid for bacteria, and, if possible, for fetal lung maturity. He will check to see if the umbilical cord has slipped down and do all the other tests listed in How Does the Doctor Confirm or Rule Out Preterm Labor? below, to check out both your and your baby's condition and readiness for delivery.

WHAT HAPPENS AFTER THE TESTS?

You will either deliver, or not, depending on how far along you are, whether there is infection or fetal distress, and whether you are in a facility with a low infection rate in the maternity ward. If you are very far away from your due date, and the hospital has a low infection rate, your doctor may keep you in the hospital and monitor you for infection while trying to keep you pregnant.

The trend in obstetrics today is to do nothing to bring on labor if the woman is between twenty-five and thirty-four weeks' pregnant, except to monitor for fetal health and signs of infection. Your vital signs and the baby will be checked every four hours to make sure both of you are still healthy. If you go into preterm labor (as most women with preterm PROM do), you may be given tocolytics to stop your contractions. You will also have nonstress tests to check the baby's health. After thirty-one weeks, an amniocentesis is usually attempted to see whether the baby's lungs are mature.

If your membranes rupture at thirty-six weeks, the doctor will probably wait until you go into labor spontaneously or induce you with oxytocin if you don't go into labor within twelve to forty-eight hours.

If I Think I'm in Preterm Labor, What Should I Do?

There may come a time in your pregnancy when you will believe that you are experiencing unusual uterine activity or have developed one or more symptoms of preterm labor. If this happens, this is what you should do.

First, remember that if it turns out that you are indeed in preterm labor, there are treatments available to help stop it and prolong your pregnancy. Take a moment of comfort in that and:

- Don't panic. Labor, even preterm labor, is a lengthy process. It is highly unlikely that the baby will pop out of you in the next few minutes.
- Empty your bladder if it is full. A full bladder can cause uterine contractions.
- Drink two twelve-ounce glasses of water. Up to 85 percent of the time, hydration and rest, on your left side, will cause your contractions to stop or slow down. Fluids increase the blood flow to the uterus, helping it to relax.
- Now, get on your bed or the couch, and lie down on your left side—*never flat on your back* (which can compress major blood vessels, block blood flow to the uterus, and cause more

contractions). Lying on your left side not only provides the most blood flow to the uterus but also may help in slowing down contractions.

- Monitor your uterus for contractions for an hour, as outlined above in How Do I Monitor Myself for Contractions? Remember to write down when your session starts, how long each contraction is, and how much time goes by between contractions.
- Check your other symptoms: Do you have a backache? Do you have intestinal or period-type cramps? Is your vaginal discharge suddenly heavier or different in color? (If you have a sudden gush of watery clear or pinkish fluid from the vagina, this may be your water breaking, and you should go immediately to the hospital.) Do you feel pressure in your vagina, upper legs, or pelvis? Do you simply feel like something is wrong?

If you have more than four contractions during the hour, stop monitoring at the fourth contraction and call your doctor. If he is not immediately available, tell his service that you have gone to the hospital. Then go, and present yourself at the labor and delivery suite. If your uterus is contracting this much, your doctor would probably tell you to go to the hospital anyway. Have someone else drive you if at all possible. Call an ambulance if you have to.

Time is going to be of the essence now, if indeed you are in preterm labor. The earlier you get yourself to medical help, the better your chances of stopping the labor and prolonging the pregnancy. If you dally, you may unknowingly pass the point of no return.

That's what happened to Kathy, who had already been hospitalized once for a tear in her placenta that caused bleeding. She was sent home on strict bedrest after two weeks and was being monitored for contractions by a home-monitoring company. At twenty-nine weeks, her nurse called her and told Kathy to get to the hospital—the last monitoring strip she'd sent to the nurse over the phone showed six contractions in half an hour. "I thought, 'Oh, I have lots of time,' " she said. "I took a shower. I packed. I didn't know that I was already seven centimeters dilated." Kathy gave birth that night to a severely premature baby. "If only I hadn't waited, they told me, my baby might have been born much later, and avoided all the problems we have with him now."

A Note About Crying Wolf: Don't Worry About It

Some women avoid taking action when they are having contractions because they don't want to be a "bother" if it's a false alarm. They worry that their doctor will be angry with them if they wake him up or disturb his leisure time.

BIG MISTAKE!!! Your doctor can enjoy his off-time another day. But you'll never be able to put your baby back inside you. Don't let your ego get in the way of your taking responsible action.

How Does the Doctor Confirm
or Rule Out Preterm Labor?

He can't unless you see him in person. Probably before your doctor even gets to the hospital, the staff will ask you to undress and put on a hospital gown. You'll be asked to climb into a hospital bed and lie down on your left side. If the staff doesn't place you on your left side, do it yourself. If you feel unbalanced or uncomfortable, ask for pillows or, if they have one, a foam wedge to place under your back to help tilt you.

Uterine Monitor

Next, a nurse or the doctor will place an electronic contraction monitor on your belly. The monitor is held to the stomach by a belt or a large elastic tube that you step into as if you are putting on a skirt. The monitor itself consists of a special microphone attached to a machine that picks up uterine contractions and records their strength and duration on a strip of paper. You will be able to see what's being recorded by watching a dial that registers when the contraction starts, peaks, and stops. Sometimes a second transmitter is also placed on the belly to pick up the baby's heartbeat. The doctor or nurse can then read the paper(s) and tell how often you are contracting and how the baby's heart is reacting to your contractions.

But this doesn't mean that you're just going to lie there like a lump. You should try to be aware of whether the monitor is catching all the contractions that you feel (it sometimes doesn't and needs to be repositioned on the belly). If that's the case, call the nurse so she can adjust the straps and the monitor.

PELVIC EXAM

You will be given a physical exam. The doctor will listen to your heart and lungs. He will also give you a gentle pelvic exam. And here's another point at which you must speak up. If you think your water has broken, this is crucial information. Tell the doctor doing the exam, *before he starts*. Instead of doing a pelvic with his hand, he will then use a sterile speculum (a metal or plastic instrument inserted into the vagina, then opened, to hold the walls of the vagina apart and provide a view of the cervix). This way, no bacteria that could migrate up into the uterus and cause infection are likely to be introduced into the vagina. He will want to be extra sure that everything is completely sterile, and he will order that only pelvics that are absolutely necessary be allowed, so as not to introduce unnecessary bacteria into the vagina later.

If you suspect your water has broken, the doctor will take a sample of fluid from your vagina and test it to see whether amniotic fluid is present. (See Premature Rupture of the Membranes [PROM], above.)

If the doctor finds that there is amniotic fluid in your vagina, he will place an order on your chart that no manual pelvic exams are to be performed on you. If he doesn't mention this to you, bring it up with him, and ask him if this will be the case. This is important information for you to have, so that you can keep tabs on your own condition and make sure that no one misses this vital piece of data on your chart.

Whether the pelvic is done with a sterile speculum or by hand, the doctor will be checking your cervix to see whether it is still long, firm, and closed (as it should be) or whether it has started to flatten (efface), soften, and dilate.

If your cervix has dilated more than two centimeters (it dilates to ten centimeters during delivery) or has effaced more than 80 percent, and your contractions are coming more than eight times an hour, you are definitely in preterm labor. Even if your cervix has not changed that much yet, but there has been some change, and your contractions are coming at regular intervals of less than fifteen minutes, the diagnosis is probably preterm labor, and you can expect the doctor to begin medical treatment to try and stop the labor process.

If I Am in Preterm Labor, How Will the Doctor Treat Me?

Your treatment will differ depending upon how far along the labor and cervical changes are and whether your water has broken. Most preterm labor, if caught early enough, *can* be stopped and the pregnancy prolonged until your baby is more mature. Frequently, it can be held off until your baby progresses to the point that she'll breathe on her own after birth.

THE FIRST PROCEDURES

Regardless of how serious or slight your cervical changes are when you reach the hospital, there are several procedures you can expect to undergo in fairly rapid succession:

- A doctor or nurse will take your vital signs—pulse, listen to your heart and lungs, take your blood pressure—to make sure that your physical condition is stable.
- A nurse will draw several vials of blood from your arm to find out your blood type and see whether you have an infection or other blood abnormality that could be the cause of your contractions, or at least be adding to your uterine irritability.
- You will be asked for a urine sample to test for bladder/urinary tract infection (remember, bladder infections can cause uterine contractions). The sample may have to be taken through a catheter—a small rubber tube inserted through the urethra into the bladder—if you cannot get out of bed or are gushing amniotic fluid that may contaminate the sample. Catheterization does hurt, but the procedure only lasts about a minute.
- The doctor or a nurse will insert an IV line into your hand or arm and start hydrating you—that is, putting fluids and nutrients into your blood system—to try to stop uterine contractions. In almost 85 percent of all cases, contractions can be stopped with bedrest and fluid therapy. The IV will also be there in case the fluids don't do the trick and you need contraction-stopping drugs.
- The nurses will continue to monitor you for contractions and fetal heart rate with the electronic monitors on your belly.

Some or all of these steps may be taken before or during the pelvic exam. In addition, there are several other procedures that you may have:

- The doctor may order an ultrasound scan of your uterus to obtain an image of the baby, to see whether she is normal size for her gestational age and to determine whether there are any unseen problems that could account for the preterm uterine activity.
- If you are more than thirty weeks along, an amniocentesis may be performed (a needle is inserted through your abdomen into the amniotic sac to obtain fluid) and the fluid examined for evidence of infection and to check that the baby's lungs are mature enough for her to breathe outside your body.
- You may take a mild sedative to help relax your body.
- Your heart activity may be monitored with an electrocardiogram (EKG), to make sure that you have no heart abnormality that would make you a poor candidate for tocolytic drugs.

TOCOLYSIS

If the intravenous fluids and bedrest on your left side don't slow down your contractions enough to stop cervical changes, your doctor will have to go to the next step: contraction-stopping drugs—tocolytics (pronounced TOE-CO-LIT-ICKS).

Some women are not good candidates for tocolysis. There are certain situations and medical conditions under which stopping the contractions with drug therapy—or any therapy, in fact—is medically unsafe. These are:

- if you are severely hypertensive (that is, have very high blood pressure) or preeclamptic (see Chapter 7, Hypertensive Disorders of Pregnancy)
- If you are bleeding a lot because of a placenta previa or placental abruption (see chapters 4 and 9)
- if you yourself are bleeding heavily (as from an accident)
- if your uterus is infected
- if the baby has severe intrauterine growth retardation (see Chapter 5)
- if the baby has died inside you

But not every situation is clear-cut. There are many cases in which the doctor and you must make a real judgment call as to whether to proceed with contraction-stopping drug therapy, taking into account all the potential benefits and disadvantages to both you and the baby. These are deliberations in which your doctor should involve you, explaining to you and your husband the up and down sides of each avenue of treatment. Ultimately, unless treating you will actually threaten your own life, it is almost always up to you what course to make the final decision.

These are hard choices to make, for both you and your doctor. There may be factors weighing in on both sides that are difficult to balance. Whatever you decide, you'll be living with the result of your choice for the rest of your life. So don't treat this decision lightly, and don't leave it solely up to someone else.

In my case, for instance, only my daughter's sac had ruptured. She seemed not to be in distress, but she was growth-retarded. My son's sac was intact, and he seemed to be developing normally. Leaving them both inside me risked Jenny's further growth slowdown, and limb disfigurement, but probably assured Dylan's future health. It also meant many more weeks of me on bedrest, IV hydration, increasing anemia for me from the bleeding, and possible serious infection. But taking them both at twenty-nine weeks meant they'd both be in the neonatal intensive care unit (NICU) for weeks, and that neither might survive.

After careful consultation with our OBs, the NICU's head neonatologist, and several other specialists, we opted for keeping me pregnant as long as possible. I held out for a month before giving birth, and only one of my babies survived. We sometimes still ask ourselves whether we did the right thing—if not waiting might have meant we'd have both our children today. But we know that not waiting might also have meant we'd have no babies now, or two severely damaged kids. What we can say with assurance is that we made the most informed decision we could and did what both we and our doctors thought best at the time. You can't ask for more than that.

If you don't have any of the conditions that make it undesirable for you to have drug therapy, and

- the baby appears to be healthy
- the baby is over twenty weeks of gestation (although tocolytics are given in some medical centers earlier than this)
- your cervix is less than four centimeters dilated

you will be given tocolytics in an attempt to stop the contractions.

The Drugs

There are several different drugs that are commonly used to stop preterm labor in the United States. The most frequently prescribed of these are called beta-mimetic adrenergic agents, or beta blockers.

The three most often used of these drugs are called ritodrine, terbutaline, and isoxsuprine. Although it has yet to be proven conclusively, there is some evidence that use of these drugs tends to enhance lung development of fetuses, which might make it less likely that they would experience respiratory distress at birth if born prematurely.

If you are diabetic, have hypertension, have asthma, heart disease, are hyperthyroid, or have kidney disease, you will not be a good candidate for some or all of these drugs, because of their side effects. If you have one of these conditions, you may, however, be able to take the other most commonly used drug, magnesium sulfate (see below).

All the drugs discussed below are usually given first intravenously—that is, the doctor puts it into your IV. The first dose is much higher than the maintenance dosage you will be put on later and is called a *bolus*—a concentrated mass of the drug given quickly to stop the contractions. The side effects of each drug (and they all have them) are most intense when the bolus hits your bloodstream and is first absorbed by your system.

With all of these drugs (except mag sulfate), you should eventually be switched from taking the drug through an IV to injections and then to pills. When the shots and then the pills start, you can expect their effectiveness to have peaks and valleys as the drugs are absorbed into and processed by the body. So, for example, if you get shaky (and most women do) taking ritodrine, you can expect the shakes to be at their worst a couple of hours after taking each pill, growing progressively weaker as the pill wears off.

What this also means is that at the start and end of each pill's effectiveness (or each shot's), you may experience some contractions—as they "break through" the drug. Sometimes the contracting is so pronounced that the doctor will have to increase your dosage and/or frequency of medication, or place you back on intravenous administration of the drug to quiet your uterus back down.

Now, this won't be fun.

Nobody in the hospital is likely to tell you this, but you ought to know: Every single one of these drugs feels extremely unpleasant at first, and you can expect to have strong reactions to them. These side effects will lessen over time, and what may feel intolerable to you initially will be easier to take within the first few hours.

Remember—and ask your partner to keep telling you—why you are taking these drugs. *For your baby.* Keep telling yourself, *You can do this. It's for the baby.* You'll only be miserable for a few hours. You'll get to keep your healthy baby for the rest of your life. This drug may help you carry this baby to maturity. That's the goal.

Remember this as you read the rest of this section, and keep it uppermost in your consciousness if you have to take tocolytics to prolong your pregnancy.

Ritodrine (Yutopar)

Ritodrine is the only beta-adrenergic drug approved by the Food and Drug Administration (FDA) for use as a tocolytic. It works directly on the walls of the uterus, causing them to relax. It also helps the mother's system increase blood flow to the uterus and placenta.

With careful administration and monitoring, it is considered safe for both mother and fetus, although it does cross the placenta. Long-term studies have been performed on babies born to mothers who used ritodrine to stop preterm labor, and no ill effects have been detected as these children grow and mature.

As do all beta blockers used to stop contractions, ritodrine has numerous side effects on the woman. It increases her blood glucose level and insulin output and therefore can cause diabetic women (gestational or long-term) to lose control of their blood sugar. For this reason, most doctors don't give their pregnant diabetic patients ritodrine or any other beta mimetic.

Although it does not do so in every patient, the drug also can cause the following side effects:

- heart palpitations
- rapid pulse
- tremors in the hands and legs
- nausea and vomiting
- headaches
- nervousness
- inability to sleep well
- feelings of depression, anger, or anxiety

- hot flashes
- heat intolerance
- chest pain or tightness
- shortness of breath
- rashes
- constipation or diarrhea
- bloating

Most women will have only one or two of these side effects, if any. Each of these symptoms occurs with different degrees of frequency and intensity. The most commonly felt effects are the trembling, headaches, and palpitations. The drug is excreted by the kidneys into the urine.

For Joanie, it was the nervousness that got to her. "That stuff is miserable," she told me. "It's like a hyper drug. You feel like you want to clean the house. It makes you shake like you're an alcoholic and you need a drink. It made me feel extremely warm. I kept the house set on sixty-two degrees in order to be comfortable. Those effects lasted about three weeks. Then the shaking subsided. The shortness of breath stayed with me, though.''

After the initial bolus goes into the bloodstream, continuous infusions of ritodrine are given by IV until the contractions come under control. Thirty minutes before the woman is taken off the IV ritodrine, she starts taking the drug by mouth in pill form. For the first twenty-four hours of pill therapy, she takes one or more pills at intervals around the clock. Then, if possible, the dosage is lowered and given less frequently, around the clock until the baby is at term.

Isoxsuprine (Vasodilan)

Like ritodrine, isoxsuprine acts directly on the uterine muscle to relax it. Isoxsuprine, like all other beta mimetics, also relaxes smooth muscles all over the body, including those in blood vessels, and may therefore create very low blood pressure in the mother.

The side effects of isoxsuprine on the heart and vascular system are greater than those of ritodrine, and many doctors therefore prefer ritodrine or terbutaline for that reason. Other common side effects of isoxsuprine include:

- tremors
- palpitations
- restlessness
- skin rash

The drug is excreted by the kidneys.

After the contractions have been brought under control, therapy continues by injection for forty-eight hours. The woman is then switched to isoxsuprine pills taken at intervals around the clock until the baby is at term.

Terbutaline (Brethine)

As far as many doctors are concerned, terbutaline is the drug of choice to stop premature labor contractions. Very few patients develop side effects so severe that therapy has to be discontinued. And the side effects that do develop tend to lessen over time so as to be more easily tolerated by the woman. Still, terbutaline has yet to be approved for tocolysis by the FDA, although it is approved for the treatment of asthma during pregnancy and has been used widely in Europe and the United States for stopping preterm labor.

Terbutaline can create numerous side effects. It increases the woman's blood glucose level and insulin output and therefore can cause problems for diabetic women. Thus, most doctors don't give their pregnant diabetic patients terbutaline.

Terbutaline's common side effects are similar to ritodrine's:

- rapid heartbeat
- palpitations
- headaches
- nausea and vomiting

- sweating/hot flashes
- ringing in the ears
- anxiety
- tremors of the limbs

Most women say that of this list, they most often experience increased heart rate, headache, shaking of the hands, and anxiety or restlessness while taking the drug.

"Both times when I started on terbutaline," said Marie, "they started it with IV, then injections, then oral. I was on pretty high doses of it. I felt absolutely miserable. My head hurt real bad. I didn't want to open my eyes. It was like having a horrendous hangover. I felt nauseated. My hands were trembling like I had DTs or something, with the headache and all. Then, each day I felt a little bit better. I finally got adjusted and coped quite well with it. The worst part is the headache and shaking. You want to jump right out of your skin. You feel like you want to get up and scrub the walls, but they're telling you to stay in bed. The first week is definitely the roughest. By the time I went off it both times, I wasn't feeling miserable. I didn't enjoy getting up in the middle of the night to take the drug. It's all in what you have to do, and to have my kids I would have done anything."

Like ritodrine and isoxsuprine, terbutaline acts directly on the uterine muscle to quiet and relax it. It is excreted through the kidneys in the urine.

In recent years, a new technology has emerged that allows a woman to receive a constant, subcutaneous (that is, under-the-skin) dosage of terbutaline, which greatly reduces the peaks and valleys usually experienced on pills or injections. The device is called a *terbutaline pump,* a portable, computerized gizmo that automatically delivers just the right amount of terbutaline in tiny doses, all day and night, into the fatty tissue beneath the skin.

Pump therapy (as other tocolytic therapy) is almost always begun in the hospital. It usually starts with a seventy-two-hour stint on intravenous mag sulfate (see below) to quiet the uterus completely. Then the patient is weaned from the intravenous mag sulfate as she is placed on the terbutaline pump. A nurse skilled in pump therapy now teaches the woman how to use the pump herself. Essentially, it goes like this:

The woman inserts a very fine needle into the skin of the upper thigh. Attached to the needle is a small, hollow tube, which in turn is attached to the machine. The needle is withdrawn, but the tube—

called a catheter—remains in place and is taped down so it cannot move. The drug is then pumped through the catheter into the tissue under the skin, where it is absorbed by the body. Of course, the injection site must be changed several times a week, and the woman must become used to and comfortable with this procedure, or have a nurse do the changing for her.

The beauty of the pump, say the women who have used it, is that it makes the side effects less noticeable, lets them sleep through the night instead of getting up to take the pills, and allows them to be at home with their families (much of the time . . .) once they've learned how to use the device. Women on the pump do need careful medical supervision, and most doctors will not put a woman on the pump unless she lives in an area where a nursing service can make frequent home visits. These nurses deliver the drug to the patient, monitor the woman's heart rate, and check the infusion site (usually the upper thigh) for infection and swelling.

"The pump worked out fine for me," said Sheryl. "After I got used to putting in the needle myself, it was okay. The side effects weren't as bad. It controlled my contractions better. And I really enjoyed the daily contact with the nurses from the monitoring service. It's good to have that one on one."

Unfortunately, the pump is still not universally available in the United States. Many medical centers and small hospitals either do not have it or are only using it experimentally.

Magnesium Sulfate

Called *mag sulfate* by most hospital personnel, this is the drug of choice for women who have another medical problem that makes them poor candidates for the other tocolytics. And, as noted above, it is often part of the protocol for using the terbutaline pump. It can also be used when the other tocolytics fail, but tends not to have the longevity of action that the other drugs do. Many women who have to take mag sulfate do not succeed in staying free of contractions long-term.

Mag sulfate works directly on the central nervous system as a depressant and lowers the excitability of muscle fibers, which keeps muscles from contracting. It is also the drug of choice for controlling seizures in women who have hypertensive disorders during pregnancy. (See Chapter 7, on hypertension, for a full discussion of the advantages and disadvantages of magnesium sulfate.)

For tocolysis, mag sulfate is delivered intravenously. First, a bolus is administered, which takes effect virtually immediately. Then continuous but lesser amounts of the drug are added to the IV drip to keep the body relaxed. The body excretes unused mag sulfate through the kidneys.

If you have to take mag sulfate, it's likely that you'll have only the more common reactions to the drug. Unfortunately, it is considered the most uncomfortable drug of all the tocolytics to experience. So say nurses and social workers I have spoken to in the field. It makes you feel unbearably hot as it dilates the vessels.

The extremes of sensation dissipate after the first twenty to forty-five minutes of administration of the drug, although you will continue to feel feverish. Mag sulfate also makes the muscles feel weak, and you may feel lethargic and woozy.

"I remember feeling very, very hot," said Jodi. "Mag sulfate is really nasty stuff. It makes your eyes cross. You can't focus on anything. You feel kind of out of it. Numb. You know things are going on around you, but you don't care much."

"God, I was sicker than a dog on that," said JoAnn, an obstetrician who ended up having bad preterm labor. "I felt like my whole body was going down the tubes. I lost tone in my muscles. My mouth became extremely dry. My teeth were actually numb. I couldn't feel my mouth. It's terribly scary when you have these weird neurological symptoms and no one prepares you for it. I remember my eyes burning like they were on fire. I don't remember my patients ever complaining of these weird neurological symptoms. This is definitely going to change the way I basically practice medicine. From now on, now that I know firsthand, I'll let these women know what to really expect."

A Note on Constipation

Almost all tocolytics will slow down your digestive system somewhat. Also, some tocolytics, such as ritodrine, require that the woman take in less fluid, to guard against kidney and lung problems, and that can make constipation worse.

If your doctor does not suggest it, ask him to prescribe stool softeners such as Colase or Metamucil for you while you are in the hospital, and then continue them once you go home. Whatever you do, *do not use an enema* to loosen your stool. Enemas can cause contractions of the uterus, the very thing you are trying so hard to avoid! And, if you want to take some kind of over-the-counter laxative, discuss it with your doctor first to make sure what you want to do will not adversely affect your uterus or the baby.

Monitoring Your Condition While You're on Tocolytics

Even though you'll be in the hospital while your preterm labor is first being treated, and you will feel like things are a little out of your control, you still have a very important role to play in your treatment.

You should be continuing to monitor yourself, both your contractions and, equally important, your heart rate. Ask your doctor or a nurse to teach you how to take and record your pulse rate. Then take and write down your pulse twenty to forty minutes after taking each pill, and just before taking the next dose. This information will help your doctor fine-tune your dosage to your particular needs.

Your pulse will be a little higher than you are used to, most likely. It should sit between ninety and one hundred ten beats per minute, but certainly no more than one hundred twenty beats per minute, or fifteen to twenty beats per minute above what was normal for you before you became pregnant. If your pulse is higher than these rates before your next dosage, *don't* take the pill. Call your doctor (or get the nurse to do it), let him know your heart is beating a little too fast, and ask him when or whether you can take the next dose of medication.

You should continue this regime at home, no matter how often a nurse practitioner comes in to see you or how often you visit the doctor.

How Preterm Labor and the Drug Experience May Affect You Psychologically

All pregnant women are prone to mood swings and are sensitive—it comes with the territory. But once a complication like preterm labor is added to this normally heightened emotional state, only a stone would remain completely calm and unperturbed. You are no exception. Expect to experience a wide range of feelings and emotions during this time, whether you are merely at risk or you actually go into preterm labor. It's okay to be depressed, scared, weepy. We all are.

JoAnn: "Even though I was on tocolytics and everything seemed to be going along okay, I had this fear that my cervix would dilate suddenly. I could not wait each week to hear them say, 'No change in the cervix, JoAnn.' Then I'd relax a little bit."

Jodi: "I was only in the hospital two days and I cried the whole time I was there. I went in for my regular monthly checkup. I asked my doctor what was happening when my stomach got hard. And her eyes got real big. I just couldn't figure out how this could happen to me. I'm never sick, I was walking three miles a day. At the time, you want to blame somebody, and the only person you can blame is yourself. I understand now that it wasn't anything I did."

Sheryl: "Being back home was harder than being in the hospital. My husband works long hours. We were kinda at each other's throats a lot in the beginning."

Laura: "I was terrified that I'd lose the baby."

The best advice I can give you is not to be too hard on yourself. You're going to feel rotten some days; okay on others. You may even feel elated on the days that you get to go to the doctor and, like JoAnn, are told "no change in the cervix."

The thing to keep in mind is that this is a temporary situation— no matter how endless it seems at the moment. And also remember that a lot of the anxiety, crabbiness, and moodiness that you may experience is a direct result of the drugs you may be on. These are common side effects of tocolytics.

Then, of course, there is the tedium and pain of prolonged bedrest that you will probably have to contend with. Chapter 15, Bedrest: Keeping Yourself from Going Bonkers, is *must* reading for you.

Can I Go Home Once the Contractions Are Under Control?

Maybe. If your doctor feels that your home environment can be tailored to allow you to get the rest and attention you will need to keep your condition under control. There is always the possibility that in your case you will be best off staying in the hospital until you deliver— an upsetting proposition (I know. I was there a month and a half!).

More than likely, if you are allowed to go home, bedrest will be a big component of your home treatment. You may be told that you must rest in bed at all times, or you may be able to be up and around part of the time. In some cases, you may even be allowed to return to work part of the time—although this is unusual.

Most likely, your doctor will require you either to self-monitor and have frequent contact with his office or to be on home monitoring with one of the several services available. You may also need health care at home by a nurse practitioner and/or a social worker. Some of the home-monitoring companies provide this service as well.

Home-Monitoring Companies and Nursing Services

The home monitoring provided by commercial companies has several facets to it. The two most critical are daily contact with a registered nurse assigned to your case and electronic monitoring of your contractions up to several times each day. The electronic monitor is a smaller version of the electronic monitors used in the hospital. Although each company's machine is slightly different, they all consist of a transducer which you strap on your belly to pick up contractions—even those that you cannot feel—a unit that stores up to several hours of monitoring data, and a modem or acoustic coupling device through which you send the information to your nurse over the telephone.

In order for home monitoring to be successful, you have to participate both willingly and actively. You will spend some time (up to four hours per day) every day wearing the monitor. You have to strap the device on, follow directions, and phone in the data daily to the home-monitoring center nearest you. This can seem like a nuisance, especially when you are feeling no symptoms. But it can be a lifesaver. Literally.

"After my experience," Marie told me, "it is so important to me to have the benefit of monitoring when it's available. Monitoring wasn't available when I was pregnant. They told me I had the flu. Then they said I had a urinary tract infection. In fact, I was eight centimeters dilated. I lost both my babies, and I had no symptoms. I didn't feel any of those contractions. Now how nice it is to have that reassurance that a monitor would pick my contractions up."

There are four national companies that provide the monitoring service, as well as some smaller regional or local firms. They all have a number of services in common. Each employs only registered nurses with between one and five years' labor and delivery work experience. They all provide an initial home visit, during which the nurse gives you a complete physical exam, including a pelvic, if necessary. She will teach you how to use the monitor and transmit the data to the company. If your doctor orders them, your nurse will visit your home to conduct nonstress tests and physicals and take blood and urine samples from you.

You will also be checking in with her daily by phone. Aside from discussing your monitoring results, your nurse will discuss your other symptoms (if you are having any) with you and answer any questions you might have about your condition and activity levels. She will talk to you about your medication and work with your doctor to make sure you are receiving the right dosage. Most of the firms provide twenty-four-hour-a-day access to each nurse. But if you have to send a monitoring strip in at night, some companies have you transmit to a regional center, where someone other than your nurse will read the strip.

If your uterus is contracting more than four times in an hour, your nurse or the service will call you back and tell you that you may be in preterm labor and will advise you on what to do next.

Each of the national companies also provides other services, such as home visits to do nonstress tests that determine the baby's activity level and well-being, intravenous hydration therapy and feeding, diabetes monitoring, and terbutaline pump therapy.

The four major firms (at the time of this writing) are:

CARELINK
205 Technology Drive
Suite 100
Irvine, CA 92718
1-800-333-5341

PDS (PHYSIOLOGIC DIAGNOSTIC SERVICE, INC.)
500 Northridge Road
Suite 690
Atlanta, GA 30350
1-800-888-8672

HEALTHDYNE PERINATAL SERVICES
1850 Parkway Place
Marietta, GA 30067
1-808-456-4060

TOKOS MEDICAL CORPORATION
1821 East Dyer Road
Santa Ana, CA 92705
1-800-234-0599

AVAILABILITY

The four national companies have new offices opening all the time all over the country. Your doctor can check with each firm to see which one(s) is (are) available in your area and the services that they can provide to you.

You should ask your doctor which national or local company he uses for this service. If he has never used one (and many doctors have not), and you feel that you might benefit from the daily contact and the electronic monitoring, ask your doctor to contact one of the firms for you. At this time, only a doctor can obtain these services for you, and an insurance company will not pay for the service unless it is ordered for you by a physician.

Cost and Insurance Reimbursement

According to the American College of Obstetricians and Gynecologists (ACOG), the cost of using a home-monitoring service averages about $80.00 per day (1990 dollars), and overall, about $5,616 per patient. While this seems like a lot of money, the alternative is in-hospital monitoring, which is much more costly. The same types of services in hospitals, depending on your location, can run up to more than $1,000 per day, including the cost of your room.

Nonetheless, many insurers still simply refuse to reimburse the cost of the at-home monitoring. The monitoring companies and the doctors to whom I've spoken feel that insurance companies are less familiar with home monitoring and have no set policy about it or will only go with what they know: hospitalization. Also, the FDA has yet to approve home-monitoring equipment for contraction monitoring, and many insurers won't reimburse anything that doesn't have the government's seal of approval.

And even though the doctors and women who do use these companies' services swear by them, ACOG has not yet endorsed home uterine activity monitoring devices for clinical use. In other words, ACOG isn't sure yet, based on a number of studies that have been done, whether it is the daily contact with the woman, or the monitoring device itself, that helps the woman avoid preterm birth. This may be another reason that some insurers don't want to reimburse patients for the home-monitoring expense.

But this doesn't mean that you should give up on the idea of home monitoring. Check with your insurance company, and ask whether they will cover this expense if your doctor orders the service for you. If the company says no, dispute the decision. Your doctor should be willing to help you in this. And so should the monitoring company you might choose. Economically speaking alone, the insurance company ought to be anxious to provide coverage. Home monitoring, where available and used, may save the insurer over nine hundred dollars per day.

What Happens if the Tocolytics and Other Regimens Don't Work?

You'll deliver prematurely. Needless to say, this won't exactly be the birth you envisioned. You should be prepared for that. If the baby is under thirty-six completed weeks of gestation, she will be taken almost immediately to the NICU. She may have trouble breathing. She won't look like the baby you've imagined—she'll be smaller, redder, more wrinkled. You may very well have a c-section. I don't mean to frighten you—just to make you aware that this will be serious business and that people will be working their hardest to give your child the best shot at making it.

It is reasonable to expect that you may have:

- continuous electronic fetal monitoring, when it's available
- a cesarean section if the baby exhibits any sign of distress at all
- a big episiotomy if you deliver vaginally, to reduce the stress on the baby's delicate head

- rapid intervention after birth if the baby is having trouble breathing

Generally, if the baby is under twenty-six weeks' gestation, you will deliver her vaginally. Unfortunately, the mortality rate of babies born at this level of immaturity is 30 to 40 percent, and therefore the risks to you from cesarean section are considered to outweigh its benefit to the baby.

If the baby is between twenty-six and thirty-two weeks' gestation and is coming out head first, most doctors will also allow a vaginal birth, treating the baby as gently as possible. You'll probably have epidural anesthesia (see Chapter 13, Cesarean Section, for a description of this type of anesthesia). There is some controversy over whether cesarean section gives the baby a better chance at survival when the baby is this premature. No conclusive study on this point has yet been done.

But if the baby is coming into the birth canal feet first, many doctors will do a cesarean section, with a low vertical incision (that is, the incision runs up and down under your belly button, not side to side). Any time a vertical incision is made in the uterus, there is a chance that the scar will rupture in subsequent pregnancies (see Chapter 13, Cesarean Section). The possibility of future harm to you may militate against your having a cesarean now.

After thirty-two weeks' gestation, you most likely will be allowed to give birth vaginally if the baby presents herself head-down. The doctor will track the baby's heart rate with an electronic fetal monitor during the entire labor and will intervene with surgery if the baby shows signs of distress. If the baby is coming down feet first, the doctor will deliver her by cesarean (85 percent of the time), to avoid the possibility that the baby's head will become trapped in the cervix.

Remember, your doctor, the pediatrician, and the neonatologist—all of whom will be present at delivery—will be working their hardest to make sure that your baby has the best chance possible of surviving, and surviving well.

Will My Baby Be Okay?

Unfortunately, no one can guarantee that she will. The inescapable fact is that premature babies are born before they were designed by nature to enter the world. Sometimes that means that they aren't ready to breathe air, or digest milk, or live in regular room temperatures. And sometimes that means that they'll die. It can also mean that they'll survive, but with mental or physical handicaps. Fortunately, the odds that premature infants will survive get better every year.

Preemies are always at risk for certain diseases and difficulties. But not every child who is born prematurely will have these problems. Their risk of them is simply higher than the child born at term. The single biggest killer of preemies is respiratory distress syndrome (RDS, in hospital parlance). Other problems include bleeding into the internal organs, heart, and brain; cessation of breathing, called *apnea;* and blindness.

It is the babies who are born extremely early—at between twenty-four and twenty-eight weeks of pregnancy—who weigh the least and do the worst. The less the baby weighs, and the younger she is, the more likely the baby will be to suffer complications, and, sadly, the more likely she is not to survive at all, or to survive with serious physical and/or mental impairment.

But, if your baby is born prematurely, her odds are good. In 80 percent of these instances, the baby survives with no long-term after-effects. Of the 20 percent who suffer birth accidents or permanent damage from their own prematurity or the treatments necessary to save their lives, most babies will grow up with a good to excellent quality of life.

But it would be unfair of me not to touch on the sad minority in these statistics. And it would be unrealistic for you to ignore the possibility that your baby, if she is born premature, may not be one of the lucky ones. Some babies, like my daughter Jenny, just cannot make it no matter what anyone does—no matter how brilliantly the doctors do their jobs. Chapter 10, Pregnancy Loss: When the Worst Happens, provides complete information on what to expect in the tragic event of your baby's death.

If you are at risk for premature delivery, you may want to know more about what to expect from the delivery, the NICU, and your baby as she grows and develops—both at the hospital and once you bring her home. I recommend you read *The Premature Baby Book,* by Helen Harrison. It is an excellent source of information for you to have, and one that will give you heart.

A Note on Corticosteroids

Many institutions now recommend injecting the mother in preterm labor with glucocorticoid drugs, twenty-four to forty-eight hours before delivery, to speed fetal lung development. The drug usually used is betamethasone, a steroid. Chapter 7 contains a discussion of these drugs and the questions surrounding their use. You should discuss the use of these drugs with your doctor until you are satisfied that all your questions about them have been answered.

A NOTE ABOUT THE LEVEL OF CARE YOUR HOSPITAL CAN PROVIDE FOR THE BABY

If you have received a diagnosis of preterm labor and/or preterm PROM, most medical authorities urge that you deliver in a medical center equipped with the highest level of neonatal intensive care possible—a level-3 NICU (short for *neonatal intensive care unit*). Such hospitals are prepared to administer the most complicated treatment to newborns, including chest surgery if needed. At a facility with a level-3 NICU, you can be assured of the best care for your baby.

This is crucial, since experts agree that immediate excellent neonatal care is necessary for the best outcome when treating severely preterm infants. Very premature babies have problems that are optimally handled only in the NICU. For instance, they become cold easily and must be kept in incubators to maintain a proper body temperature. Preterm infants may have respiratory distress from inhalation of meconium and/or from immature lungs. And all preemies must stay in the NICU for as long as it takes to bring them up to a weight of at least five pounds.

Also, studies have shown that preemies born in medical facilities with level-3 NICUs survive more often and with less residual damage than premature infants born elsewhere and then transferred to a medical center that has a level-3 NICU.

If you are planning to deliver in a facility that does not have a level-3 NICU, many authorities suggest that you change where you are going to have the baby, even if it means changing doctors—for the baby's sake. Should you wish to consider such a change, you should discuss your thoughts and reservations about your current facility with your doctor. Every case of preterm labor is unique, and you should make your decision based upon as much information and input from your OB as possible.

TREAT THIS AS AN OPPORTUNITY TO TAKE CONTROL AND TO PLAY AN ACTIVE ROLE IN YOUR CARE.

When you are having a complicated pregnancy, it's common to feel out of control of your body and your situation. And who could blame you? Your body is doing things that you have very little say about. It's normal and natural for this to upset you. You desperately want to do something, anything, to help yourself and your baby.

When it comes to preterm labor, you can. You can monitor yourself. You can keep written records that will be helpful to your doctor. You can tell your doctor how you feel and work closely with him to construct a routine that is the least disturbing to your uterus and, at the same time, as unrestrictive for you as possible (keeping in mind, of course, that sometimes total bedrest is the *only* answer . . .). You can enlist your loved one(s) in helping you monitor your uterus, and, by doing so, you can create a reality check system for yourself.

If your doctor does not recommend it, you can ask for and be placed on a home-monitoring service, to have daily human contact with medical personnel and the reassurance of good, constant care. You can comply fully with medication requirements and treatments such as bedrest and hydration.

In short, your uterus may have a will of its own, but that *does not* mean that *you* are out of control. The reality is that there is much that you can do for yourself and for your baby. In the end, there is always the chance that you may not be able to get all the way to term. But, if you participate actively in your care, you will have the satisfaction of knowing you did everything humanly possible to hold on to that baby for as long as you could. Through your actions, you will be increasing your odds of having an excellent outcome. Becoming actively involved in monitoring for preterm labor and working closely with your doctor to prevent preterm birth of your child is not only an opportunity for you to take a measure of control over a potentially overwhelming situation, it is your responsibility.

Sheryl's attitude is the one that you should adopt. She went into preterm labor at nineteen weeks. She was in and out of the hospital several times, placed on tocolytic drug therapy and on a home-monitoring service. She complied fully with doctor's orders and worked daily with the nurses, adjusting her dosages, keeping records, and staying put in bed. Her son, Sean, was born only ten days early, with high apgar scores and no problems whatsoever.

"I had headaches, and a rapid heartbeat," she told me. "I felt like my heart was going to leap out of my chest. I was anxious the whole time. I was ornery. That's the way my husband puts it. I had to keep reminding myself that the reason why this was happening was because I was doing everything in my power to make sure my baby was okay—that he'd be able to breathe and not go into the NICU when he got here. Every time I didn't want to hang in there, I'd think: You can do this. You're doing this for your baby. Every day I make it through means it's that much more likely that he'll make it.''

9

Bleeding, Hemorrhage, and Placental Abruption

The day before Lennette's birthday had been a taking-it-easy day. She was four months along in her third pregnancy and was anticipating having to go on full bedrest in a few weeks to prevent the preterm labor she had had in her other pregnancies. She'd had a cerclage (a stitch) placed through her cervix the previous month to help it stay closed as the pregnancy progressed. Everything had been going well, and her OB was optimistic that Lennette would make it to term.

Then, in the middle of the night, Lennette woke up bleeding. "It was as much as the first day of my period (my heaviest day), but all in one spot. It was very scary. I was convinced I was having a miscarriage." In the back of her mind, Lennette told herself: "Forget it, the baby's dead. You're bleeding to death." She immediately called her doctor and described the situation in detail. The doctor told her that she was okay. It did not sound as though she had passed any tissue, and Lennette was not having contractions. She should lie perfectly flat until 6 A.M., then call the doctor again.

By the time 6 A.M. rolled around, the bleeding had tapered off to spotting, and what blood there was had turned darker—a sign that fresh bleeding had stopped. She arranged to visit her OB's office later that day. "The nurse and doctor were so upbeat and positive and were very supportive," said Lennette. "The nurse laid me down and said, 'Okay, let's find this baby.' Hearing her say that infused me with hope, hope I hadn't had since I woke up bleeding." The nurse found the baby's heartbeat easily: The baby was still there, alive and well.

If she wasn't miscarrying, what caused Lennette to bleed so much? A blood vessel rupture in her cervix, brought on by the cerclage suture.

The vessel healed by itself within two days without any medical intervention, and the baby was never in any danger. "But seeing all that blood," Lennette said, "I would never have believed that the baby was still inside me." Lennette did not bleed again for the rest of her pregnancy.

Yet the incident really shook her. "Even with all the other stuff I went through in that pregnancy—my amniotic fluid leaking, premature rupture of the membranes, and an emergency c-section—nothing was as scary as the bleeding."

BLEEDING IS NOT ALWAYS A SERIOUS COMPLICATION . . .

Bleeding during pregnancy *is* scary, but not all that unusual. Between 10 and 20 percent of all pregnant women bleed or stain during some part of their pregnancy. Bleeding can occur at almost any time during pregnancy, from the first few days, right up to the last few hours. Some bleeding problems are associated with a particular stage of pregnancy: Some women bleed when the fertilized egg first attaches to the uterus (called *implantation bleeding*); others may experience placental abruption (premature separation of all or part of the placenta from the uterus), which only occurs after the twentieth week of pregnancy.

No matter at what stage the bleeding commences, like Lennette, up to half of those women who do bleed reach term without further complications brought on by the bleeding, so that neither mother nor child is permanently affected. There are also a number of minor, nonuterine problems—such as hemorrhoids, bladder infections, and polyps or lesions of the vagina and cervix—that can cause bleeding during pregnancy. If you have bleeding due to one of these problems, you will need treatment, but none of them will adversely affect the outcome of your pregnancy.

. . . AND COMPLICATIONS CAUSED BY SERIOUS BLEEDING DO NOT NECESSARILY DOOM THE PREGNANCY.

Even some of the most serious complications—placenta previa (where the placenta forms too low in the uterus—see Chapter 4), placental abruption, and threatened abortion (in which bleeding could progress to miscarriage)—do not necessarily doom you to losing the baby or having a severely damaged child. The bleeding of what is called *threatened abortion* has a 75 percent chance of resolving itself and the pregnancy continuing to term with a healthy outcome—if you follow doctor's advice and allow treatment. In other words, if you take immediate action and receive good medical care, even if you have these grave bleeding problems, the odds are in your favor.

Of course, not every story has a happy ending. Sometimes the baby dies; and yes, sometimes the mother does, too. There are also several complications which cause bleeding that always result in the loss of the pregnancy. Fortunately, these conditions are the exception rather than the rule. This chapter will discuss both the exceptions and the more common causes of bleeding. Placenta previa and miscarriage are discussed in separate chapters elsewhere in the book.

Cardinal Rule Number One: If You Bleed, You Call

Let's begin with the basics. If you start to bleed, you are not going to know why you are bleeding, what the source of the blood is, or whether you or the baby is in danger. You will probably be frightened (who wouldn't be?), and you may want to deny the possibility of anything drastic being wrong. But don't let that keep you from making the phone call. *No matter when bleeding starts, immediate action and prompt medical attention are crucial to good results.* No bleeding in pregnancy is to be taken lightly. Any time you bleed, your doctor needs to know so that he can start treatment at once, if necessary. What that treatment will be depends on the source of the bleeding, your stage of pregnancy, and the severity of the problem. Like Lennette, you may be asked to stay at home, in bed, until the bleeding slows or stops. You may have to go directly to your doctor for an examination and an ultrasound to determine the cause of the bleeding. Or you may have to go immediately to the hospital for supervised care.

Cardinal Rule Number Two: Make That Call, No Matter the Time

Don't stand on ceremony or worry about waking the doctor; calls in the middle of the night come with the territory of being an obstetrician. Call your doctor even if all you see is a little blood. Remember, bleeding is not normal any time during pregnancy, except when you expel the mucus plug just prior to a full-term labor.

If you are not bleeding heavily, your doctor can tell you whether he wants to see you immediately, whether you can wait to see him, and whether he'll see you at his office or in the hospital.

A Word About Describing the Bleeding

Your doctor is going to want to know whether you are bleeding slightly, moderately, or heavily. The sight of bright red blood coming out of your body is truly frightening, and you are likely to overestimate how much blood has passed. Nonetheless, try to be as objective as you can when describing the problem to your doctor. Are you just spotting, like you would at the beginning or end of a period? Is it every time you go to the bathroom? Are you soaking through pads every few hours or every hour? (If it's every few minutes, go to the hospital immediately.) Is the blood bright red, like from a cut? Or is it darker? Try to estimate amounts and whether you feel that it's subsiding or not. Are you passing tissue or clots along with the blood? Your OB is going to make his judgment based on what you tell him. So try as hard as you can to avoid minimizing or dramatizing your observations.

If you are bleeding heavily (a cup of more at a time, or persistently soaking through pads at a rapid rate), or if you wake up in the middle of the night in a pool of blood, call the doctor's office or service and tell them you are on the way to the hospital because you are bleeding. Don't wait for the doctor to get back to you, just get to the hospital as quickly as you can. If you are truly passing this much blood you *must* be seen immediately. The doctor's answering service will tell him to meet you at the hospital.

If you haven't been instructed earlier to go directly to the labor and delivery or maternity section of the hospital, go to the emergency room. Don't wait for your husband or neighbor to park the car. If the ER is crowded, for heaven's sake, don't stand on line or wait around for others to take their turn. Get yourself attended to *right away*.

Kathy did not know these rules when she started bleeding heavily in her twenty-third week. "I was only twenty. I didn't even know there was anything called a 'high-risk pregnancy.' I thought you either had a miscarriage or you had a baby. And I thought I was having a miscarriage." Kathy did the right thing initially. She called her doctor, who told her to meet him at the emergency room. But, when Kathy got there, the doctor had not yet arrived. She waited patiently, for forty-five minutes, before insisting that someone else look at her.

That wait nearly cost her the pregnancy—and her life. Kathy was bleeding from a partial premature separation of her placenta—called a *partial abruption*. The hemmorrhage was so bad that she had to be flown to a fully equipped medical center, where she stayed for two weeks, receiving blood, fluids replacement, and contraction-stopping drugs.

"The doctors there told me that if I'd stayed in the other place even one more hour, I would have died," she told me. "Next time, I'll know better than to wait around an ER bleeding." When Kathy told me her story, her baby girl was eight months old, developing normally.

If I Wind Up at the Hospital, How Will They Treat My Problem?

If you rush to the hospital with profuse, bright red vaginal bleeding, you should be prepared for intense intervention on the part of your doctor and the hospital staff. Exactly how they will treat you will depend on how many weeks along you are, whether you have also started having contractions or are in active labor, just how badly you are bleeding, whether your baby is in distress, and what the exact cause of your bleeding is.

Essentially, for any serious bleeding complication, there are two standard courses of treatment: immediate delivery by cesarean; or what doctors call *expectant management*—that is, strict, in-hospital bedrest and frequent monitoring until the baby is mature enough to live without a respirator outside the womb. Either way, you can expect some rapid initial testing and procedures when you reach the hospital:

- The doctor will examine your abdomen to determine whether the uterus is soft, or contracted, and to assess the position of the baby.
- He will listen to your heart and check your blood pressure (which can help to tell him how much blood you've lost).
- He will check you for shock.
- He will place a fetal monitor on you to find your baby's heartbeat and assess the baby's condition.
- The doctor will insert one or more intravenous lines into your arm(s) and start infusing you with fluids to replace the blood you've lost, to prevent shock, and to ready a vein in case you need a transfusion or drugs to stop contractions.
- The nurse will draw several blood samples from you to type your blood and check it for infection and composition (another way to tell how severe the blood loss is).
- You will have an ultrasound scan of your uterus to assess the exact position of the placenta and the baby and determine whether the placenta is really the cause of the bleeding.
- If you are in labor, the doctor may start you on tocolytic

drugs to stop the contractions. With some complications, contractions can worsen the bleeding.
- The doctor may also perform an amniocentesis to assess the lung maturity of your baby.
- If the lungs are immature, and your condition can be stabilized, you may receive injections of drugs called corticosteroids that speed fetal lung development.

All of these procedures and tests will probably happen in rapid succession if you come in bleeding heavily. More time can be taken if the bleeding is slowing down or has stopped. You'll probably be asked to use a bedpan if you need to urinate, on the theory that the more you move around, the more likely you are to provoke more bleeding. Or the doctor may order the insertion of a catheter (a plastic or rubber tube) into your bladder to drain urine, so that you don't have to move at all.

A Note About Your Feelings

If you go to the hospital with a bleeding emergency, it will be absolutely normal for you to feel overwhelmed and frightened. The rapid change of scene, the frenetic pace of the treatment you'll be receiving, your concerns about the well-being of the baby are likely to scare and disorient you.

Remember that the staff will be working fast to give you and your baby the best chance of making it to term, and while most labor and delivery suites in hospitals are warm and friendly places these days, the urgent nature of your problem may make staff dispense with the niceties.

This doesn't mean that you should give up all your say in the matter. If you have questions, ask them. If you have concerns about some procedure, say so. Don't assume that, just because you are in the hospital now, everybody who enters your room is going to know all the details of your condition and the treatment or advice you've received thus far. You must take responsibility for informing people about what's going on with you, including what your obstetrician has said to you, for your own sake.

Transfusions and Autotransfusion

If your doctor discovers your condition early enough in your pregnancy, you may be able to take advantage of a recent advance in treatment: storage of your own blood for later transfusion. Many women with severe or even moderate bleeding require transfusions as part of their treatment.

The technology also exists to recapture blood lost through vaginal bleeding, clean it and replace it intravenously in the woman's body. This is called *autotransfusion*. Autotransfusion is still limited in obstetrics and gynecology practice—principally because of lack of training in its use for obstetric purposes and unfamiliarity with or lack of the proper equipment. But a growing number of physicians are beginning to view the practice as the wave of the future.

However, autotransfusion does have its limitations: It isn't recommended for women whose blood is contaminated with bacteria, or for women with cancer (because blood-carried cancer cells could cause cancer to develop in other areas of the body). And, with severe hemorrhaging, it's likely that at least some banked blood or blood products other than one's own will have to be used.

These are options that you should definitely discuss with your obstetrician.

What Can Cause Bleeding During the First Half of Pregnancy?

There are many conditions that can cause bleeding before the first half of pregnancy is through. In fact, vaginal bleeding is one of the most frequent complaints of early pregnancy. If you are bleeding, and do not have abdominal pain, you can take heart: It's usually not an emergency requiring intervention. Many causes of bleeding *do not* result in loss of the pregnancy.

But don't let that fact keep you from calling the doctor, *immediately*. Remember the cardinal rule:

IF YOU BLEED, YOU CALL.

Most likely, your doctor will want you to come into the office, so that he can rule out acute problems either right away or when the bleeding slows down. Once you meet with him, there will be certain things your doctor will ask you and test you for:

- He'll take your medical history. Be prepared to tell him the date of your last period (date it began, not ended); whether you've taken a pregnancy test, and if so, which kind (blood or urine test). He'll ask whether you've passed tissue along with the blood. He'll ask whether you have a predisposition to bleeding disorders or a history of them in your family.

- He will do a physical, checking your blood pressure, your heart, and your lungs for signs of abnormality. He'll look to see how badly you're bleeding and examine you internally to see if the source of the blood is your vagina, cervix, or uterus. He'll check your cervix to see whether it is closed (closed is more indicative that you are not miscarrying), check the size of your uterus, and feel your abdomen and around the cervix to determine whether there are any masses inside your uterus or around your ovaries and tubes.

- He will take blood samples. One will be a pregnancy test to confirm the pregnancy (if you haven't had one yet). Other samples will be to screen the blood for infection, to do a red blood cell count to tell if you're anemic or have a clotting disorder, and to type your blood.

- He may order an ultrasound examination to rule in or rule out problems like placenta previa, premature separation of the placenta from the uterus (abruption), or ectopic pregnancy (pregnancy outside the uterus).

- He may admit you to the hospital, depending upon the amount of bleeding and how far along you are.

Ultrasound can be inconclusive when performed before you are eight weeks' pregnant (dated from the first day of your last menstrual cycle). Although ultrasound can detect fetal heart motion (a sure sign that things are okay so far) by seven to eight weeks of pregnancy, it does not always find the baby this early in the pregnancy. If you have not passed tissue through your vagina with the bleeding, and the technician cannot find the baby's heart and see it moving, this does not necessarily mean that the pregnancy has been lost or is in jeopardy. In short, when that happens, no news is no news. You'll need a retest after the eighth week, to confirm that you are still pregnant, and that the fetus is inside, not outside, the uterus.

IMPLANTATION BLEEDING

Implantation is the term used to describe the attachment of the embryo to the uterine wall and its connection with the mother's blood supply. Implantation bleeding is one of the most common causes of early pregnancy bleeding. In all likelihood, you will not be hospitalized for it and will probably have to do nothing more than rest for a day or two, if that, before it stops.

When the fertilized egg attaches to and invades the cells in the uterine wall, it destroys some of the small blood vessels carrying the increased blood supply, as well as other tissue around the attachment. Occasionally, the process causes the uterus to bleed at this site. Small amounts of bright red blood or brownish stain escape through the cervix. The bleeding lasts one or two days, stops when the uterine lining heals at the implantation site, and is not accompanied by pain.

Implantation bleeding that follows this pattern is not a signal that something is wrong with the pregnancy. But as this happens so early in the pregnancy, it's easy to think you're having an early miscarriage or a late period—especially unsettling if you've been trying to get pregnant. When I started bleeding three weeks after I started fertility drug therapy, I was very upset. I had been sure that I was pregnant, but there I was bleeding.

When I saw the blood, I was just as sure that my period had started, only a little bit late. But the next morning, the bleeding had almost stopped. That wasn't normal for me, so I called my doctor's office after I got to work. "What are you doing at work?" his nurse demanded. "Come up here right now and let's do a pregnancy test. I think you may be pregnant. Then we're sending you home to bed until forty-eight hours after the bleeding has stopped." Sure enough, the urine test was positive. I was pregnant. It was implantation bleeding, and it stopped completely just a few days later.

My experience is not uncommon. In cases like mine, going to the doctor to check out the cause of the bleeding can make a real difference in the outcome of the pregnancy. Many women, when they feel their period coming on, take painkillers or alcohol to avoid cramps. Both in excess might harm a developing embryo. If you've started bleeding or staining and you have any reason to suspect you might be pregnant, call the doctor and set up a pregnancy test before you take any painkiller. That just might not be your period; it might be your future child making its first real connection to you.

CERVICAL OR VAGINAL SORES, LESIONS, AND POLYPS

Sores, cuts, or lesions and polyps (small tumors attached to the body or internal organs by a fleshy stem) inside the vagina or on the cervix are another source of bleeding that almost always has no effect on the pregnancy or the baby. In pregnancy, the cervix and the vagina are full of blood vessels, and these can be easily damaged, even by active intercourse.

When your doctor examines you to determine the source of your bleeding, he will be able to see any damage to the vagina or cervix. He'll swab your vagina and cervix with cotton, to pinpoint the source of the blood. Once he finds it, he may leave it alone to heal on its own.

He may apply pressure with a cotton swab, or he may cauterize (seal) the vessels with a silver nitrate stick.

If the source of bleeding is a lesion or a polyp, the doctor will examine the area to determine whether the sore is benign or malignant. The doctor may remove part or all of the lesion or polyp surgically (a process called a *biopsy*) and send it to a lab for examination. This is usually done under local anesthesia in the office or on an outpatient basis at the hospital. The vast majority of such biopsies show no malignancy. The procedure is considered minor, and most pregnancies continue undisturbed by it until term. The doctor may also simply cauterize the site to stop the bleeding and create a clean wound that will heal up by itself with no further intervention. Again, the baby will not be harmed, and you will have minimal discomfort.

HEMORRHOIDS AND BLADDER INFECTIONS

Sometimes the bleeding is not from the vagina at all, but from the anus or the urethra. You might think that you'd definitely know the difference, but you'd be surprised how many women are fooled by such bleeding, especially as pregnancy advances and sensations in the pelvis change.

During pregnancy, all women are more prone to bladder infection and to hemorrhoids. (See Chapter 11, Other Fairly Common Medical Complications During Pregnancy, for an explanation of urinary tract infections and their symptoms.) Such infections are often accompanied by cramplike pain and can cause bleeding and involuntary release of urine. Blood-tinged urine that leaks out is easy to mistake for amniotic fluid from the vagina, because you may not feel it escape. The urine can become very bloody if the infection remains untreated.

And even though it's a minor condition, left untreated, bladder infection can jeopardize a pregnancy.

Whether or not you bleed, if you suspect a bladder infection, call the doctor and tell him. He'll want you to make a urine specimen to be tested at a lab. He may put you on antibiotics (several used to treat urinary tract infections do not cross the placenta and therefore do not affect the baby). He may also have you increase your fluid intake and could even ask you to go to bed for a few days to give your bladder a chance to calm down (sometimes the jarring motions of walking or running can further irritate an infected bladder). And in severe cases, treatment in a hospital could even be prescribed.

Hemorrhoids are also common during pregnancy. The extra hormones and blood supply that the body creates to sustain pregnancy increase the blood supply to the rectum (lower part of the large intestine) and anus (the outlet of the rectum to the outside of the body through which bowel movements pass). Peristalsis, the wavelike motion of the intestines that pushes food through the digestive system, slows down. Stool becomes dense and hard and thus more likely to cause the woman to strain when moving her bowels. Straining causes the already swollen blood vessels of the rectum and anus to bulge and bleed as stool rubs against them.

This bleeding is bright red and can be surprisingly profuse. It's possible to mistake this bleeding for vaginal bleeding. If you have bleeding after moving your bowels, telephone the doctor. He may or may not ask you to go to the office for an exam.

Either way, he can prescribe a stool softener and fiber therapy that often eases the problem. In addition, you should try to drink more fluids and increase the amount of fresh vegetables and fruits in your diet. In some cases, your doctor may suggest that you see a specialist to treat severe anal bleeding. Ask your doctor's advice before using any over-the-counter hemorrhoid drug. Some hemorrhoid salves may contain ingredients that can affect the fetus. And finally, don't worry about the baby if you have bleeding hemorrhoids: She won't be affected by your problem.

Threatened, Inevitable, Complete, Missed, or Septic Abortion/Miscarriage

The mere mention of possible miscarriage strikes terror into the heart of any woman who wants to have the baby she's pregnant with. Medical texts, and most physicians, call early pregnancy loss caused by the uterus expelling the fetus *abortion.* It's an unfortunate term, especially because of the negative emotional, religious, and political connotations that surround surgical abortion (removal of the pregnancy by D&C or suction curettage) in the United States. Most of us call it *miscarriage,* and that's what I'll call it for the rest of this discussion.*

Three-quarters of all miscarriages occur before the sixteenth week of pregnancy, most before the end of the eighth week. In fact, many more pregnancies than most of us believe actually end in miscarriage: Up to one-third of all pregnancies spontaneously abort before the end

*Miscarriage is defined as termination of the pregnancy before the fetus is viable. The definition of viability is a hot issue in many states. Legally, some states place viability (when the baby can survive outside the womb) at as early as twenty weeks' gestation; other states say a fetus is not legally viable until twenty-four weeks. No matter what the legalities, the fact is that continuing medical advances keep rolling back the dates of viability. Babies weighing as little as five hundred to six hundred grams and who have only developed to twenty-three to twenty-four weeks' gestation have been known to survive premature birth. Just a few years ago this was impossible.

of the eighth week. Many times, the woman won't even know she was pregnant and will think that she simply had a heavier-than-normal period.

Different labels are given to miscarriages and the bleeding they cause, depending upon the stage at which the woman arrives requesting medical help and/or what has happened medically. For example, *threatened miscarriage*, is the condition in which bleeding has begun, but the fetus is still alive and might continue to thrive. *Inevitable miscarriage* is the label used when the rejection/expulsion process has progressed too far for anyone to turn it back. The fetus is usually already dead, and it's only a matter of time before the uterus sheds its lining and the pregnancy. *Complete miscarriage* refers to total expulsion of the pregnancy, with no tissue left behind. *Missed miscarriage* is the condition that occurs when the fetus dies before the twentieth week of gestation but is not expelled by the uterus for eight weeks or longer. *Septic miscarriage* is miscarriage in which infection sets in either before the pregnancy is lost or after expulsion of the fetus.

The symptoms of impending or actual miscarriage are:

- vaginal bleeding (bright red and/or dark red, which may start as staining)
- cramps—usually mild at first, but they can be quite severe
- passage of tissue or blood clots

If you begin to bleed without cramping or with very mild pain, you may be in danger of miscarrying. This is threatened miscarriage, and prompt action is required if it will be possible to keep your body from expelling the pregnancy. Now's the time to ignore what you've heard numerous times in your life—that there's nothing you can do.

There *is* a course of action that can be taken. Treatment does not work every time, but, in up to 75 percent of all cases of threatened miscarriage that show up as bleeding without pain, the condition resolves and the pregnancy continues uneventfully to term and results in a healthy infant. The key is prompt recognition of the problem and faithful adherence to treatment once it's started. *Call the doctor.*

If threatened miscarriage is the problem, as with virtually any bleeding of early pregnancy, your doctor will perform certain tests. He'll do a blood test to check for anemia from blood loss, a blood pregnancy test to make sure you are pregnant (if pregnancy has yet to be confirmed) or to check and see if your pregnancy hormone levels have dropped—an indication that you may be miscarrying—and an ultrasound exam to make sure the baby is still alive inside you and that you do not have an even more serious problem. If the ultrasound picks up fetal heart motion inside the uterus (remember, this is possible as early as eight weeks of pregnancy), there's better than a 90 percent chance that the pregnancy will continue to term.

In early pregnancy—before the second trimester—treatment for threatened miscarriage is:

- bedrest until forty-eight hours after bleeding has stopped
- abstinence from sexual activity (intercourse as well as orgasm from other means)
- mild sedation to help you relax and to keep your uterus relaxed

This regimen may not sound like much. But if the fetus is not malformed or genetically damaged, it usually does the trick. If the fetus is defective in some way, your body is likely to continue the process and miscarry. Chromosomal abnormalities exist in up to 60 percent of all early miscarried fetuses.

Later in pregnancy, threatened miscarriage tends to announce itself by contractions without bleeding (see Chapter 8, Preterm Labor and Premature Rupture of Membranes).

HYDATIDIFORM MOLE

Unfortunately, there are some causes of bleeding during the first half of pregnancy that virtually always result in the loss of the pregnancy. Hydatidiform mole is one of these. It is the most common of the group of disorders called *trophoblastic diseases*—diseases caused by the abnormal formation of tissue or excessive production of normal placental cells. (Another trophoblastic abnormality is the *blighted ovum*—a condition in which a chorionic sac forms, but contains no fetus. These pregnancies abort early on. The first symptom: bleeding.)

Hydatidiform mole, also called *molar pregnancy,* begins at the stage of pregnancy before the developing embryo becomes a fetus. It happens quite rarely—only once in about seventeen hundred pregnancies. The condition tends to affect women under twenty or over forty. No one knows why.

The good news about this disorder is that for eight of ten women, there is no recurrence. There is an excellent chance that if you choose to become pregnant again, you will have a normal pregnancy that goes to term.

There are two types of hydatidiform mole: complete and partial. With complete hydatidiform mole, a sperm fertilizes an abnormal egg. The result is that no fetus develops. But the villi—tiny branching structures that, in normal pregnancy, later become the placenta—continue to form and attach to the uterine walls. Cells continue to reproduce, and a tissue mass of many cysts forms. Eventually this tissue begins to die; bleeding ensues, clots form, and the uterus tries to expel the products of the blighted pregnancy.

With a partial hydatidiform mole, the normal egg is fertilized by two sperm or by one abnormal sperm. In this case, a fetus does develop, but some of the villi form abnormally into a cyst-filled tissue mass. Even though parts of the placenta develop normally, these are not enough to sustain the pregnancy. The fetus usually dies before the end of the ninth week of pregnancy. Rarely, the baby survives to term. Almost always, bleeding ensues, and the pregnancy must be terminated.

Both types of mole announce their presence through vaginal bleeding. Most women are unaware of the condition until bleeding starts. Other symptoms include:

- anemia
- preeclampsia (also called toxemia. See Chapter 7, Hypertensive Disorders of Pregnancy)
- hyperemesis gravidarum (severe and repeated vomiting. See Chapter 3, Hyperemesis Gravidarum)
- A uterus that is larger than it should be for the length of the pregnancy

Most likely, if you have this complication, you won't know until your doctor tells you the results of an ultrasound scan, the diagnostic test that definitely rules hydatidiform mole in or out as the cause of bleeding. What you will know is that you are bleeding and having cramps or contractions as your body tries to expel the tissue. You may pass clots and pieces of tissue, some of which will be grape-shaped.

As with any bleeding in pregnancy, it's important that you let the doctor know right away that you've started to bleed. With this particular problem you may actually have a lot more blood loss than either you or the doctor thinks at first, because blood can become trapped in the uterus behind the tissue mass.

The only cure for the bleeding is the removal of the pregnancy—which, you must remember, in all likelihood cannot sustain itself. With complete hydatidiform mole, no fetus will form, so there is no baby to save. If you have a partial mole, the ultrasound scan will tell your doctor if there is even the remotest chance that there is enough normal placenta to nourish the baby until she can survive outside the womb. This would be extremely rare.

If you have this disorder, your doctor will, in most cases, want to perform a D&C—dilation and curettage. Under general or regional anesthesia, the doctor dilates your cervix and gently scrapes the walls of the uterus with a sharp instrument, called a curette, to remove the remains of the pregnancy and ensure that no tissue stays behind to cause infection or hemorrhage.

Before you have the D&C, you can expect some extra testing on top of the normal drill for women who come to the hospital with bleeding (see above, If I Wind Up at the Hospital, How Will They Treat My Problem?). The nurse will draw blood to detect anemia caused by the bleeding, to check your hormone levels, and to ascertain whether your kidneys and liver are functioning normally (potential complications of this complication). Chest X rays may also be taken.

ECTOPIC PREGNANCY

Ectopic pregnancy is the complication that many women fear most, and for good reason. So let's start with the worst of it and get the scary stuff out of the way.

Ectopic pregnancy—the attachment and growth of the embryo outside the womb—is an extremely serious complication. It virtually never has a good outcome for the fetus, is the leading cause of maternal death in the United States (between 1 and 2 percent of all ectopics are fatal), and is one of the most frequent complications (happening in one to two of every one hundred pregnancies). It always needs surgery to correct and can compromise the woman's ability to conceive again later, and the odds of it happening to the same person twice are fairly high. Ectopics are becoming more common, rather than less: Their incidence has nearly tripled in the past two decades, in part because of the rise of venereal diseases and *pelvic inflammatory disease,* or PID for short (infection of the structures in the pelvis, usually brought on by use of intrauterine devices—IUDs), that scar the fallopian tubes (see Chapter 11, Other Fairly Common Medical Complications During Pregnancy).

That said, having an ectopic does *not* mean that you'll never be able to conceive or have a normal pregnancy again. Some studies say that nine out of ten women—even those who lose a fallopian tube as a result of an ectopic—can still have a successful pregnancy later. I know. I'm one of those women. I had an ectopic when I was twenty-six. I had surgery to remove the pregnancy, and I also lost one fallopian tube. At the time, I was sure I'd never conceive again. I was wrong.

Ectopics happen most often to women in their twenties and thirties. The problem can be caused by a number of things: fallopian tube abnormalities that the woman was born with, scarring of the tube due to previous infections or abdominal surgery, pelvic tumors, using an IUD for birth control, DES exposure when the woman was a fetus herself, endometriosis, or even an egg that migrates from one ovary to the opposite side's tube.

Just what is an ectopic pregnancy? It's defined as the implantation of a fertilized egg outside the uterus—most often in the fallopian tube (90–95 percent) or in the abdomen (far less than 1 percent). Except for the rarely successful abdominal pregnancy, in which the fetus develops in the abdominal cavity, ectopics always result in the termination of the pregnancy, by surgery, to save the mother's life. Often, in the tubal ectopic, the tube is so damaged by the time the problem is discovered that it, too, must be removed.

One reason this damage occurs is that up to half of all women with ectopics are misdiagnosed initially. The symptoms of ectopic pregnancy set in very early—within the first eight weeks—and they can mimic nearly fifty other medical conditions, such as appendicitis, a ruptured ovarian cyst, or an early miscarriage, to list just a few. To make matters more difficult, some ectopic pregnancies do not produce enough of the hormones of pregnancy to register on standard urine pregnancy tests, and levels may be misleadingly low even in blood pregnancy tests. When these diagnostic tools fail, and the physician does not recognize the pregnancy from other symptoms, he may treat the woman for another suspected ailment. Thus, the pregnancy grows in size, further damaging or possibly rupturing the tube.

By the eighth week of pregnancy, 80 percent of all women with ectopics are diagnosed as having them, even if the initial diagnosis was an incorrect one. But, usually, by the eighth week, there is significant damage to the tube.

Because it's so difficult to recognize an ectopic, it's important for you to know the symptoms of ectopic pregnancy and how they are likely to set in, so that you can seek prompt treatment. The symptoms are:

- pain, which may be stabbing and fleeting, or constant; it may be in one spot (particularly on one side or the other) or all over the abdomen; this pain may or may not be accompanied by
- bleeding, bright red or brown, that can be profuse or slow, spotting or steady
- the sensation of rectal or bladder pressure
- shoulder pain caused by the enlarging fallopian tube putting pressure on nerves

The way symptoms crop up is different for every woman. For me, my period was about two weeks late. I felt queasy and thought I had a stomach bug at first. Then I got what I thought was my period. But it stopped and then started again one day later, with constant, bright-red bleeding; not a lot, somewhere between spotting and staining. As this happened, my "queasiness" got worse and I started having pain on my lower right side. I also came down with a low-grade fever.

I knew that none of this was normal, so I called my gynecologist, who, much to my dismay, insisted I come in for a pregnancy test. If I'd had my period, how could I be pregnant, I wondered. (With an ectopic, you can.) The test came back a low positive, and when my doctor did a pelvic exam, the slightest touch hurt. He put me in the hospital, did a D&C and abdominal surgery to remove the fetus, and I lost my severely damaged left tube.

Most women (about 60 percent) will have symptoms that are some variation of what I experienced. They begin gradually and increase in intensity. For between 50 to 95 percent of women, the first symptoms will be bleeding with abdominal pain within seven or eight weeks after they've missed a period. For some, there will be no vaginal bleeding, but there will be abdominal pain. It may start as a feeling of gas in the bowels, or a stitch in the side. It may come and go. But as the fetus grows and distends the tube, nerves are irritated, there is internal bleeding, and the pain grows steadily worse and more constant. A fever may also begin.

If you have the gradual onset of any of the symptoms of an ectopic, it may be tempting to wait around and see if the pain subsides, or slight bleeding stops. Don't. *It is crucial that at the very first sign of bleeding or abdominal pain, you call the doctor.* If you're wrong, and all you really have is gas, you may feel embarrassed, but there's no harm done. If you're right, and you are having an ectopic, early detection will save your life and possibly your fertility. If an ectopic is allowed to proceed untreated until you are in an extreme medical crisis, you are likely to develop infection and hemorrhaging that can scar your other tube or your ovaries, or kill you.

For four out of ten women, there will be no temptation to make the mistake of waiting around and seeing if the symptoms go away. For these women, the symptoms are overwhelming. There may be knifelike pain in the belly and/or back. Bleeding from the vagina may be profuse, just a little, or nonexistent. If there is internal hemorrhaging, the woman may feel suddenly weak, thirsty, or starved for air. She may vomit. The pain in the abdomen can even be so severe that she cannot walk. If any of these acute symptoms happen to you, *call your doctor and go directly to the hospital.* Failure to act quickly can cost you dearly.

Doctors classify ectopics as subtle presentation or catastropic, according to your symptoms when they first see you. Subtle presentation means you have pain and some bleeding, but have not suffered a rupture or catastropic bleeding. Catastropic presentation is when you don't seek medical help until you are in shock from blood loss and pain. Both require surgery.

If you go to the doctor or the hospital with subtle presentation, you will be asked the standard questions and have the usual blood and urine tests that you can expect with any bleeding during pregnancy. Your doctor will also perform a pelvic exam. During the exam, he will gently move your cervix back and forth with one or two fingers. This is one way that he can discern whether you are bleeding because of an ectopic, as a classic symptom is pain when the cervix is moved. He will feel your uterus and around your ovaries and tubes to see whether there is a mass. This may also be uncomfortable.

A procedure called *culdocentesis* may also be part of the exam. For this, the doctor inserts a hollow needle through the vaginal wall close to the cervix. The needle is attached to a vacuum tube (much like that for a blood test), allowing it to draw off fluid. If you are bleeding internally, it tends to pool behind the vagina in the peritoneal cavity, which is where the needle penetrates. So, if blood can be drawn from the cavity, it usually means that a bleeding ectopic is in progress.

Preparations for culdocentesis are much the same as those for a regular pelvic exam. You'll be on an examination table with your legs in stirrups. The doctor opens your vagina with a speculum, swabs with antiseptic the area to be penetrated, and may numb the spot with a local anesthetic. If one isn't offered, you can ask for it. Once the area is cleansed and numbed, he will insert the needle through the vaginal wall.

Something else you'll probably be slated for is an ultrasound exam to rule out intrauterine pregnancy. If no pregnancy can be found in the uterus, and if your human chorionic gonadatropic (pregnancy hormone) levels test above a certain level, it again points to an ectopic.

If the doctor definitely rules in an ectopic as the cause of your problem, the doctor will schedule you for surgery, probably that day or the following morning. If you come to the hospital with catastropic presentation, you'll be in surgery within hours.

In either case, it's likely that you won't have the option of choosing what type of surgical procedure will be used, although you can discuss options with your OB to see whether there is any leeway in your treatment. Don't forget, whether the surgery is done on an emergency basis or can be put off until the next day, it is being performed to save your life.

There are several ways that the surgery may be performed, depending upon the amount of damage your internal organs have suffered and the extent of the bleeding. Often, rather than just proceed directly to major surgery, the doctor will first perform a diagnostic laparoscopy to determine the extent of the damage. Most doctors do this while the patient is under general anesthesia.

Once the woman is anesthetized, a small incision (rarely noticeable postsurgery) is made in the navel. The abdominal cavity is inflated with carbon dioxide gas to give the surgeon plenty of room to view the ovaries and fallopian tubes with a fiberoptic instrument called a *laparoscope*. Sometimes it's too hard to see everything that needs to be viewed through the one incision, in which case, the surgeon must make another small incision through the lower abdomen (at the line where bikini panties would sit—also called a *bikini* cut or incision). If the pregnancy is small enough, it can sometimes be removed through these small openings.

Most of the time, if ectopic pregnancy is confirmed, the doctor will proceed to do a laparotomy—a larger bikini incision that allows him free access to the fallopian tubes and uterus. Depending upon the amount of damage the tube has sustained, the surgeon may take the fetus and the tube, or he will try to preserve the tube and thus the woman's fertility for future pregnancy. He will also repair any damage to other internal organs that the ectopic may have caused. And he may do a D&C as well.

If you have catastropic presentation, you will already have lost a lot of blood before getting medical treatment. You may have to have blood transfusions and fluids replacement even before surgery starts. The doctor may dispense with the laparoscopy and proceed right to a laparotomy to reach the bleeding quickly and stop it.

Recuperating from the surgery will take from several to many weeks, depending upon the amount of blood you've lost, the size of the incision(s), and the amount of internal stitching that was required to close you up. Generally, you can expect your recovery to be similar to that of a cesarean section (see Chapter 13, Cesarean Section); both procedures require the same restriction on activity, and both manifest the same physical discomfort during the healing process.

But an ectopic is very different from a cesarean in one important aspect. An ectopic results in a pregnancy loss, and you must not be surprised if you feel sad, angry, or simply depressed by what has happened to you. It's normal and natural to grieve this loss just as anyone else who has suffered the death of their unborn child. Those feelings may come months after your loss—particularly around the time the baby should have been born. Don't be too hard on yourself if you find you're behaving oddly right after the surgery or six or seven months later. All of us who have had ectopics have residual feelings to deal with.

My ectopic surgery was in April. That December, I could not fall asleep without holding a small, soft pillow close to my chest—something I'd never done before. I cried uncontrollably over sentimental television commercials. I felt awful and I really couldn't figure out why, until a friend pointed out that it was the month my baby would have been born. The connection helped me tremendously. After that, I found a professional counselor to help me cope.

Everyone's level of need in handling pregnancy loss is different. Chapter 10, Pregnancy Loss: When the Worst Happens, offers numerous suggestions to help women deal with their loss and provides the names and addresses of support organizations around the country.

What Causes Bleeding During the Second Half of Pregnancy?

Many of the causes of bleeding during the first half of pregnancy can create bleeding during the latter half as well. But there are two major causes of bleeding during pregnancy that occur most often after the twentieth week: placenta previa and placental abruption. Placenta previa, the most common cause of second and third trimester bleeding, is covered separately in its own chapter, Chapter 4. Placental abruption—the premature separation of the placenta from the uterine wall—which occurs with less frequency, is discussed below.

PLACENTAL ABRUPTION

Placental abruption—premature separation of the placenta from the uterine wall—is considered the gravest of all complications in pregnancy. The key reason is that when the placenta detaches too early, the hemorrhaging that follows has the potential to kill both the mother and her child at a time when most infants could otherwise survive outside the womb. It is a condition that requires quick recognition and immediate medical intervention for a good outcome to be achieved. Despite this danger, up to 75 percent of all abruptions result in no permanent harm to mother or baby.

Jane's is a typical story. She was twenty-five weeks' pregnant with her third child when her placenta started to separate. "The pregnancy had been perfect until then," she said. "That day in particular, I'd helped a friend move some furniture at an auction, and then carried my four-year-old son in from the car. When I got in, I felt fluid leaking. When I checked, it was blood red. I also had some abdominal tightening, coming more often than I remembered with the other two pregnancies. I called the doctor, who wanted to see me right away. We met at his office, and he did a very careful, long ultrasound, which found what looked like a black blob. Everything else around it on the screen was gray. The placenta was tearing away from the uterus. My doctor wouldn't let me go home and pack or anything. He took me in his own car to the hospital, telling me that there was a chance that nothing more would happen and it would not get worse, or it could tear away completely. There was no way to tell.''

At the hospital, Jane went on a regimen of total bedrest and anti-contraction medication to prevent preterm labor and contractions that could worsen the tear. She spent only six days there. The bleeding slowed down, then stopped, and Jane was sent home. She spent another six weeks on bedrest, then was allowed to resume some activity. A weekly ultrasound showed the ''black lake'' of blood diminishing, until it was gone. There were no further complications, and Jane delivered her healthy, normal eight-pound, seven-ounce baby girl vaginally, just five days before her due date. She told me ''it was the best delivery I'd ever had. The other two were cesareans!''

Only one of every one hundred to two hundred pregnancies is complicated by placental abruption. It can happen any time after the twentieth week, but occurs most often after the twenty-eighth week— that is, during the third trimester. The separation can be partial or total and can vary greatly in severity depending upon the size and location of the area that detaches from the uterus.

Abruption is triggered by a sudden disturbance to the uterine blood supply, which can be brought on by a number of conditions. For instance, if a woman who is near term lies flat on her back for any length of time, the weight of the uterus lying on the major blood vessels that supply the placenta can temporarily press them closed. The sudden compression can actually cut off blood supply to the placenta and cause the placenta to partially or totally shear away from the uterine wall. Or, if the woman suffers a violent blow to the abdomen (like the steering column hitting the belly during a car accident), the force can be transmitted to the placenta and cause it to rip away from the uterine wall.

Premature separation of the placenta can also be due to chronic poor blood supply to the area. This can be caused by a number of medical conditions, such as diabetes, chronic kidney disease, and hypertensive disorders (high blood pressure and its complications—see Chapter 7) predating or brought on by the pregnancy. Rapid decrease in uterine size can also be a culprit—just after the birth of the first baby in a multiple pregnancy or when hydramnios (overabundance of amniotic fluid) spontaneously drains. In addition, uterine tumors or other uterine abnormalities can bring on abruption.

When these events take place, they can cause part or all of the placenta to pull away from the wall of the uterus. The blood vessels in the wall lose their connection to the placenta and begin to bleed into the uterus.

If the tear is at the edge of the placenta, the blood drains from the uterus through the cervix into the vagina. If the separation is in the center of the placenta (a *central abruption*), the blood cannot escape to the outside and is called a *concealed hemorrhage.* The uncontrolled bleeding builds up pressure behind the placenta, forcing more and more of the placenta away from the uterine wall, until the separation reaches an edge and blood comes rushing out through the vagina. This is the most dangerous type of placental abruption. The woman is usually unaware that she is bleeding and thus does not seek medical help before she is in shock. Because the doctor cannot see it, he may underestimate the amount of bleeding that has occurred. The baby often dies before the physician can intervene. Fortunately, concealed hemorrhage only happens in about 15 percent of all abruption cases.

The medical community grades or ranks abruptions depending on the mother's symptoms, the degree of blood loss and placental separation, and fetal and maternal distress. Some physicians rate abruptions on a scale of 0 to 3; others use the terms *mild, moderate,* and *severe.*

About 75 percent of all abruptions are considered *mild* (or a 0–1 on a number system). In fact, with 30 percent of all premature separations, no symptoms are present and no one knows it has even happened until after delivery (grade 0). No medical intervention is necessary, as these minimal abruptions remain undetected until after birth.

Another 45 percent of abruptions announce themselves with vaginal bleeding that may or may not be accompanied by uterine pain or tenderness and contractions. These involve only a small portion of the placenta. The baby is not endangered, and the bleeding is not so profuse as to produce shock. The tear often heals spontaneously and the bleeding stops. If no further bleeding occurs, vaginal delivery is probable.

About 15 percent of all abruptions are considered *moderate* (or grade 2). These involve a greater portion of the placenta and may or may not show up with external bleeding. The uterus becomes *tonic*— that is, constantly contracted and painful. When this happens, the fetus goes into distress from lack of oxygen and may die inside the mother before intervention is possible. If the baby dies, most doctors will work for a vaginal delivery, both to spare the mother from surgery, and to protect her from further hemorrhage. If the baby is alive and continues to be distressed, the doctor usually performs a cesarean to get her out of the hostile environment that the womb has become.*

---

*With all levels of abruption, the prevailing wisdom used to be that a cesarean was in order if the woman did not deliver within six hours of arriving at the hospital. This is no longer always true. Some doctors now opt for continuous replacement of lost blood. As long as they can keep up with the rate of hemorrhage, these physicians will allow labor to continue—unless, of course, the baby is in too much distress.

Then there are the 10 percent of abruptions that are *severe* (or grade 3). Bleeding is massive and may be concealed. The uterus is unremittingly contracted and hard. The mother goes into shock from blood loss, and her blood's ability to clot (coagulate) is disrupted. The major hemorrhage within the uterus becomes uncontrollable, and other organs also begin to bleed. This syndrome is called *disseminated intravascular coagulation*—or DIC, for short.

Although DIC occurs most often in severe abruptions, it can occur in moderate cases as well. DIC is reversible through intravenous infusion of platelets, fresh whole blood, and other coagulation-encouraging products. But DIC-related bleeding can continue for some time after delivery.

Tragically, in severe abruption cases the baby always dies. Once the coagulation deficit is corrected, vaginal delivery of the dead fetus is usually attempted within six to twelve hours. Sometimes a cesarean is necessary both to retrieve the baby and to stop the bleeding.

You will know that you may be having an abruption if you have some or all of these symptoms:

- slight, moderate, or profuse bleeding from the vagina that begins suddenly after your twentieth week of gestation
- uterine contraction that makes your uterus hard all over and does not stop
- abdominal tenderness or pain
- a sudden feeling of thirst, faintness, or inability to ''get enough air''
- nausea

Again, and I cannot stress the importance of this enough, *if you bleed, call the doctor, no matter what the time. Don't wait around to see what's going to happen. Get to the hospital immediately!* With abruption, early diagnosis is essential: With proper diagnosis and intervention, the likelihood of fatal complications for you is extremely low—between 0.3 and 1 percent. For your baby, quick action reduces mortality from a 60–80 percent probability to 4 percent.

Rosalie told me that when she had her abruption, her doctor said to 'give it an hour, then call me back.' I sat around and waited the hour. There was blood all over the kitchen. Every time I stood up, blood ran down my legs. When I finally got to the hospital, my doctor said, 'Thank God you got here!' Looking back, I think I should have gone in right away. And he should have told me to. I could have lost the baby. As it was, when my son was born, his apgar score [a test done on a 1–10 scale after birth to judge the health of a newborn] was three, which is low. If I could say one thing to other women in a similar situation, it would be: *Go! Don't* wait around for that hour." Rosalie's baby recovered completely. He's now eight years old, healthy and normal.

No matter what degree of placental separation you may have, you can expect fast, aggressive intervention on the part of the hospital medical team:

- The doctor may insert several IVs—one or more for fluids, one or more larger line(s) for blood transfusion.
- Nurses will draw numerous tubes of your blood. Among other things it will be typed and matched to donor blood for transfusions, tested for anemia (an indicator of unseen hemorrhage), and tested for DIC.
- There may be blood transfusion(s) to reverse DIC and anemia and to prevent shock.
- The doctor may order that a catheter be inserted into your bladder to closely monitor the output of your kidneys, which can shut down when there is massive blood loss.
- To support the baby, you will breathe oxygen from a mask, a hood, or an under-the-nose tube.
- There will be an electronic fetal monitor tracking the baby's progress to detect the smallest signs of distress. And, if you are in labor, your contractions will also be monitored.
- If you are going to deliver, the doctor may rupture your water (the fluid in the amniotic sac) to speed the delivery. This procedure can manage the bleeding and decrease the release into your bloodstream of the amount of substances that interfere with clotting.

If the doctor determines that neither you nor the baby is in immediate danger, and you don't deliver right away, you will be managed expectantly—that is, nursed along until your baby is capable of surviving outside the womb. This will probably mean total bedrest, in the hospital. Under certain circumstances, you may be allowed to be on bedrest at home. In general, those circumstances are that you must live within fifteen to twenty minutes of the hospital, have reliable and constant adult supervision in case you begin to hemorrhage again, have access to reliable and fast transportation, and adhere faithfully to bedrest instructions. You may also be placed on a monitoring service to check you daily for contractions. I suggest that you read Chapter 15, Bedrest, for ideas on how to keep yourself occupied and sane during this time period.

The one thing you *must* hold on to while this is happening is that even though having an abruption is painful, terrifying, and awful, you are much more likely than not to come through it okay, with a healthy baby at the end.

Colleen went through the wringer, but she told me it was worth it. She was hospitalized at twenty weeks with what became a chronic abruption. She lived in the hospital for ten weeks, during which she was in the labor and delivery suite a total of fifty separate times. She had DIC and pain so severe that she couldn't see. She had bloodwork done every half hour for hours at a time, for days on end. When I spoke to her, her little boy was eight weeks old—still two weeks away from his original due date. But the baby was healthy and tested normal, with no problems anticipated. "While it was happening, I just wanted the nightmare to be over. But now, I look back, and I have this wonderful, beautiful baby. It's a very happy ending to a long, sad story."

10

Pregnancy Loss: When the Worst Happens

I was in the recovery room no more than an hour, with my husband by my side, when the neonatologist came to see us. "How are my babies?" I asked him hopefully. He had a look on his face that I didn't like. He seemed unhappy. And he had an X ray in his right hand. I could see a tiny rib cage outlined there. Before I could form my next thought, he told us that our son seemed fine; in a couple of weeks, when he'd gained enough weight, we could take him home. Then, the words that forever changed my life: "But your daughter is a very sick little girl. Her lungs. . . ." Jenny's lungs. In the X ray. No!

Numbness immediately set in. The words that penetrated were snatches of the doctor's assessment—"one hundred percent oxygen and still not getting enough . . . brain dying . . . joints frozen . . . if she were to live . . . never be able to use her arms and legs . . . a matter of time . . . absolutely no hope."

My God! He was telling me that my daughter was dying! I'll never get to see her alive, I thought. They'd rushed her to the NICU as soon as she was born. Since I'd had a c-section, I probably wouldn't even get to the NICU before she died. I remember choking out requests: Don't let her feel any pain. No heroic measures. Let her die with dignity. I want to see her as soon as she's gone.

That last request, I must have said it over and over like a mantra. I'd read only one article about infant death, in some women's magazine, and it had said it was important for the mother to see the baby. Otherwise, the article stressed, the mother might not believe that she'd given birth or that the death had taken place.

The doctor said how sorry he was. He promised to do everything he could to make her comfortable. Then he left us to go tend to my little girl. I remember thinking that I was just too tired to cry right then. I stared up at my husband: He looked stricken and helpless.

The nurses came in and out, pushing here, poking there. A shot, a new IV fluid drip in my left arm. Then everything went fuzzy.

The next thing I remember is being in my room, numb inside. I was so excruciatingly sad. I felt like rocks were on my chest. But I couldn't cry. I asked many questions about my son. My son who would live and grow up to be a man. I sent my husband down to take Polaroids of him for my wall, until I was strong enough to go see him. I don't remember asking much about Jenny.

Later, my parents came to see me. They were with me when my husband came back. He was still in the yellow gown they make you put on in the NICU. But something was wrong. He ducked right into my bathroom. I knew somehow before he came out again that Jenny was gone. My husband was crying. My parents left the room.

Then the nurse brought Jenny. Her body was still warm. I had a hard time forcing myself to remember that she wasn't only asleep. She was so beautiful. What a gorgeous face. Such long, slender fingers; pretty feet; delicate ears. Her arms and legs were stiff, and her feet were not quite pointing the right way. But she looked just perfect to me. I only got to hold her for a few minutes. I wanted to hold her longer, but I didn't think I was allowed to. I took off her little cap and tucked it inside my nightie. It's the only article of Jenny's clothing I have. My parents came back in, looked at her, cried with us, and said their good-byes.

And then she was gone. I never saw Jenny again.

No one on the hospital staff told me I could see her again. No one told me pictures could be taken. They didn't say I could bathe her or dress her. No options were offered about how to handle her remains. No clergy visited my room. When it came to dealing with Jenny's death, we were on our own.

So we made what we believed to be the best and most reasoned decisions we could under the circumstances. We asked the hospital to take care of Jenny's remains. We told them that if they could learn from her death, they could use her body to learn from. We couldn't bear the idea of having a memorial service. We wanted to focus on our living, breathing son who needed us. We felt there was no time for grieving. Life was for the living, and we had to get on with it.

I've regretted each of our choices about Jenny ever since.

If just one person had stopped in and asked us to reconsider our decision, if anybody had told me that there are support groups all over the country for grieving parents, if anyone had said that it's *good* for parents to hold the baby, bathe her, dress her. . . . Well, let it suffice to say that we would have done it differently.

Unfortunately, our experience was all too common. Thousands of couples who lose a child before, during, or shortly after birth receive no or very little emotional or practical assistance. They are forced to endure one of life's most searing pains without support, and, because they have no guidance, they often end up making choices that are wrong for them, choices that prolong their grief.

Now, especially when it comes to pregnancy loss, I'm a big believer in being well-informed and knowing your rights. When Jenny died, we had no idea what to expect and demand of others. At no other time in my life has being ignorant of the facts cost me so dearly. I do not want that to happen to you.

If no one steps forward to walk you through the first days of grieving and prepare you for what is to follow, reading this chapter will provide a beginning guide. The Other Reading and Resources section at the back of the book and the support organizations listed at the end of this chapter can help you continue on with the difficult work that lies ahead of you.

If you are in one of the many hospitals with terrific care for parents in your situation, this text will still help you sort things out. This chapter is also for anyone who just wants to know what to expect and what some of the options are in case the worst happens. And may it *never,* ever, happen to you.

What Is a Pregnancy Loss?

In her twelfth week of pregnancy, Ann started bleeding. She knew what was coming next, she said, because this had happened to her twice before. She was losing the pregnancy. "When I got to the emergency room, the doctor wanted to do a D&C right there." (D&C stands for *dilation and curettage,* an operation in which the doctor scrapes the inside of the uterus with an instrument to remove the remains of the pregnancy.) "But I insisted on going to the operating room. Half an hour after it was done, they sent me home, at 2 A.M., in a rainstorm. It happened so suddenly and intensely, and then it was all over and no one acknowledged that I'd had a loss. This was in nineteen seventy-nine, and people weren't talking about loss and how to deal with it. I picked up on the external cues—no big deal, you can go on and have another."

Ann had had a miscarriage—the loss of a fetus before twenty weeks' gestation have passed (in many states, after twenty weeks, it's called a *stillbirth)*. All her babies died during the first trimester. Often, when miscarriage happens in the early weeks, the baby is not recognizable as a human form. Does that mean that there is no real loss? That this shouldn't count as the death of a child?

No. People who specialize in counseling newly bereaved parents will tell you that pregnancy loss is the demise of any baby, no matter how short a time that baby spent in the womb. That means that miscarriage counts. Ectopic pregnancy counts. Stillbirth counts. Babies who die within minutes of birth count. Even a blighted ovum—when a placenta with no fetus forms, and the woman's body behaves as if it were pregnant, counts. Any pregnancy that doesn't result in a living infant that you get to take home and nurture is a pregnancy loss.

And the loss is so much greater than just the actual death of the child. You had hopes and dreams for that child. You may have imagined what she looked like, whom she would take after, what it would be like on her first birthday. You were preparing for a lifetime of loving and living with this new person. These things died along with your baby.

Loss After a Complicated Pregnancy

If your baby died after a complicated pregnancy, you may feel doubly bereaved and angry. While working so hard to maintain your pregnancy, you developed a deep emotional investment in your baby. This means that your loss may feel extremely painful. This is especially true for women who have been on prolonged bedrest. You've given up all your usual activities, done everything humanly possible to protect your child from harm, and it still wasn't enough.

Keep all this in mind if you seem to feel "overly emotional," if your grief is stronger or lasts longer than you think it should. Remember, you already had a big loss before your baby died: First you lost your perfect pregnancy, then the baby herself. You should expect to have to work through these issues as well as the usual issues that surround a pregnancy loss.

Working Through the Grief

You didn't choose to go down this path, but go down it you must. There is no "normal" or "right" way to deal with the death of your baby. "Our tendency is to put mourning on some kind of scale—like this loss is worse than that loss," says Judith L. M. McCoyd, who specializes in perinatal bereavement counseling. "I've had clients come to me and say, 'But other people have had it so much worse than me. Why do I feel so bad?' ' '

The answer, says McCoyd, is that "grief is grief. It has its own scale and it's not related to length of gestation. While there may be differences in how people grieve, you don't have to grieve less if you lost your baby at twelve weeks' gestation rather than at two days after a full-term birth. Some people are more connected to their immediate feelings than others. But any kind of judgment about the appropriateness of someone's grief is *in*appropriate."

In other words, almost any way that you grieve your loss is in the realm of normal. Although each person's grief is unique to him or her, everyone does go through some arrangement of an identifiable group of feelings. But it is important to emphasize that no two people grieve in exactly the same way. There is no "proper" order or definite path. For many people, one set of feelings predominates for a while, although all may overlap. It is normal to experience each feeling or some feelings repeatedly over the course of months or even years. Your way will be your way, and it will be the right way for you.

SHOCK, NUMBNESS, AND DISBELIEF

"On December twenty-ninth," said Ron, whose son died sixteen days after birth from complications due to prematurity, "I remember, they called us at nine A.M. and said 'you ought to come down here.' It didn't dawn on me they were saying he's going to die, you should get down here. It didn't connect. We went down and they were hand pumping him with a big black balloon. I remember it still wasn't really dawning on me. They asked us to go out in the waiting room. I asked why."

Ron could not accept what the doctor was telling him. This is a common reaction to the news that your baby is dying or has died. It is too overwhelming to grasp. It's such monstrous news that you don't want to believe it.

Once it does sink in a bit, it's quite normal to feel numb or be in shock. You may find it impossible to cry or feel much of anything at all. It took me weeks even to start to come out of my emotional shell after Jenny died. Some people emerge from shock within hours. But both time periods are considered well within the range of normal.

ACTIVE GRIEVING, OR YEARNING AND SEARCHING

"One day, when the visitors stopped coming, and I ran out of things to do about the funeral, I had no more thank-you notes to write or anything, that was the day that *boom,* it hit me all at once,'' said Marie. ''I was alone, the babies had died. I started crying and I couldn't stop.''

For Marie, this was when she really began to grapple with the intense emotions she felt about her babies' deaths. At some point after the death of a baby, most people experience intense feelings—anger, sorrow, guilt—as they try to sort out what happened. You may direct your anger and sorrow outward and feel angry at God or at your doctor for not preventing this terrible loss. Or you may lash out at loved ones with little or no provocation. This might be described as ''active'' grieving, or yearning and searching. And it may last anywhere from weeks to years.

The Hardest Question: Why Did This Happen?

At some point during this time, you'll feel compelled to ask this question. Why, why my baby? Why did this happen? You'll ask your doctor. You'll ask the nurses. If you are a religious person—and often, even if you're not—you'll ask God. You'll ask your clergy. And you'll ask yourself. Why *my* baby? Why me?

Sometimes the medical answer is quite clear; but many times, it is not easy to find. If your doctor cannot readily ascertain why the baby died, you may request an autopsy to find out. Often, though, even an autopsy won't tell you exactly what went wrong. Sometimes, as hard as it is to grasp, no one can tell you why.

Even when there is an adequate medical explanation for your loss, you may find yourself grappling with the greater whys. Why did such a terrible thing happen to you, to your baby? If only one in however many pregnancies end this way for this medical reason, why is yours that one? Why has life been so unfair?

You probably already know that there are no pat answers to these questions. And because of that, you may find yourself examining every tiny detail of your own behavior, searching for the one thing you did to cause this awful tragedy to happen. The truth is, you probably did nothing to make your pregnancy result in the death of your baby. More likely, you did everything you possibly could to keep the pregnancy going. The truth is that there are events in life over which no one can have control. This is one of them. But what you know in your rational mind can't always overrule what you feel inside.

THE "EMPTY ARMS" SYNDROME

"Three weeks after my baby died, my arms and my heart literally hurt," said Nancy. "My arms felt so heavy that I kept looking down and expecting to see her there. But of course, she wasn't. It was just my imagination."

What Nancy described to me are common sensations for many women whose baby dies: They feel a terrible emptiness, physically. You may have these feelings—aching arms, a heaviness or soreness in the chest over your heart. And you may daydream or dream at night about your baby. It is also not uncommon to think you hear a baby crying in your house. This is a normal part of wishing that this hadn't happened to you, of yearning for the baby you still should have.

During these times, it is also common to have other physical symptoms. Your sleep patterns may shift, or you may feel exhausted, but unable to sleep. You may feel constantly winded, as if you've just been running. You may have nausea and/or poor appetite. And you may sigh a lot.

The severe stress that the loss of a baby creates can actually compromise your health. You may find yourself plagued by a series of colds or other viruses. And your inability to concentrate makes you a ripe candidate for accidents such as spraining an ankle or injuring a finger. Most bereavement specialists suggest that you get a complete physical sometime within the few months after the baby's death. Then your doctor can spot any potential problem before it gets out of hand.

DISORIENTATION, LONELINESS, AND DEPRESSION

"I remember, Susan cried every day for a year," said Harold. "She was incredibly depressed."

In the wake of all the intense emotional upheaval (or sometimes preceding it), many people feel drained, unhappy, and empty. You may lose interest in what's going on around you, feel listless, be unable to concentrate, and experience a loss of appetite. It may be hard to drag yourself out of bed in the morning. Your personal grooming habits may suffer. And grieving may seem interminable at this point.

It is also common to feel particularly susceptible to the vagaries of life. You may not feel safe going outdoors, driving, or taking public transportation because you fear that something else terrible might happen to you or to other loved ones. If you've gone back to work, this can also mean that your performance may suffer.

These feelings may be protracted, or you may have them for only a few weeks or even days. Feelings of helplessness and unhappiness may also come and go over the course of months.

ACCEPTANCE AND REORGANIZATION

"One day, I'm not even sure exactly when . . . I guess about six months after the stillbirth . . . I was watching an *I Love Lucy* rerun on T.V. You know, the one in the chocolates factory? Well, I started laughing, and my husband looked up from his paper, very startled," said Emily. "I guess I hadn't laughed since the day I delivered Benjamin. That's the day I mark as when I started to feel better."

Eventually, one does begin to feel better. How long that takes varies for each person. Sometimes it will start with a moment, like Emily's, and then just continue on. For others, the good days and bad days intermix. Either way, you begin to accept your loss, and your life takes on its new shape.

It is not realistic for you to expect that you can put life back just the way it was before the baby died. This was a true loss, and its repercussions will most likely affect both your perspective and the way you operate in the world. There will always be days—and events—that will trigger intense feelings of grief. What is important is that you find a way to integrate what happened to you into your life so you'll be able to experience the full range of emotions that the rest of your life will have to offer. You cannot face the future with a part of your past walled off inside you.

The Special Pain of Losing One of Multiples

When I became pregnant with twins, my husband and I became part of a special group. Expectant parents of twins and larger multiples are treated differently by their doctors, their families, and society in general. When the babies are born, the parents are showered with even more attention than most new parents. Everyone is eager to comment on the babies, show their appreciation, and generally make a great fuss over you and your kids.

When one or more of those babies doesn't make it, but you have a child(ren) who does, all the fuss dries up. People become confused as to what to tell you—should they congratulate you on the birth of the child who did survive or send condolences for the one who died? Do they ignore the death and tell you that you are lucky one (or more) lived? I had friends who didn't call me for several weeks or months because, they said later, they just didn't know what to say.

You may find yourself equally or even more confused than your family and friends: How can you celebrate the new life you will bring home and mourn the death of your beloved other child at the same time? How can you cleave to your newborn and let go of your other baby? Yours will be a unique kind of pain, because your living child will always remind you of the child you lost. Your sorrow reminds you of your joy, and your joy reminds you of your sorrow.

It's okay to feel your happiness—it does not demean your memory of the child who died. And it's okay to feel great sadness—that child was going to be an important person in your life, and you should not minimize that. Your living child(ren) doesn't "make up for" the one(s) who died. You cannot injure your living child(ren) by making room in your life for the appropriate and necessary grieving of your dead baby.

In time you may come to feel keenly both joy and sorrow each time the child(ren) that did survive does something new for the first time. Parents of multiples who died say that they often "see" the child(ren) that died when they look at the survivor(s). I often look at my own son and see what Jenny might have been like. I feel deeply sad still that I don't have the two I counted on when I sometimes watch my son playing or feel his gentle fingers on my cheek when I kiss him good night. And I am told that this does not stop. When he graduates from high school, when he marries . . . I will think of Jenny, then, too.

It is a difficult situation for everyone. You should be prepared when some people attempt to avoid talking about your dead baby or to downplay the significance of her death. As a society, we don't deal with infant death well to begin with. When one or more babies survive a multiple birth, it's an easy out for friends and family to focus on the life you've brought home.

Just because many people don't want to talk about it doesn't mean that you shouldn't. You *need* to talk about your dead child. You *need* to work through your grief about her. It's all right for you to bring the subject up, as often as you wish. If certain people in your life cannot deal with that, then save these conversations for those who can allow you to share your pain with them.

At the end of Chapter 12, Multiple Pregnancy, there is a listing of the national support groups for parents of multiples. Call them, and find out what local chapters are in your area. Many local groups have bereavement support for people in just your situation. Also, call the Our Newsletter organization listed at the end of this chapter. It is a national bereavement support group for those of us who experience the unique pain of losing one of a multiple pregnancy.

You Will Make Many Choices

"All these little issues come up that you never dream you have to encounter in your life, and you're supposed to have some knowledge— like the etiquette for a funeral," said Marie. "The pastors came to our house after the graveside services—we didn't know if we were supposed to pay them something after, like you would after a wedding. We didn't know what to do as far as a monument, inscriptions, how much you pay for the funeral home, pay for the plot, pay for the marker. All this was new and overwhelming."

As numb as you feel, just like Marie, you're going to be asked to make a number of decisions in the first twenty-four to seventy-two hours after your baby dies. These include:

- Hospital personnel should ask you if you want to see, hold, bathe, dress, photograph, and name your baby. (Some babies miscarried as early as eight weeks' gestation may be recognizable as tiny little humans and should be available for you to see and hold if you want to.)
- You'll be asked if you want an autopsy on your baby.
- You may be asked if you wish to donate the baby's organs and/or corneas for transplant or research.
- You will be asked for a decision on how you wish your baby to be handled: Do you want a funeral, a memorial service, cremation, a religious ceremony, and so on.
- You will have to start planning your baby's funeral or cremation arrangements, if you choose to have any kind of service. (In some hospitals, it is a requirement that the parents be responsible for the disposition of their child's body if she was over a certain number of weeks' gestation—often twenty.) That will mean choosing a funeral home and the type of memorial service you wish (religious or secular) and choosing a final resting place.
- Someone from the hospital will require information for a birth and/or death certificate if the baby was over twenty weeks' gestation (these requirements vary by state).
- There may be other forms to fill out at the hospital.
- You will probably want to inform those closest to you of your baby's death and will need to decide how you'll do that.
- If you and your husband work, you will want to let your employer(s) know what has happened, and you should arrange to take time off. You may have to inquire about your company's maternity and paternity leave policies regarding infant death: Many companies allow the bereaved parents to take their planned-for leave of absence or parental leave regardless of the pregnancy's outcome. If leave is still offered, take it. You're going to need the time together. Unless you feel it would be *good* for you, it's much too soon to go back to your old routines.

- You may need to arrange for child care if you have other children at home, and you will have to decide how to tell your other children that their brother or sister has died and won't be coming home.

LETTING THE HOSPITAL "TAKE CARE OF EVERYTHING"

You may also be given the option of having the hospital "take care of everything." This usually means that you give the baby over to the hospital and allow the administrative staff to deal with the baby's remains according to hospital procedure. The loss of the baby can be so staggering for the parents that dealing with the baby's remains can feel like more than they can handle. Thus giving control of the baby to the hospital can seem very appealing, and many people accept this offer of "taking the burden off" them.

The problem with giving away control over what happens to your baby is that it often feels like a big mistake later on. You may discover in a few weeks or months—or even years—that you wish you knew what had happened to your child. But hospitals do not routinely inform parents of the location of the baby's final resting place. You may long for remembrances you could have had if you'd arranged the funeral and a memorial service. And you may feel remorse about letting your child go to strangers.

This is a decision you cannot take back once the hospital has carried out its offer. It you have any question whatsoever about whether you are doing the right thing by giving the baby over to the hospital, then take time to think about it. You don't have to rush into making this decision. You may be better off enlisting support people to hold your hand while you make the arrangements yourself.

We're all different: It may be that allowing the hospital to take care of the baby *is* exactly right for you. If so, there's nothing wrong with letting the hospital do everything. But you should be given the opportunity to make this decision after getting all the facts and after serious reflection and with the guidance of a counselor, social worker, clergyperson, or other support person(s).

NO MATTER WHAT ANYONE SAYS, YOU DON'T HAVE TO MAKE ALL THESE DECISIONS THIS SECOND.

It may seem monstrously unfair that you have to make all these choices so soon. In the first twenty-four hours, you've barely had a chance to absorb the fact that your pregnancy is over and there is not going to be a baby for you to take home.

"I was having a hard time dealing with all these questions and choices that were there," said Marie, whose twin son and daughter were born at twenty-four weeks, each living only hours. Her son died first. "The nurse asked, do you want to hold him? I hadn't even dealt with their birth. I felt really overwhelmed. . . . In my room, my pastor came and gave us choices, and people told me what had worked for them. We needed to make decisions about where to have a service, whether to have an autopsy, how involved should I be. I was feeling number and number."

What Marie did not know is that some of the choices she had to make need not have been made in those very first hours.

Obviously, some choices do have to be made immediately. For instance, if your child was born alive but is now dying, you need to think quickly about whether you wish to be with her and hold her during her last moments. (For some people, watching their child die is far too much to bear; for others, being able to share their love with, provide comfort to, and have contact with their baby at the end is of utmost importance.) If you want to participate in the bathing of the baby after her death, you need to let your wishes be known right away; otherwise, the nurses will do this task as a matter of course.

You can put off decisions on almost everything else for at least a few hours and, in some cases, for as long as a few days.

You shouldn't get only one chance to see and hold your baby at the hospital. If you decide you don't want to hold her right away, the hospital should accede to your wishes and make the baby available to you again. The hospital does not have to send the baby out of the facility right away. And your option to see and hold your baby should not end once she is taken to the funeral home. There, her body will be prepared or embalmed. Her body and her looks will remain basically unchanged for days. Most infants, no matter how prematurely born, can be viewed and held again and dressed at the funeral home.

In fact, because the baby's remains have been prepared, it is possible to put on hold making the funeral arrangements for as long as days or even weeks. That means that even if you've had a cesarean, you should not have to be absent from your baby's funeral. (Some religions prohibit delaying the burial. If you wish to have a religious ceremony, you need to find out what the requirements are, and then if you need to, work out compromises with your clergy.) If you cannot avoid missing the funeral, plan to have someone stay with you during that time. You can even hold a little service of your own.

If you can't decide about whether you want photos right away, you have not lost the option of having pictures taken of your child. Your baby can be photographed any time before the burial or final disposition of her remains.

Many—but not all—hospitals these days are very good about giving newly bereaved parents as much breathing space as possible when it comes to making these decisions. It's possible that you may feel pressed by staff to make every decision almost immediately. If this happens, you can always ask for more time, and it should be given to you whenever possible.

What You Have a Right to Expect from the Hospital

It may be difficult for you to stand up for yourself if you need to in the first hours and days after your child's death. When your baby dies, you may feel so diminished, exhausted, or numb that just about the last thing you want to do is complain or make requests. At facilities with good bereavement programs, you won't have to. Many hospitals know exactly what to do to help you through your first days of mourning.

Unfortunately, it is still true that many other hospitals are not strong in this department. So it will be important for you to know what you have a right to expect of the staff and then to ask for these things if or when they are not provided. These are the *minimum* services that facilities should provide and you shouldn't be at all embarrassed if you must be insistent to get them:

RIGHTS OF PARENTS WHEN A BABY DIES*

- to be given the opportunity to see, hold and touch their baby at any time before and/or after death
- to have the opportunity to have a photograph of their baby
- to be given as many mementos as possible, i.e., crib card, baby beads, ultrasound picture, lock of hair
- to name their child and bond to him/her
- to observe cultural and religious practices
- to request an autopsy
- to be given information regarding their baby's status
- to be cared for by empathetic staff who will accept their feelings, thoughts, beliefs

*Reprinted from "Considerations for Perinatal Bereavement: Rights of Parents When a Baby Dies and Rights of the Baby," Women's College Hospital, Perinatal Bereavement Team, Ontario, Canada.

- to be with each other during hospitalization
- to be informed about the grieving process
- to plan burial or cremation according to their religious or cultural tradition

Rights of the Baby

- to be recognized as a person who was born and died
- to be named
- to be seen, touched, held by family
- to have life ending acknowledged

Seeing and Holding Your Baby

"We lost the heartbeat at the hospital while I was in labor," said Janis. "My baby was stillborn. The nurses were really good about letting me hold her. But back then, they didn't take pictures. But because I got to hold her, I have an indelible memory of her."

It's been well-established that parents—the mother, especially—should be encouraged to see and hold their baby before death, if possible, but certainly after the baby has passed away. This may sound incredibly morbid to you at first. But it really isn't: This was your child. Seeing her will help make her death real for you, an important first step toward healing.

Also, seeing her will help dispel any fantasies you may have about what was wrong with her, if anything. (Many babies die from internal complications, or from birth accidents, not because they are deformed in some way.) And, if she had a physical defect, your imaginings of what the deformity looks like will almost always be worse than the actual defect. Most likely, when you do see the baby, you will find yourself focusing on the baby's perfect features rather than the imperfect.

Usually, when people mourn, part of what sustains them is their fond memories of the individual who is gone. But your baby's time with you ended before she even arrived, or just afterward. You do not have that rich past to draw upon for support. Seeing and holding your baby, and allowing grandparents, siblings, or other close family members to do so (if they wish and you approve), will help you create special memories of your child that you will never forget. Don't give these up, and if the opportunity to create them isn't offered, ask for it. It is your right.

BATHING YOUR BABY

Before funeral homes were widespread in this country, it was considered part of the normal course of things for the family to bathe and dress the deceased for the funeral. Today, all that is often done by the funeral home. But in your baby's case, it needn't be. You were planning to give this child baths for years.

Again, it may at first seem unnatural to you to contemplate handling your dead child, especially in such an intimate way. But when you think about it, this is one of the few things you will ever get to do *for* her. It is one of the few opportunities you will have to be with her before you must let her go for the last time. It is a memory that you may cherish in the years ahead.

If you are unsure of how to start, the nurses should be able to show you how to handle the baby. Some premature infants' skin is quite fragile, but in most cases, you won't harm the baby in any way by sponging or dabbing her off and cleaning her.

Of course, this is a personal decision that only you can make. Bathing the baby may be too hard for you emotionally, or, if you had a c-section, you may not yet be physically able to bathe her. Just remember that bathing the baby is an option to consider. If you want to give her the bath, and you are not asked if you would like to, make your wishes clearly known to the staff, and don't be dissuaded. This is *your* baby. You can bathe her if you want to.

DRESSING YOUR BABY

Dressing your baby is another option that should be offered to you by the hospital staff. Depending on how far along you were when your baby died, you may already have had a little outfit all picked out to bring her home in. This outfit belongs to this baby, and it is reasonable and natural to want her to have it in death.

If you have no special little clothes for the baby, or if the baby was too premature to fit into regular infant or preemie clothing, you may be able to find doll clothes that fit her or someone who makes tiny gowns just for these circumstances. Members of bereavement support groups and churches and synagogues sometimes provide this service for newly bereaved parents.

Some parents find that it helps them feel closer to each other and to the baby to go shopping together for a special outfit for the burial. "Our son didn't have anything that was white in all the clothes that we had already received as gifts while my wife was pregnant," Ron told me. "So we had to go shopping to get something white to bury him in. We looked forward to that. I remember how picky we were, like we were buying him something for his first holy communion.''

Photographing Your Baby

"If our house ever catches fire," Marie told me, "after making sure the kids, my husband, and the animals were out of the house, the next thing I'd go for is the box where I keep Nicholas's and Danielle's keepsakes and pictures."

While seeing, holding, bathing, and dressing your baby create memories of her to treasure in your mind, you may later find that you also want tangible things to remember her by. Photographs are often the most important of these.

You would be surprised at the warmth and softness such pictures can convey if they are well-taken. Hopefully, a staff member at the hospital is well-versed in taking photos of babies who have died. If the hospital does not offer to take pictures of the baby for you—and they *should*—you can take them yourself.

If you find it too difficult to photograph the baby (and you might; this, as do so many other facets of this process, depends entirely on the individual), you can ask a friend, hospital staffer, family member, or professional photographer to do so. If you then find that you cannot bring yourself to look at the baby's pictures, you can ask that these be put in an envelope and placed with the baby's records, or ask someone you trust to put the photos somewhere secure. You can then choose the time and place you want to view them. The same can be done with a videotape.

My husband took pictures of Jenny while she was still alive in the neonatal intensive care unit (NICU). To this day I have not looked at them, but it gives me great peace of mind to know that someday, if I want to, I will be able to look at my little girl. I have no photos of her after death, when she was pain-free and without hardware attached to her. I regret this deeply.

Other Remembrances

There are many other mementos that you can have to remember your baby. The hospital should, as a matter of course, offer these to you. They were your child's, and it is your right to have them. But sometimes hospitals don't offer them, and if not, you should ask for them. These include:

- the cap the baby wore in the NICU
- the blanket she was wrapped in

- her NICU undershirt
- her wrist bracelet
- a lock of her hair
- her isolette card
- any crib toy the hospital may have provided
- her comb
- her pacifier
- her hand and/or footprint (almost all hospitals make these for identification purposes shortly after birth)
- Her birth and death certificates
- Blessing or baptismal card
- Her hospital records
- X rays or sonogram pictures of the baby

If your baby was stillborn, or if you miscarried, many of these items may not be available to you. Still, you can ask for and expect to receive any and all items connected with your baby that the hospital has in its possession. These are the only mementos you will have of your son or daughter. Don't leave them behind.

Changing Location Within the Hospital

After your baby dies, or you have miscarried, you may wonder if you will find it quite difficult emotionally to remain on the maternity floor. Some women find it excruciating to listen to the sounds of the newborns as they are wheeled in to see their parents. The happiness and laughter of other families' visitors when they come to see the new mothers may serve only as painful reminders of what the bereaved parents do not have. On the other hand, some women find the sounds, smells, and cheerful atmosphere of the maternity ward comforting. Also, nurses on the maternity floor are better skilled in helping the newly bereaved mother cope with physical aspects of postpartum care.

The hospital should offer you the choice of staying on the floor, or moving to another section of the hospital that is not connected to maternity. If staff do not mention this option to you, and you feel that it would be easier on you to be off the maternity ward, request that you be moved. There is no reason that you cannot continue to receive the care you need on another floor.

Bending Normal Visitation Rules

The night Jenny died, I could not bear to be alone. I never wanted company as badly in my life, preferably my husband's. Even though it was against the hospital's usual policy, my husband stayed with me through the night every night after I had the babies until I went home. The nursing staff never even questioned it.

When your baby dies, it often helps in the early days to have someone with you at all times. Even if you don't talk, it may give you comfort just to know they're there.

For many couples, this is a time of needing to be together, to support each other, to offer comfort and share their loss. Especially at night, when you are used to the warmth and safe feeling that being with your partner gives you, it may be very hard to be alone.

Every hospital's visiting hours and rules are different. Some hospitals' policy is to allow spouses to remain overnight with their wives if birth is imminent or has just occurred. Some hospitals have policies against spouses rooming-in, especially if the woman is sharing a semi-private or multiple-bed room.

Under normal circumstances, these policies are understandable. But your circumstances will not be normal. Your baby just died. You may feel empty enough as it is, without having to face the prospect of being alone during the long hours of the night. If you feel that the two of you need to be together through the night, tell the hospital staff. Ask if a cot can be provided for your husband (or another family member if you are a single parent or your husband cannot be there).

You shouldn't, but if you do meet with resistance, enlist your doctor's, clergy's, social worker's, or counselor's assistance in persuading officials that this is what is best for you right now. This is one time that the hospital should be willing to bend the rules.

SEEING COUNSELORS AND CLERGY

These days, many hospitals have on-staff social workers, nurses, or other professional counselors specially trained in perinatal bereavement counseling. Most facilities also have a chaplain on staff, or at least on call, who may be trained in the art of pregnancy-loss counseling. If the hospital provides such people, you should expect them to visit you in your room shortly after you return from delivery.

If no one comes to you, or if you feel a need to talk to someone, ask the nurse on duty whether such a person is on staff at the hospital, and request that they come to see you as soon as possible. If there is not a counselor on staff at the hospital, ask whether there is a bereavement support group allied with the hospital with which you can be placed in touch. Failing that, call one of the national organizations listed at the end of this chapter (see, Outside Support, below) and find out whether there is a support group in your area. Most of these organizations provide immediate telephone support. And most of them will be able to help you connect with someone who can listen to and address your concerns and feelings.

What You Have a Right to Expect from Your Clergy

"I have always felt I was a good religious person," said Aliene, whose only son died four days after his birth at twenty-eight weeks' gestation, because of complications brought on by severe prematurity. Aliene was a regular churchgoer, and she still has a strong faith in God. "I never blamed the Lord. I questioned Him, but I never blamed Him. He had a reason, and someday I'll know what that reason is. . . . But I don't go to church anymore," she told me. "Not since the day the pastor at my church gave me 'comfort.' The things he said to me were not the things I needed to hear. All he told me was 'You should be grateful you had four days.' That really bothered me. A pastor, of all people, should know that I had a lifetime planned for my son, not four days! His other suggestion was to write a letter to my ex-husband, who left me after I became pregnant, and ask him to forgive me for losing the baby. I've had a real hard time finding and going back to a church since then."

Many people turn to their religious leader for solace and guidance after a pregnancy loss. No matter what your religion is, or whether you still practice your faith, in times of crisis, it is a common impulse to seek out the comfort that religious conviction and/or ritual can provide. We rely on our pastors, priests, and rabbis to be stronger than we are, to be more knowledgeable about the processes of death and grieving than are we, and to say the right things to bring us relief.

While oftentimes this expectation is well-founded, you must be aware that it also often is not. Chaplain Jim Cunningham at Fairview General Hospital in Cleveland, Ohio, whose own son was stillborn at term, says that in a survey he has done of bereaved parents, more than 50 percent felt that their pastor, priest, or rabbi had been unhelpful after the death of the baby. Over 66 percent thought that their congregations were also unhelpful.

"There's a world of possibilities in the way you will be treated," says Chaplin Cunningham. "You end up taking care of a lot of other people's needs in this process. That's unfair, but that's how it is. And sometimes," he says, "you have to do that with clergy. You, the bereaved parents, become their teachers, and hopefully they will become the learners."

Which is why it is important for you to know, at least generally, what your religion's conventions are when it comes to the death of a baby in utero, or very shortly after birth. Most religions have shorter or no specific services and rituals for miscarried or stillborn babies. Even babies who die shortly after birth (days or weeks), receive little religious recognition in some instances. And, despite religious teachings, in some congregations children baptized before death forever have a different status than those who receive the blessings after dying.

Depending on your religion, there will also be different requirements in timing of the funeral. In the Jewish tradition, burial of the dead usually comes the day after death. Some churches prefer the dead to be interred within forty-eight to seventy-two hours. In others, the burial need not be for some days after that. And within each of these traditions there is often some flexibility, depending upon the receptivity of the parents' clergy.

At a minimum, your priest, rabbi, or pastor should be willing to provide you with full information about your denomination's customs and should explain in detail all your possible options. He should allow you to choose what you feel and think is best for you and should encourage your full participation in the services. In addition, he should help "walk you through" the maze of choices and requirements that go along with the religious ceremony—such as working with the funeral director and obtaining permits (when necessary). Your clergy should also willingly do what he can to support you in working through your grief, whether that means having private counseling sessions with you, referring you to religious or secular support groups, or simply offering a strong shoulder and open ear when you feel ready to talk about your experience.

And there is nothing wrong with "shopping around" to find someone who is sympathetic to your needs. Many people will go outside their usual congregation if they feel their regular clergy is not meeting their requirements or if they do not belong to one particular congregation.

"It's your baby," says Chaplain Cunningham, who has written books and numerous articles on infant death. "The issue is not what is right or wrong religiously, it's what you need. My advocacy to parents is not to get boxed in by the traditions. Insist on having the funeral or memorial service your way insofar as you can. Your clergy is not there to get their needs met; they're there to get yours met."

What You Have a Right to Expect
from a Funeral Director

If you decide not to have the hospital handle the final disposition of your baby's remains, you will most likely request the services of a funeral establishment. The funeral home and its staff should assist you in all phases of planning the service for the baby, taking care of state requirements (if there are any), arranging for a final resting place for your baby, and working out the logistics of transporting the baby and the bereaved family from funeral home to service site to gravesite (if the two are different).

How Do I Locate a Funeral Director?

The vast majority of people in your situation have never had to contact or use a funeral home before. Sometimes the hospital will have one or more funeral establishments with which it works and will call one of them to pay you a visit in the hospital when your baby dies. So start by asking whether the hospital provides such a service, and if it does, let the person come visit you and see whether you like him.

Your next best bet is to ask other parents who have lost a child (if you know such people) which funeral home they used. Talking to those with direct experience is often most helpful, since some funeral homes deal with handling dead infants much differently than they do adults. Parents who have had a loss are the most likely to be candid with you about what they liked and did not like about the services they received. If you don't know of a couple, you can also call a local bereavement support group or one of the national organizations listed at the end of this chapter for assistance in locating a good establishment.

Failing that, if your parents or other, older relatives live in your town, ask them if they know of an establishment that they've been satisfied with. Yours may be one of those families that have been in the same place for many generations, and you may be surprised to find out that a particular funeral director has had a long-standing relationship with your relatives. If the family doesn't know a funeral director themselves, perhaps they have friends who have had good experiences with a home in your area.

Finally, if you cannot get a referral, there are always the yellow pages.

ALL FUNERAL HOMES ARE NOT ALIKE

How you will be received and treated will vary widely from one establishment to another, just as protocol and empathy vary from one religious congregation to another. And just as it is okay to "shop around" and find sympathetic clergy, you should not have to "settle" for the first funeral director you contact, if how he behaves and what he offers you do not suit your needs.

"What you should look for," says Thomas Zerbel, a funeral director in Escanaba, Michigan, who frequently cares for parents experiencing the death of a baby, "is someone compassionate and understanding, who is willing to sit down with you and provide you options. If you're not satisfied in the first ten minutes, excuse yourself and contact another funeral director." Zerbel has developed and manufactures miniature baby caskets—ten-inch Burial Cradles—for infants who have miscarried, the only such caskets in the United States (see Other Reading and Resources at the back of this book for further information).

IN-PERSON VISIT

A good funeral director should be willing to come to you for the first visit, not make you go to him. The funeral director should come to your hospital room or, if you have been discharged, to your home. The initial visit need not be lengthy unless you feel up to it.

TAKING YOUR TIME

Once you've settled on the funeral establishment, planning the service and settling the details can be put off for up to several days. In the meantime, the funeral home will arrange to have your baby's body transferred to its facilities to begin preparing her remains for their final disposition. Or, in most states, you may transport the baby yourself.

Being able to hold off on details and the service itself (if you are having a religious ceremony and your religion allows the delay) can be particularly helpful when the mother has had a cesarean and may not be sufficiently recovered physically to take part for several days.

DISCUSSION OF OPTIONS

When you are ready to discuss the details with the funeral director—whether at the initial meeting or at a later time—there are a number of items that he should bring up for discussion. These include:

- a reminder that you don't have to hurry, unless your religion requires it
- a frank, up-front explanation of all costs, if there are to be any. Many funeral homes provide their services, including some type of casket, free of charge to newly bereaved parents of miscarried, stillborn, and early-loss babies. But charges of one to three hundred dollars just for the casket are not out of line. Other potential fee items include: costs to transfer the baby from the hospital to the funeral home, then to the service site and to the cemetery; embalming or other body preparation; dressing the baby; and positioning her in the casket.
- a reminder that cemetery costs (again, if any) are separate from funeral home costs. There will be the cost of buying the grave, a fee for opening (digging out) the grave and closing (filling in) the grave. These expenses can run as high as several hundred dollars. Often, the baby's grandparents offer to let the couple bury the child in the grandparents' plot, saving the expense of purchasing one separately just for the baby.
- a full explanation of options for the final disposition of the baby, including burial, cremation, and a combination of cremation and burial
- full details of choices available for the service, including: at home, in the funeral home, at graveside, or from a church or synagogue. The funeral director should bring up practical matters for discussion and not allow you to focus solely on the type of atmosphere you would like.
- legal costs and requirements (if any) in your state. The funeral director should explain and take care of any legal papers, obituary notices, death certificates, and transfer and burial permits that may be needed.
- an explanation of your options for memorializing your baby's final resting place. Many funeral homes hope that, because they do not charge for their services for the death of a baby, the parents will use the money to place a marker on the grave. Many bereavement professionals feel it is important for the parents to mark a baby's grave, to provide the parents and family with a physical place to return to. Costs for such memorials run from fifty to over one thousand dollars, with one to four hundred dollars on the average. It is not unusual to spend more on the grave marker than on all other funeral costs.
- Most important, an exploration of your wishes. He should

seek out your opinions and directions for the music, flowers, other decorations, whether you want a viewing of the baby, and an open or closed casket. He should offer you the opportunity to hold the baby again, for as long as you like, to dress her in her final outfit, to greet your guests, to participate actively in the service. He should make suggestions as to how you might be able to participate—such as writing part of a service, or reading poems or your journal (if you kept one).

Again, these services are the *minimum* that you should expect from a good professional. As hard as it is to keep in mind in this terribly trying time, *you must come first.* The funeral director is there to serve your needs, not vice versa. He should feel to you like a help and support, not another burden for you to carry. Take your time and try to find this for yourself. Later on, it will make a tremendous difference in how you remember your child's passing.

Your Family and Friends Will Be Grieving, Too

Although it will feel like the loss of your child is yours alone, your family and friends will have their own difficult feelings about the death of your child to cope with. Your own parents were probably looking very much forward to having this particular grandchild, whether she was to be the first or the twenty-first. Your siblings were looking forward to becoming doting aunts and uncles to your child. If you have other children, they were anticipating a new member of the family, too (see Helping Your Other Child(ren) Deal with This Loss, below). And your friends were eager to greet and enjoy your new arrival.

On top of that, each of these people now hurts for you, too. Their own grief, coupled with a desire to make you feel better, may be quite hard for them to deal with. You may find yourself in the odd position of having to help them give you what you need.

In her excellent book, *Empty Arms: Coping with Miscarriage, Stillbirth and Infant Death,* published by Wintergreen Press, 1982, 1990, Sherokee Ilse suggests what family and friends can do. Rather than you having to try to teach them, I suggest you offer Sherokee's ideas to them. I know a number of bereaved parents who bought extra copies of her book and passed these out to friends and relations, to help them understand what one goes through when there is an infant death. If anyone had told me about this book after I lost Jenny, I would have done the same.

Here is what *Empty Arms* suggests:

WHAT FAMILY AND FRIENDS CAN DO

Loved ones, this is for you. It is not easy to know what to do or say to someone whose baby has died. Death reminds us all of our own humanness and mortality. Most of us would rather not think or talk about death. However, at this painful time in the parents' lives, they need to talk about their baby, their feelings and their concerns. It seems even more difficult to deal with the death of a baby. All were waiting for the joyous day and now the opposite has happened.

Friends and family can aid and support the parents by encouraging them to talk. This helps them to accept the death and grieve themselves, along with sharing this intense pain with you. Ignoring the subject does not make it go away, nor does it make the parents feel less pain. Don't protect them from this pain. Instead help them face it. In most cases, it hurts more when people will not talk about it with the parents. This is often interpreted by parents as insensitivity or disinterest. They need to know that their loved ones are willing and interested in hearing about their experience. After all, this has been one of the most tragic and devastating events in their lives.

What Can I Do to Help the Parents?

Offer a tear, a hug, a sign of love and concern.

Listen, talk about the death and about their son or daughter. Ask questions if they want to talk. Most parents need and want to talk about their baby, their hopes and dreams with their child that has died, even if it was a miscarriage. Ask the parents "Do you feel like talking about it now or would later be better?"

Realize that the parents are sad because they miss this baby, this special person: he or she never can be replaced by anyone else. They had pictured their son or daughter in their minds, learning to walk, starting school, making friends, graduating, getting married and having their own children. They did not lose "just" a baby, but a whole future.

Comments such as, "I am sorry about your baby," or "I know this is a bad time for you, and I would like to help," or "Please tell me what you would like me to do," or "Can I bring dinner over?" and "I feel so sad," might seem trite, but they really do help.

Comments such as "It was for the best," "It might have been abnormal," "You can always have another baby," "Forget it, put it behind you," tend to deny the importance of this baby in the parents' lives.

Send a card, note, poem or some other personal expression of sympathy after the death, especially after a few weeks. Most cards stop coming then and that's when the shock seems to set in. Also remember anniversaries, holidays and due dates with a card, call or visit.

Bring a plate of goodies or a casserole to the family.

Offer to baby-sit the other children, wash clothes or do some other household chores.

Bring a book that might offer comfort or some understanding. . . .

Give a gift certificate for a dinner or maybe a facial or massage at the local spa or health club.

Give a plant, a living bush, a tree or flowers. Sometimes living things represent continuity and a sense of future which is so desperately needed at this time.

Pass on names and phone numbers of others who have experienced a similar loss and seem to be coping well. There is a real need to talk with others who "have been through it." Offer to make the call for them, since it is very difficult to call someone you don't know when you are hurting.

Ask parents about their preference regarding donating money and memorials. I used the money friends donated to help publish this book.

Recognize that the parents' grief and healing process will be painful and will take time, lots of time. They will not be recovered or done "thinking about their baby" after a month or even a year.

Be aware that they never again will be quite the same people you knew before they had this baby. Their lives have changed; their perspectives and goals also might be different. Recognize and respect this.

Do discuss other topics besides their loss, since life must go on. However, be prepared that they will probably look at all other life issues in light of this loss. It may be in their minds always, especially in the beginning months.

Again, recognize the importance of this baby. The loss and pain cannot be replaced with another baby. And do make the effort to talk with them about the baby and how they are doing. Months down the road a simple "How have you been doing since your baby died?" can give much comfort.

Your assistance, comfort and support can be very influential in how the parents cope with the death of their baby and how they recover. You are important, dear loved ones; they need you now more than ever.

HELPING YOUR OTHER CHILD(REN) DEAL WITH THIS LOSS

If you have other children at home, you need to assume that even a one-year-old will be able to at least sense that something is amiss. It is crucial to their well-being, and yours, that you find a way to include them in your grief process, that you explain to them what happened and allow them to react however they will to their loss of their sibling.

Professional counselors who specialize in child grief say that when you do not help your children, no matter how young, to understand what happened to the baby, they are likely to have fantasies about the loss that will be much more hurtful to them than the truth. For instance, your other child may believe that his normal feelings of ambivalence about sharing you or his room and toys with a new sibling somehow killed the baby. If you don't share your feelings with your child, he is also likely to feel that you are withdrawing from him because you are angry at something *he* did, or that *you* blame him for the baby's death.

One good way to explain what happened is to use visual aids. Show your child pictures of how babies develop. Say, "This is how big the baby was." Children take things literally and need concrete examples. Don't tell your child that the baby "went to sleep" or was "so sick that she died." Your child will be likely to assume that *he* or *she* won't wake up.

Some psychologists and other bereavement professionals feel that children over the age of two to three are mature enough to benefit from actually seeing and even holding the baby after she has died and attending the funeral. Although this is not a settled question among helping professionals, many parents I have spoken with have done this, without apparent harm to their child(ren). If you feel that you wish to include your living child(ren) in this way, you may want to talk to a counselor about the best way to approach it.

Encourage your child(ren) to share their feelings with you. Be aware that children may express their grief differently than you do. They may not seem upset by the news, or they may cry openly. Their behavior may regress, returning to activities such as bed-wetting or thumb-sucking. Young children especially may not be able to grasp the full details or impact of the loss and may express their feelings through play, rather than by direct emotions. Try to answer all questions factually and directly.

Just as you need to accept their emotions, your child(ren) needs to accept yours, notes specialist McCoyd. Explain to them that Mommy and Daddy are sad because they miss the baby. Be sure to use the baby's name; it helps make the baby real for your remaining child(ren). Also, be certain to assure your child(ren) that Mommy and Daddy won't be this sad forever. Again, be concrete: You can say things such as "When the flowers come up in the spring, I don't think that Mommy will be crying this much anymore."

Your tears and other emotions will not frighten your child(ren) if you explain what's going on. And it may actually be beneficial to your child(ren) in another way: You are teaching them that it's okay to cry and that you can get better after being sad. Your own example will help them to grow.

Thoughtless Remarks and Inept Comforting

"All the nurses in the hospital would say that 'it was meant to be,'" said Deb, who lost her daughter at twenty weeks' gestation because of an undiagnosed incompetent cervix. "We finally started telling them that we didn't want to hear that anymore. My daughter was perfect: It was a condition that I had that caused her death. This wasn't 'meant to be'—it was preventable!"

There probably isn't a parent alive who has suffered through a pregnancy loss without enduring the added pain of thoughtless remarks and inept attempts at comforting. And these are hardly confined to health care workers: Family and friends do it, too.

Some of the most common verbal atrocities are:

- "It was God's will."
- "It was meant to be."
- "You can have another one."
- "Thank goodness you never really knew her."
- "You need to just get on with your life now."
- "Don't you think you've been depressed about this long enough?"

It is as certain as the changing of the tides that someone is going to say at least one of these things to you during the coming weeks and months.

It's important to realize that people are not saying these things to be deliberately cruel. Almost always, they are having trouble with their own feelings about the death of your child. They are speaking from their own discomfort, and they probably are not thinking their comments all the way through. Unless they have lost a child, they really cannot imagine what you feel like right now, even if they have children of their own.

Also, family, friends, even strangers feel compelled at a time like this to *do* something. In order to help, they feel they must be active. Giving a word of comfort is one small way that they can be. So they say something they think is comforting, but it comes out insensitively. They don't usually understand that what you need most right now is a good listener, not a talker or an advice giver.

So if you have the strength (and you may not right now), it's going to be up to you to teach them what you need. Tell them you need a listener most of all. Give them materials on grief to read. Tell them that their comments are not helpful, and tell them why. Even a simple ''That's not how I see it'' or ''Your comment doesn't help me'' may be enough to interrupt their stream of discussion so that you don't have to be further exposed to inappropriate comments.

Outside Support

''The support group [SHARE] was really terrific. I don't think I could have made it without them.''—Aliene

''The support group was of great help. I knew it was always there. I would go to meetings and just listen. It helped me to hear that other people had the same feelings. Knowing others shared my pain was good.''—Janis

I just can't stress this enough: *Take advantage of any help that you can find.* This is no time for you to be alone. There are tens of thousands of parents out there who know exactly what this experience is like. And while only you can work through your own pain, having the support of others who can understand your feelings and who are willing to listen to your story can make a world of difference in how you weather this early period following your baby's death.

Here is a list of the national or regional offices of the main bereavement support organizations in the United States and Canada. These contact people will help you find counselors, one-to-one, parent-to-parent contacts, and/or local support groups in your area. In addition to these national organizations, there may be one or more strictly local bereavement groups based in your region. Usually, your local hospital can help put you in touch with them.

A.M.E.N.D. (Aiding A Mother & Father
    Experiencing Neonatal Death)
Maureen Connelly
4324 Berrywick Terrace
St. Louis, MO 63128
(314) 487-7582

A free counseling service supported by The Life Seekers, and available to parents who have experienced the loss of an infant through miscarriage, stillbirth, or neonatal death. The main purpose of A.M.E.N.D. is to offer support and encouragement to parents having a normal grief reaction to the loss of their baby. Although A.M.E.N.D. is based in the Midwest, the group will work with any parent who calls, regardless of location in the United States.

BEREAVED FAMILIES OF ONTARIO
Diane Oakes Foster, executive director
214 Merton St. Suite 204
Toronto, Ontario M4S 1A6
Canada
(416) 440-0290

A provincewide self-help organization staffed by professionally supervised, trained volunteers who have experienced a loss themselves. Started in 1978 under the auspices of the Hospital for Sick Children, the group now has fifteen affiliates throughout Ontario and welcomes inquiries from bereaved parents on both sides of the U.S./Canadian border. Bereaved Families offers a number of programs. It provides a monthly newsletter, as well as a series of pamphlets on bereavement, and holds monthly "family night" meetings. The group also has an extensive library, a professional referral system, and a public education program.

OUR NEWSLETTER
(a Multiple Birth Loss Support Network)
Jean Kollantai, founder
P.O. Box 1064
Palmer, AK 99645
(907) 745-2706

A national network of parents who have experienced the death of one or both of their twins, or one or more of their higher multiple birth children. The groups offers a bimonthly newsletter and parent-to-parent support for those suffering the special grief of a loss of one or more of multiples. For a minimal fee, the group will send you a parent contact list, a 120-page packet of information and support articles, a supplemental reading list, and a twins club packet.

PREGNANCY AND INFANT LOSS CENTER
Sherokee Ilse, president and founder
1421 East Wayzata Blvd. #40
Wayzata, MN 55391
(612) 473-9372

This national nonprofit center offers the newly bereaved parent support and provides a referral service to support groups nationwide. The center also provides professional training on loss, holds workshops on perinatal bereavement, and offers consultation for professional care providers. The center publishes a quarterly newsletter and offers for purchase an extensive line of literature.

RESOLVE THROUGH SHARING
Rana Limbo, R.N., M.S., director
Lutheran Hospital
1910 South Avenue
La Crosse, WI 54601
(608) 791–4747, Ext. 3675

A national group that began in 1981, Resolve Through Sharing is a hospital-based perinatal bereavement program that now has over five thousand certified counselors in eight hundred hospitals in the United States, Ireland, England, Canada, and the Philippines. The group holds one- to four-day courses to provide professionals with the skills they need in responding to families who have lost a baby. The group also publishes written and audio materials on these topics for parents. Call or write the above address and telephone number if you wish to be trained as a counselor, want to know if there is a Resolve Through Sharing–trained professional in your hospital, or wish materials to be sent to you.

SHARE (Source of Help in Airing and Resolving Experiences)
Sister Jane Marie Lamb, founder
St. Elizabeth's Hospital
211 South Third Street
Belleville, Illinois 62222
(618) 234-2415

SHARE is a network of mutual-support groups, helping parents and others work through the grieving process after the loss of a very young baby. There are over two hundred local SHARE groups in the United States and abroad. The national office functions as the clearinghouse for requests for information about the local groups and provides telephone support. The national office also publishes a bi-

monthly newsletter, provides resources for adults working with bereaved children, and offers assistance to perinatal professionals. The
group has a wide array of printed and audiovisual materials and will
help parents begin their own local SHARE groups.

UNITE, Inc.
Janis Heil, M.Ed., director
7600 Central Avenue
Philadelphia, PA 19111
(215) 728-3777 (tape)
(215) 728-2082 (social services)

This is a nonprofit bereavement support organization, founded in
1975 and serving Delaware, New Jersey, and Pennsylvania. Local
UNITE groups hold support group meetings, and there is a one-to-
one support network with trained parent counselors. UNITE provides a quarterly newsletter and holds hospital inservice meetings,
communication education programs, and conferences for bereaved
parents, professionals, and the community, trains bereavement counselors, will make referrals to other professional counselors, and will
assist parents in forming their own UNITE, Inc., groups.

11

Other Fairly Common Medical Complications During Pregnancy

There are a number of complications in pregnancy other than those to which I've devoted full chapters. In this chapter you will find descriptions of the more common of these, their treatments, and their likely outcomes.

Rh Incompatibility

Rh incompatibility is a complication in which the mother's and the fetus's blood are incompatible. Undiagnosed and untreated, this problem can be catastrophic for the fetus or newborn. However, with modern screening methods and treatment, the problem can be avoided altogether, and, if the blood incompatibility does arise, the baby can usually be saved and have a healthy, normal life.

Your blood, just like everyone else's, is one of four major types—A, B, AB, or O. In pregnancy, there is another blood factor, or antigen, with which the doctor is concerned: the Rhesus (or Rh) factor—named for its similarity to a substance found in the blood of rhesus monkeys. Everyone, both men and women, carries an Rh factor. You are either Rh positive (Rh +) or Rh negative (Rh –). About 85 percent of all people are Rh + .

Problems may arise only if you are Rh – and your husband is Rh + , and he passes the Rh + gene on to the fetus. (The problem doesn't arise if you are Rh + and your husband is Rh – .) It is the man who determines the baby's Rh factor. Your husband may have both Rh – and Rh + genes, meaning that the fetus has an even chance of being either Rh − or Rh + ; if your husband carries only Rh + genes, the fetus will be Rh + , and thus incompatible with you.

During pregnancy, a small number of red blood cells from the fetus always enter the mother's bloodstream. If the mother is Rh − , and the baby is Rh + , the mother's body will react to the Rh + red blood cells as if they were foreign bodies and form antibodies to them.

This is not a problem for the first pregnancy. But, in any subsequent pregnancy in which the fetus is Rh + , the mother's antibodies will be activated to destroy *all* blood cells carrying the Rh + antigen. That is, her body will treat the fetus as a foreign object and destroy the baby's red blood cells. This can lead to anemia, jaundice, and even death before the baby can be born. If the fetus survives until delivery, the newborn may still suffer such severe anemia and jaundice that she develops cerebral palsy, mental retardation, or dies.

This used to happen quite often. In recent years, the incidence of complications for Rh incompatibility has dropped dramatically, in large part because of the development of screening tests and a drug called RhoGAM—short for rhesus gamma globulin.

Rh incompatibility screening should be done during your first prenatal checkup, when your doctor takes a blood sample from you. This sample is tested to see whether you are Rh − or Rh + , and, if you are Rh − , whether you have the Rh antibodies that might harm your unborn child; this is called the Coombs' test. If you show no antibodies in the first test, then during your twenty-eighth week, the Coombs' test will be repeated. If you still have no antibodies, the doctor will inject you with one shot of RhoGAM to make sure that any fetal cells that enter your bloodstream will be destroyed. If you have amniocentesis at any time before you deliver, you will probably be given a RhoGAM shot as well, since the procedure can release some fetal cells into your bloodstream.

Then, as soon as you deliver the baby, the doctor will take a sample of her blood from the umbilical cord. If she is Rh + , you will receive another RhoGAM injection, within seventy-two hours after the birth, which will kill all the fetal red blood cells in your body and prevent you from forming the antibodies that could hurt your next baby, should you choose to become pregnant again. After every subsequent pregnancy, you will also receive RhoGAM, even if your next pregnancy ends in miscarriage or is ectopic or otherwise blighted. This will keep you from developing antibodies that might harm your next child, if you get pregnant a third time, and so on with each pregnancy thereafter.

If you already had one Rh + baby and are now pregnant with another, but never received RhoGAM after your last pregnancy, it does not automatically mean that your fetus will be badly harmed or die. There are treatments to help your fetus. First, your doctor will keep a close eye on your baby's progress in your womb. Your OB will give you a Coombs' test every two to three weeks to make sure that your antibodies don't exceed a level that would permanently damage the fetus. If the level stays under the critical mark, you will deliver at thirty-eight weeks (when the baby is presumed mature enough to survive outside the womb), either by cesarean or by induction.

If the tests show that your antibody level is too high, the doctor will perform an amniocentesis to assess the baby's condition and lung maturity. Amnios will be repeated every one to three weeks until either the baby's condition has deteriorated too much to wait any longer for delivery or her lungs have matured, whichever comes first.

Should the amniocentesis tests show that the fetus is suffering from anemia or her condition is worsening, and she is too young to survive outside your body, the doctor can perform an intrauterine blood transfusion—that is, a blood transfusion while she is still inside you. The transfusions can be repeated every ten days to two weeks. This will give the baby enough new red blood cells to allow her to develop to a point where she can breathe on her own outside you. At that time (usually between thirty-two and thirty-four weeks' gestation), you will either be induced and have a vaginal delivery, or the doctor will take the baby by c-section.

If, after the delivery, the baby develops severe anemia or jaundice, the neonatologist can give her one or more transfusions to help stem the problem. In all probability, with good care, your baby should do quite well.

Hydramnios

Amniotic fluid is the liquid in which the baby floats all during your pregnancy. It is made of water and secretions from the amnion (the membrane enclosing the fetus in fluid inside the uterus) and the fetus during the first half of pregnancy. By the second half of pregnancy, the amniotic fluid is also thought to contain fetal urine. The fluid itself is clear, usually odorless, and is constantly replenished. However, as the pregnancy advances, the fluid accumulates small bits of debris, such as vernix (the thick greasy coating that covers the baby in the latter half of pregnancy). The fluid acts as a cushion for the fetus and prevents her from adhering to the walls of the amniotic sac; it also allows the fetus to move about freely and helps her to maintain a constant temperature. In addition, amniotic fluid acts as a place where hormones, fluids, and electrolytes can be exchanged.

The normal amount of amniotic fluid is between five hundred millileters (ml) and one thousand ml, or one liter. This volume should decrease after the thirty-sixth week, as the infant grows larger and gets closer to term; by delivery, there may only be a few hundred ml. But sometimes, too much amniotic fluid develops inside the amniotic sac. This complication is called *hydramnios,* or *polyhydramnios.* It occurs in about 1 percent of all pregnancies—meaning that about thirty-six thousand women in the United States have it every year. About 80 percent of the time, the amount of extra fluid is not extreme; 15 percent have moderate amounts of extra fluid; and 5 percent are severe. In mild cases, 80 percent of women deliver full-term, healthy infants.

In the moderate and severe cases, the cause, unfortunately, is almost always that the fetus has some physical abnormality. Hydramnios also occurs more frequently in multiple pregnancies and in those complicated by diabetes.

There are two kinds of hydramnios: *chronic,* that is, the slow accumulation over time of excess amniotic fluid, which most women tolerate fairly well; and *acute,* where the buildup is over the course of hours or days. Acute hydramnios tends to set in early in pregnancy, between the sixteenth and twentieth weeks, and can become so severe that the mother is unable to breathe when lying down. In these cases, pregnancy is usually terminated early by the spontaneous onset of labor caused by the inability of the uterus to accommodate the extra size and weight of the fluid. And it is the acute buildup that usually portends fetal abnormality.

If you have hydramnios, your uterus will become distended, and as a consequence, you may have one or more of the following symptoms:

- shortness of breath (from pressure on the diaphragm)
- swelling of the lower limbs and the vulva (again from pressure, this time on vessels)
- increased indigestion (from pressure on the stomach and intestines)
- preterm labor (from overstretching of the uterus)
- spontaneous preterm premature rupture of membranes (breaking of the waters)

If this last problem occurs, because of the quick expulsion of the excess fluid, you run the risk of other complications. You may suffer from some degree of placental abruption (when the placenta pulls away from the uterine wall prematurely); the uterus then may contract poorly; and you might have a postbirth hemorrhage.

There are no drugs to take for hydramnios and no real lasting treatment. When the fluid accumulation becomes too severe, the doctor can draw off the excess amniotic fluid through a catheter, which is passed through the abdominal wall by a needle, under local anesthesia—a procedure known as *amniocentesis*. Relief is immediate, but not lasting, as the fluid is likely to build up fairly rapidly. Also, the procedure sometimes initiates labor, and pregnancy can't be continued. (See Chapter 8 for a discussion of preterm labor and delivery.)

Oligohydramnios

This is the flip side of hydramnios—that is, it means you have too little amniotic fluid. This is considered a rare complication. Usually, it occurs when your pregnancy goes well past the due date (in which case your OB may induce labor) or when the fetus has urinary tract or kidney problems and does not excrete enough urine. Sometimes it happens early in pregnancy, which almost always means that the fetus will not make it to term; those who survive usually have severe physical problems.

If there is not enough amniotic fluid, the baby may actually adhere to the amniotic membrane. Without a fluid cushion, pressure from the womb on the fetus may misshape her, causing structural problems. Also, there is a greater likelihood that the baby will press on the umbilical cord and cut off her own nutrient and oxygen supply. Lung growth may also be impaired by the compression.

There is no treatment for the disorder itself, although some medical centers have successfully corrected some fetal urinary tract abnormalities in the womb, thus allowing the fetus to excrete urine properly. There is no indication that, if you have oligohydramnios in one pregnancy, your risk of it in subsequent pregnancies is higher.

Viral Infections During Pregnancy

In about 5 percent of all pregnancies, the woman contracts one or more viral infections, ranging from the common cold or flu to rubella (German measles), cytomegalovirus (a herpes-type infection), genital herpes, and HIV (human immunodeficiency virus—AIDS). Any virus during pregnancy can cause problems for both the mother and the fetus. Most common viral infections—such as colds—are mild and have little to no effect on the fetus or her development. But certain more potent viruses can do serious damage to the unborn baby, either by causing the mother to spontaneously miscarry or by directly infecting the fetus in the womb.

Common Colds and Flu

It's hard to avoid catching a cold at any time when you are exposed, whether you are pregnant or not. Once exposed, you usually come down with symptoms such as stuffy nose, sore throat, cough, and perhaps fever, within forty-eight to seventy-two hours. When these symptoms are accompanied by body aches, vomiting, diarrhea, headaches, and high fever, the diagnosis is usually influenza.

Both colds and the flu are viruses and therefore cannot be wiped out by antibiotics, which are used to kill bacteria. When bacterial infection sets in on top of a cold, the doctor must prescribe drugs to eliminate the secondary bacterial infection. Because of this, some physicians prescribe antibiotic therapy as a preventive measure when their patients first get a cold or the flu.

All pregnant women are considered high-risk for catching the flu during outbreaks, and the Centers for Disease Control recommend that pregnant women obtain flu shots if they have chronic underlying medical problems, such as kidney and heart disease or diabetes. Pregnant women have a heightened chance of coming down with pneumonia as a result of the flu, and flu also increases their risk of spontaneous abortion.

The good news is that getting the flu or a cold during your pregnancy will not cause your baby to have birth defects. There are no studies linking the flu or colds with congenital malformations.

If you get a cold or the flu during your pregnancy:

- Let your doctor know that you think you've come down with a cold or the flu. He may want you to come in for an office visit to make certain that you don't have a bacterial infection.
- Check with your doctor before taking any medication to relieve cold or flu symptoms. Some over-the-counter drugs may have ingredients that are not recommended for use during pregnancy.
- Rest in bed as much as you can.
- Drink plenty of fluids.
- If you are nauseous, eat light, small meals six times a day instead of your usual three larger meals.
- Call your doctor if you develop a fever over 101 degrees, a severe cough, diarrhea (which can stimulate preterm uterine contractions), vomiting, a rash, or pain in your joints. These are all symptoms that should be watched closely.

RUBELLA (GERMAN MEASLES)

Rubella is no big deal for a woman who is not pregnant: a few days to a week of discomfort before it's over and forgotten. Unfortunately, the same does not hold true if you catch the virus while you are pregnant, particularly if you get it during your first trimester. About 15 percent of women are still not immune to the disease by the time they become pregnant. That is, they have not had sufficient exposure to the disease to develop the lifelong immunity that comes with having had rubella once.

If you are exposed to rubella during pregnancy and catch the virus, within fourteen to twenty-one days after exposure, you'll have one or more of the following symptoms lasting from a few days to two weeks:

- a rash that starts on the face and spreads downward, fading in time
- fever
- cough
- sore eyes
- headaches
- body aches

These symptoms are all transient and disappear over time. It's unusual for symptoms to be worse than these. Bedrest, fluids, and an over-the-counter pain reliever usually suffice to relieve rubella's discomfort for you.

The same cannot be said for the fetus. For the unborn child, rubella is a very serious pregnancy complication. If the woman is in her first trimester when she is exposed, between 50 and 80 percent of the time the fetus will also contract the infection. In the second trimester the percentage of infection goes down, and it drops even further in the third trimester.

While infection does not necessarily mean that the baby will be injured by the disease, the younger the fetus is when exposed, the greater the chances that this will occur. According to most medical authorities, all fetuses exposed before eleven weeks of gestation will suffer defects; between twelve and sixteen weeks, up to four in ten babies will be affected. For the 60 percent of fetuses exposed between thirteen and sixteen weeks who show no immediate defects at birth, up to one-third may develop serious or deadly diseases later in life, such as diabetes or progressive panencephalitis—a degenerative brain disease, which ultimately causes death.

The list of known birth defects directly attributable to rubella infection is lengthy. It includes:

- eye damage—cataracts, glaucoma, blindness
- heart abnormalities and disease
- deafness and hearing impairment
- blood abnormalities, including anemia
- enlarged liver and jaundice
- chronic pneumonia
- bone changes
- intrauterine growth retardation
- nervous system abnormalities
- chromosome damage

Exposure of the fetus to rubella in the first trimester of pregnancy is so certain to cause one or more serious defects that all medical authorities recommend that the woman with rubella consider therapeutic abortion as a real alternative.

If you are not yet pregnant, you can avoid having to make this difficult choice. Go to your doctor and take the simple blood test for rubella antibodies. If the test shows that you have not developed immunity to the disease, you can have yourself innoculated. Then, when you later become pregnant, you will not run the risk of contracting rubella and bearing a damaged child as a result.

If you are already pregnant, but do not have rubella, it is not recommended that you take the vaccine at this point, because the vaccine is made from the live virus and theoretically could infect the fetus. The American College of Obstetricians and Gynecologists (ACOG) views the risk associated with exposure to the vaccine virus to be much lower than exposure to the wild virus; nonetheless, vaccination against rubella is not normally given to the pregnant woman.

What that means is that if you are not immune to rubella when you become pregnant, the best you can do is to *studiously* avoid contact with anyone you know who has the virus or who suspects that they may have been exposed. This includes children. Rubella is highly contagious, and you would do well to inquire about the health of all children whose homes you plan to visit during your pregnancy.

GENITAL HERPES

Genital herpes is one variant of a family of viruses known as the herpes viruses. The two forms of the virus with which you are mostly likely to be familiar are *herpes simplex virus type one* (oral herpes) and *herpes simplex virus type two* (genital herpes). Type one—oral herpes— usually shows up as sores around the outside of the mouth. Most people call these lesions *cold sores,* although you certainly don't have to have a cold to get them.

Herpes simplex virus type two is genital herpes, characterized by painful sores on the labia, vulva, anus, cervix, and in the vagina. The initial outbreak of the virus usually lasts from ten days to three weeks, with itching, reddened skin, followed by wet, oozing, painful sores that eventually heal and go away. There may also be a low-grade fever, tiredness, and swollen glands.

Although the sores and other symptoms disappear, the virus does not leave the body, but rather retreats along nerve pathways to the base of the spine. It stays there, dormant, until some event reactivates the virus, causing another outbreak of sores. Repeat attacks of the virus are usually not as bad nor as long lasting as the initial outbreak.

The herpes simplex viruses are classified as sexually transmitted diseases. They can be passed from partner to partner with unfortunate ease. It is also possible to infect another person through contamination on the hands. For instance, if you have genital herpes and do not wash your hands thoroughly after urinating or touching your genitals, the virus can remain on your hands and you can then pass it along to the next person you touch. Similarly, herpes simplex type one can be passed on from kissing, or simply by touching the face and then touching another person. Fifteen percent of all genital herpes infections are caused by herpes simplex type one.

If you come down with an active genital herpes infection while you are pregnant, it is unlikely that your baby will be affected by the virus, *unless* she is contaminated by it during or after the birth. Generally, infection is transmitted to the baby during her passage through the vagina at birth. Contamination can also take place if the amniotic membranes are ruptured for a number of hours before delivery, because the virus can then travel up the cervical canal into the uterus and reach the now-unprotected fetus. After the baby is born, if you do not practice meticulous hygiene, you can inadvertently pass the virus on to her while holding, playing with, or breastfeeding her.

When a baby is infected by the mother's herpes virus—and 50 percent who are delivered vaginally when the mother has a first-time, active outbreak of the virus will become infected—the consequences are devastating. About 60 percent of the infected newborns die by six weeks of age. Half of the remaining 40 percent of infected babies will suffer from one or more serious disabilities:

- mental retardation
- visual problems (including blindness)
- spinal and brain infection
- spastic muscles
- breathing difficulties
- coma

As the effects of herpes infection can be so severe for the newborn, the premium on treatment of your infection will be to keep it from contaminating the baby. That means that if you have an active outbreak of herpes close to or at the time you are expected to deliver, you will deliver by cesarean, to avoid passing the baby through the zone of the infection. Some obstetricians recommend that any pregnant woman who has had genital herpes in the past deliver by cesarean, just in case the virus is present in the genital tract but has not yet caused the visible lesions that are the dead giveaway of the infection. Other authorities say that if there is no evidence of active infection at the time of birth, then vaginal birth is safe for the baby.

Once the baby is born, she will probably be isolated from other infants in the nursery, whether she shows symptoms or not, until it is clear that she has not caught the virus. Hospital staff will approach both the baby and you with protective gear—gloves, gowns—so that they don't pass the virus on to other women and newborns. You will still be allowed to breastfeed your baby, if you desire to do so. You can handle her and hold her as much as you want. You won't pass the virus on with your milk, and if your hands are clean and you don't allow your sores to touch the baby, you won't give her the virus when you hold her. However, you can pass it on if you do not practice excellent hygiene. The hospital staff will show you what you must do to prevent the virus from infecting your child after birth.

You may have heard that there is a drug that prevents repeat outbreaks of herpes and makes new infections less painful and shorter. The drug is called acyclovir. It is an antiviral agent that is taken orally. Although the drug is safe for the woman taking it, studies have not been done on its use during pregnancy. Effects on the fetus are unknown, and the drug is not recommended for use during pregnancy for that reason.

CYTOMEGALOVIRUS

Cytomegalovirus is a herpes-type virus. Although it is a systemic infection, it is commonly found in the genital tract and shows up in all bodily fluids and mucous membranes. You can catch it in a number of ways, from sharing the same water glass to sexual contact.

From 4 to 13 percent of pregnant women have active cases of cytomegalovirus. It's a common virus, and by the time we are adults, up to seven in ten of us have had it and antibodies to it are detectable in the blood. You probably won't even know you have it, because nine out of ten times it doesn't manifest itself through symptoms you can see. For the 10 percent of people who actually come down with symptoms, most feel like they have mononucleosis—they're tired, have a sore throat and swollen lymph glands, and may have a low-grade fever or joint pains. Occasionally the symptoms set in acutely, with a spiking fever of up to 104 degrees. There is no known treatment for the disease.

If you get a cytomegalovirus infection during your pregnancy, you may pass it on to your baby, either through the placenta or when the baby passes through the infected vagina at birth. ACOG reports that up to fifty thousand babies in the United States are born with the virus each year. But, just like adults, only about 10 percent of these infants show clinical symptoms after being infected inside their mother. However, those babies who do show symptoms can be very seriously affected. Complications for these infants include:

- mental retardation
- poor motor coordination
- fever
- enlargement of the liver and spleen
- visual problems (including blindness)
- hearing loss
- anemia
- jaundice
- stillbirth

But, nine times out of ten, the baby is just fine, and may never show any symptoms at all—or not until later in life, when the virus is reawakened by pregnancy, blood transfusion, or immunosuppression therapy.

HUMAN IMMUNE DEFICIENCY VIRUS (HIV)—AIDS

No text on viral infection is complete today without a discussion of human immune deficiency virus (HIV). HIV causes AIDS (short for *acquired immune deficiency syndrome*), a progressive disease that slowly destroys the body's immune system. Eventually, the victim's body is too weak to combat even the most minor opportunistic infections, and the person dies.

Although researchers around the world are working to find a cure and create a vaccine against HIV infection, there is no cure or vaccine yet. There are drugs available now that can effectively beat back some of the worse opportunistic infections, for a time. In fact, some doctors who specialize in AIDS treatment say that within a year or two, medical science will have advanced so far in treating AIDS that victims will have a long life after onset of the disease—in much the same way that diabetics live with diabetes, a disease that also has no cure. For now, however, those infected with HIV still face an extremely poor prognosis.

You get HIV from contact with the body fluids—blood, semen, and possibly vaginal fluid—of another infected person. The main avenues of infection are coming into direct contact with infected blood during sex or sharing contaminated hypodermic needles when injecting illegal drugs. You can also contract the disease from infected blood given to you during a transfusion. The American College of Obstetricians and Gynecologists (ACOG) reports that now that all blood in the United States is screened for HIV, the chance of this happening is very small. For fetuses, infection is passed from mother to fetus via blood in the umbilical cord, during birth or through the mother's milk after birth.

Once anyone is infected with HIV, it may be months or years before they come down with any symptoms at all. Researchers are not certain why, but HIV apparently can "hide" in the body's cells for up to eight or more years. The blood test that tells you whether you have antibodies to HIV (a sign that you have been infected) may not show your infection for up to three years after you have been exposed. If you have reason to suspect that you have been exposed to the virus, you should discuss this immediately with your obstetrician.

If you have HIV, and you are pregnant, it is likely that you will have a tragic outcome, even if the baby is born apparently healthy. Although you may have no outward symptoms of the disease, there is between a 20 and 50 percent chance that you will pass the disease on to your baby before she is born. And most of the infected children die before they reach their second birthday. If the baby is born without becoming infected, you can still pass HIV to her—through your breast milk. Obviously, for this reason ACOG strongly recommends that women with HIV not breastfeed.

Although there is still very little data on the effect of pregnancy on a woman with AIDS, or HIV, it is thought that pregnancy can speed up the progression of the disease, or make it worse. ACOG, in its excellent educational literature on HIV and women, points out that abortion is always an option for a woman with HIV.

ACOG makes available to the public its materials on HIV. Contact ACOG at: 409 12th Street, S.W./Washington, D.C. 20024-2188

Other Sexually Transmitted Diseases

CHLAMYDIA

Chlamydial infections are the leading cause of venereal disease in the United States, affecting 1.6 million women in this country each year. Chlamydia can infect any or all of the genital organs (cervix, vulva, fallopian tubes, ovaries, and so on), as well as the urethra, the anus—even the eyes. It has a long incubation period before it manifests itself in symptoms. Some women have the infection for years without having any idea that they've got it. Often, chlamydia infections occur along with gonorrhea (see below), another venereal disease that has reached epidemic proportions in the United States.

Symptoms, when they do occur, often are mistaken for other infections. For instance, chlamydia creates the same burning, pain, and urgency during urination that cystitis and other bladder infections do (see below). Other symptoms of chlamydia are swelling of the cervix and cervical oozing of white pus; pain during intercourse; and fever with abdominal pain if the infection reaches the organs inside the pelvis. Or you may have no symptoms at all—a "silent" infection.

That is why most doctors now do a test to check you for chlamydia during your first prenatal visit. The doctor swabs your cervix or urethra to obtain a sample and sends it to a lab. The results come back within a day or two.

When a routine test is not performed and you develop symptoms of urinary tract infections during the pregnancy—*and* your urine culture turns up negative—your doctor may also do a chlamydia screening.

Although it has not yet been proven conclusively, several studies indicate that when chlamydial infection goes untreated during pregnancy, the woman is likely to have preterm labor or preterm premature rupture of membranes, resulting in premature birth of the baby. Even if the baby is born at term, she may have pneumonia or conjunctivitis (eye infection).

The Centers for Disease Control have determined that a woman is at highest risk for this infection if she is under the age of twenty, unmarried, poor, lives in a large city, has numerous sexual partners, and/or has another sexually transmitted disease. It is also likely that if you have the disease, your partner(s) do(es), too.

Untreated, the mother's infection can become acute and, in some cases, render her sterile by damaging her fallopian tubes. Luckily, the infection usually clears up easily with antibiotics. If you are infected, your doctor will most likely prescribe erythromycin (considered quite safe to use in pregnancy) for you to take by mouth for seven to ten days. It is important that your partner also take the drugs, to prevent him from reinfecting you. If your infection is detected after you have given birth, the antibiotic of choice is tetracycline. Tetracycline is not safe to take during pregnancy.

Gonorrhea

Gonorrhea is widespread in the United States; the number of infected individuals has climbed steadily over the last decade. Almost always (98 percent of the time), infection is "silent"—that is, there are no symptoms. Contracting the infection during pregnancy will usually be limited to the cervix, vagina, urethra, and glands in the lower genital tract. This is due to the mucus plug in the cervix.

However, if you had the disease before you became pregnant, it can spread to the membrane lining the abdominal and pelvic walls (the peritoneum), the fallopian tubes, and other reproductive organs. When the infection is severe, permanent scarring of the tubes may occur, causing infertility or ectopic pregnancy (when the fertilized egg attaches inside the tube instead of the uterus).

Gonorrheal infections often coexist with chlamydial infections—the most prevalent form of sexually transmitted disease in the United States today (see above).

If you have gonorrhea when your baby is born, there is a high probability that she will become infected as she passes through your vagina at delivery. This infection manifests itself quickly in the eyes and can cause permanent scarring of the surface of the eye—the cornea. That's why the eyes of virtually all infants are treated with silver nitrate drops at birth. Babies of mothers with active infection also receive an injection of penicillin and are isolated from the other infants in the nursery for at least twenty-four hours. The newborn should also be seen by an eye specialist during this time.

Your doctor will do a routine screening of you for gonorrhea during the first prenatal visit. The test may be repeated later in pregnancy as well. If you test positive, it is important that your partner(s) also be tested and receive treatment at the same time you do.

There are several regimens recommended for treatment of gonorrhea. During pregnancy, treatment usually involves injection with penicillin, or, if you are allergic, with another antibiotic called spectinomycin. In addition, you will take another drug, probenecid, by mouth. The probenecid helps make the other antibiotics more effective by preventing the kidneys from excreting them. If injections are not used, then you'd take ampicillin or amoxicillin—both in the penicillin family—by mouth, along with the probenecid.

If the type of gonorrhea that you have is resistant to penicillin treatment, or you are allergic to penicillin, you may receive ceftriaxone—a broad-spectrum antibiotic that is safe to use during pregnancy.

SYPHILIS

Syphilis is less common in the United States than are chlamydia and gonorrhea (see above). But, like the other sexually transmitted diseases discussed in this chapter, the number of cases has risen steadily since the 1970s. You get it through sexual contact with an infected partner, and, if you have it, you can pass it to your unborn child through the placenta.

Symptoms of syphilis appear and then disappear in stages, according to the length of time you harbor the disease without treatment. Stage-one symptoms—or primary syphilis—appear between ten and ninety days after exposure. Average length of time between exposure and onset of symptoms is six weeks. A painless, hard, red sore, called a chancre or lesion, develops on the vulva, labia, or anus. Sometimes there is more than one sore, and sometimes the chancre is inside the vagina on the cervix, and so it goes unnoticed. The lymph glands in the groin may also become enlarged, but, as with the chancre, there will be no pain.

The chancre heals within two to six weeks after it first appears. Six to eight weeks after that, if you remain untreated, secondary syphilis appears. A rash will cover some part of your body—the palms of the hands, soles of the feet, or the trunk. You may also develop a fever, headache, joint aches, and enlarged lymph nodes. You may feel tired and lose your appetite. There may be gray-white patches inside your mouth. At this secondary stage, the infection has spread throughout your body, and all your sores are highly contagious. Even if untreated, these symptoms will resolve themselves and go away within a few weeks. It's unusual for syphilis to reach the third, or tertiary, stage in the United States. Most cases are caught and treated before stage-three symptoms manifest themselves.

Syphilis has terrible effects on the fetus. It causes the placenta to enlarge and the number of blood vessels in it to decrease. The baby may be deprived of nutrition and may die of this and other complications caused by the disease. Syphilis can permanently damage the fetus's spleen, liver, or heart. It can also damage her hearing.

If the baby shows no symptoms of the disease at birth, she may, a few weeks later, develop a runny nose, a fever, skin lesions, and deafness. Treatment with antibiotics will cure the infection, but will not undo the physical damage the disease has caused.

Luckily, syphilis is easily detected and treated. Doctors are required by law to screen a woman's blood for evidence of infection at the first prenatal visit. If the test comes back from the lab as positive for syphilis, the doctor does a second, more sensitive blood test, to confirm the diagnosis.

Once diagnosed, treatment with antibiotics is usually quite effective. Both the woman and her partner should receive treatment at the same time, to prevent him from reinfecting her. For women with evidence of syphilis in the blood, but no overt symptoms, an injection with a high amount of penicillin is given. If the woman has had the disease for less than one year, she receives either two injections of penicillin or erythromycin by mouth for fifteen days.

If the doctor suspects from the woman's history and symptoms that the infection is of long standing—more than one year—the woman takes double shots of penicillin once a week for three weeks or, if allergic to penicillin, erythromycin by mouth for thirty days.

The problem is that while erythromycin works to get rid of the disease in the mother, it tends not to reach the fetus in high enough doses. So, when the woman is allergic to penicillin, some medical centers recommend either desensitizing her to penicillin, then giving the penicillin therapy; or her taking tetracycline by mouth—despite the fact that under normal circumstances, this drug is not used during pregnancy, because it causes permanent staining of the fetus's baby teeth, may cause retardation of bone growth, and can damage the fetus's liver. But in cases of syphilis infection, these risks are outweighed by the benefit of preventing syphilis's catastrophic effects on the fetus.

Non-Viral Infections During Pregnancy

There are some infections that you might contract while you are pregnant that are caused by bacteria or parasites. These are usually treated with antibiotics or other drugs and in some cases are avoidable altogether if you practice good hygiene and are sensible about avoiding sources of contamination. Some, like urinary tract infections, are easier for you to contract because of your pregnant state. Almost all infection in pregnancy can affect your unborn child, so it is important to follow suggestions for avoiding infection and minimizing symptoms if infection does set in.

TOXOPLASMOSIS

Toxoplasmosis is a parasitic infection. Primary carriers of this bug are mammals, including mice, livestock (such as sheep and cattle), and domestic cats. Humans become infected when they eat the under-cooked meat of infected animals or handle cat feces from an infected cat. The American College of Obstetricians and Gynecologists (ACOG) reports that up to 40 percent of the U.S. population have antibodies to *toxoplasma*—meaning that four in ten people have at one time or another been infected by the parasite.

Usually, if you have toxoplasmosis, you don't know it, meaning that you are infected but show no clinical symptoms. Symptoms of toxoplasmosis, when they are apparent, can include swollen lymph nodes, fever, fatigue, sore throat, a rash, and liver and spleen enlargement. The infection is treatable with a combination of drugs—sulfadiazine and pyrimethamine. However, these drugs are considered toxic for use during pregnancy and so are not prescribed.

Unfortunately, although infection rarely causes severe problems in adults, the same is not so for a fetus whose mother contracts the parasite for the first time during pregnancy. When the mother becomes infected, she has a one-in-three chance of infecting her unborn child. Studies show that the infection is most likely to spread to the fetus when it's contracted in the third trimester; the worst fetal infections, when they occur, happen in the first trimester. One-third of all fetuses infected show clinical symptoms at birth.

Babies who are infected in the mother's womb can have severe problems, including:

- visual abnormalities
- abnormal spinal fluid
- enlarged spleen
- jaundice
- fever
- diseased lymph nodes
- convulsions
- lime salt deposits in the brain
- fluid on the brain (hydrocephalus)

You have it in your power to prevent these problems. Toxoplasmosis is an avoidable complication. ACOG suggests that you simply do four things:

- Make sure that all red meat that you eat during pregnancy is well done—that is, is not at all pink when you eat it.

- Be extra careful when you handle cats or change cat litter—wash your hands thoroughly each time you touch a cat.
- Change your cat's litter every day, so that parasites have no prolonged time in which to multiply in the litter.
- If you own a cat that you allow outdoors, keep it indoors while you are pregnant. If you let it go out, it may attack an infected rodent, catch the parasite, and spread it to you.

URINARY TRACT INFECTIONS

Of all the bacterial infections possible during pregnancy, urinary tract infections (UTIs is the medical shorthand) are the most common. This is thought to be due in large part to the physical changes in the urinary tract during pregnancy, which, to some degree, predispose the woman to infections and inflammation.

During pregnancy, the kidneys enlarge somewhat. More waste products pass through the kidneys because the woman takes in more liquids and passes waste from the fetus through her own blood system. Pressure on the ureters—the tubes leading from the kidneys to the bladder—increases, because of the development of extra blood and vessels in the pelvis and the enlargement of the uterus.

As the fetus grows and the uterus and soft tissues in the pelvis stretch and swell, the bladder is pushed up and flattened somewhat. In late pregnancy, as the fetus settles into the pelvis, the part of the baby that is lowest in the womb puts pressure on the base of the bladder, which hampers the drainage of blood and lymph. Increased pressure also means that some urine stays in the ureters and bladder at most times, making them susceptible to bacterial growth and inflammation.

Another predisposing factor has to do with increased vaginal secretions that are normal during pregnancy. These serve as a good medium for bacterial growth and the transmission of bacteria from the anus to the urethra—the opening of the tube from the bladder to the outside of your body. Once bacteria invade the urethra, it's a short trip to the bladder.

Some urinary tract infections are painless, a condition called *asymptomatic Bacteriuria*. Between 2 and 12 percent of all pregnant women have bacteriuria during pregnancy. Doctors screen their pregnant patients for this infection at the first prenatal visit. Infected women receive antimicrobial drugs— considered safe during pregnancy—to kill off the bacteria. The usual course is ten days of pills, taken two to four times a day, which usually does the trick.

One out of four times, if this infection goes untreated, the woman will develop acute pyelonephritis—a serious kidney infection. She comes down with high fever, chills, the shakes, and pain to the touch around the kidneys. Her urine output also drops or stops—a very dangerous condition. Treatment for acute pyelonephritis includes hospitalization for intravenous hydration and antimicrobial drugs.

The other typical urinary tract infection or inflammation is *cystitis.* Cystitis is inflammation of the bladder and urethra and can be caused by a number of things. The symptoms are:

- pain or a burning sensation before, during, or after urination
- urgency—you feel like you have to ''go'' all the time, but little or nothing comes out when you do
- pain above the pubic bone
- blood or pus in the urine (may or may not be present)

Often, bacteriuria or pus in the urine is what inflames the delicate tissues and creates the pain or tenderness. These can be introduced into the urinary tract by poor hygiene (wiping from back to front after urination or bowel movements), sexual intercourse, and vaginal creams or jellies which provide breeding grounds for bacteria.

But cystitis can be the result of nonbacterial irritation as well. Causes include:

- drinking too much acidic liquids—like grapefruit juice and coffee
- food allergies
- stress
- wearing too-tight pants
- bubble baths or irritating soaps
- douching
- feminine hygiene sprays
- sex that irritates the urethra—rear-entry positions and penetration of an overly dry vagina are culprits here.

No matter what the cause, passing urine when you've got cystitis can be so painful that you dread the next trip to the bathroom. It's a pain that you can't, and shouldn't, ignore. When you are not pregnant, it's okay to wait a couple of days, treat the condition yourself, and see if the symptoms subside. But when you're pregnant, you cannot afford to do this.

The reason is quite simple. When the urinary tract is infected or irritated, the uterus may also become irritable and begin contracting. The contractions can easily turn into premature labor and preterm birth, which should be avoided at all costs. Kidney infections that are allowed to become acute or chronic may also contribute to low birth-weight babies. And as you will not know whether your bladder tenderness and painful urination are due to the new bath soap you've tried or due to real infection, it's imperative that you see your obstetrician as soon as symptoms set in.

To diagnose bladder infections, the doctor sends some of your urine to a laboratory for analysis. Sometimes the doctor will wait the forty-eight to seventy-two hours for the result before treating. But often he will start you on drugs right away to eliminate the risk of the infection worsening while test results are awaited.

Even if the culture comes back negative, it's no guarantee that you don't have an infection. So if your culture is negative, and your symptoms worsen or persist, see the doctor for a repeat test. You should also be retested once the course of treatment is over, to make sure the bacteria were destroyed.

Cystitis is easily treated with antimicrobial drugs, and once you start treatment, your symptoms will ease noticeably within the first twenty-four to forty-eight hours. Untreated, the infection can travel up the ureters and start to involve the kidneys—a condition that is much more serious.

While you are under treatment for any urinary tract infection, there are several measures that you can take to ease your symptoms:

- Get extra rest.
- Drink a full glass of water every two to three hours. (The idea is to take in enough fluid to ensure a good stream of urine each time you pee.)
- Urinate often, and try to pass all the urine you are holding each time you go.
- Drink cranberry juice, which is acidic enough to discourage bacterial growth without irritating the bladder (although some doctors now maintain that cranberry juice neither helps nor hinders your getting rid of the infection).
- Stop drinking caffeinated beverages (such as coffee, tea, or colas) and alcohol. These tend to irritate the bladder.
- Wear loose-fitting clothing that puts no pressure on your urethra—that is, no tight jeans. Skirts are ideal.
- Be scrupulous about your hygiene. Wipe from front to back when you pee or defecate. Wash your vulva using warm water and mild soap several times a day—again wiping from front to back. Change pads—if you use them—frequently. They are breeding grounds for bacteria.

- Eat yogurt or take acidophilus capsules to restore in your intestine the natural flora that the drugs you're taking destroy.

Unfortunately, up to 40 percent of women who have one infection will get another one within two weeks to six months. Here's what you can do to avoid that:

- Do everything listed above for easing symptoms. These measures also help prevent irritation and infection.
- Make sure you and your partner wash your hands before having sex. Never allow him to touch your vagina or clitoris after touching your anus or penetrating your anus, since this is a surefire way to introduce bacteria into your urethra.
- Get up to pee after having sexual relations of any kind. It will help keep the urethra clear of bacteria.
- Avoid activities that can put pressure on the urethra, such as bike riding.

12

Multiple Pregnancy: The Complications of Having More Than One

"There they are," the ultrasound technician told me. "What do you mean 'they'?" I asked. "They." She pointed to two pulsing blips on the screen. "That's your uterus," she said as she outlined a fuzzy gray shape with her finger. "And here are your babies. One here," she pointed—"and one here."

I grabbed her labcoat lapel. "You mean I'm having twins?" I think I yelled it. "Are you sure there aren't any more? You didn't miss any, did you?" No, she assured me, it was "just" the two.

I was stunned. Twins! I had been dimly aware of the possibility. Twins run in my family—my mom had twins (lost to severe prematurity), and an older sister has twins, my eighteen-year-old niece and nephew. I had taken Clomid, a fertility drug, for that one month, but . . . I just never considered that I would have anything more than a "normal" singleton pregnancy.

A hundred thoughts flashed through my mind in the time between my chat with the technician and the entrance of the radiologist to confirm that the twins were in my uterus, not outside it. By the time he was finished, I was practically leaping off the table with excitement.

The radiologist gave me privacy in another room to break the good news to my husband. They ushered him into the office, and I said, "Honey, you'd better sit down." When I told him, his mouth dropped open. He reached for me, and we started laughing. We laughed and hugged and joked and cried until a nurse came in to hint that the room was needed. And then they sent us home.

I was already having bleeding problems. (Two weeks later we discovered the bleeding was from the lower twin's placenta, which was too low in my uterus—a condition called *placenta previa.*) So I had to stay in bed until the bleeding stopped. That meant I had plenty of time on my hands, so I asked my husband to buy some books that would tell me what to expect. What I found in those texts upset me. The books said that the medical community considered being pregnant with twins a *complication* of pregnancy! Multiples are automatically categorized as a high-risk situation. I thought that hideously unfair. Weren't twins twice the joy? Twice the blessing?

Yes, they are, once they've come into the world and are safe and healthy. But getting twins, or triplets, or more to make that journey in good health and end it at term can be fraught with pitfalls for both the babies and their mothers, much more so than a singleton pregnancy. And while many women who carry multiples have absolutely normal pregnancies, a significant number of us do have complications, which is the short version of why physicians treat multiple pregnancies as a high-risk affair. Now the long version. Let's start with the basics.

Why Am I Having Twins, or Triplets, or Quadruplets, or . . . ?

You are carrying more than one baby for one of two reasons: Either two or more of your eggs were fertilized by sperm and have successfully implanted themselves in your uterus; or one egg delayed in development just long enough after fertilization to cause the egg to divide into two or more identical fetuses.

No matter how it happened, your multifetal pregnancy is rare. Twins occur only once in 90 deliveries in the United States; triplets once in about 8,100 deliveries; quadruplets are more unusual still, at one in 792,000 deliveries. Almost all medical literature confines itself to discussion of twins, since greater multiples are so highly unusual.

The reason the statistics appear as one in X many deliveries is that researchers now believe that many more pregnancies begin as multiple gestations than was once thought. With routine use of ultrasound as a diagnostic tool, up to half of all pregnancies viewed before the eighth week show two gestational sacs in the uterus. (Mind you, the vast majority of all pregnancies are *not* viewed by ultrasound this early in the pregnancy—so this percentage sounds deceptively large.) But in up to two-thirds of these observed cases, only one sac and healthy developing fetus remains after the tenth week of gestation. Doctors believe that the other fetuses are simply resorbed by the body or expelled with bleeding. Most of these remaining pregnancies go to term uneventfully.

If you are having twins, you have a 70-percent chance that they will be fraternal (dizygotic)—that is, from two separate eggs, and therefore, not identical (monozygotic). Half of all fraternal twins are the same sex—two boys or two girls; half are one of each. Although all fraternal twins have genetic makeups that are different from each other, fraternal twins of the same sex may look so similar that only blood tests and examination of the placentas can confirm that they are not identical. Other fraternal twins look so dissimilar that they look like regular siblings.

Which is really what they are—regular siblings who happen to be born at the same time. They will grow and develop at different rates and have different likes and dislikes as they mature. But whether your fraternal twins (or triplets, or quads . . .) are physically alike or not, they will always have the special relationship unique to multiples.

On the other hand, 30 percent of all twins are identical—that is, the same sex, with exactly the same genetic makeup. They may look absolutely alike or can be mirror images of each other. Throughout the world, the incidence of identical twinning and ''supertwinning'' (triplets, quads, and so on) is the same no matter the race or age of the mother.

The same is not true of fraternal twinning. You have a greater chance of becoming pregnant with fraternal multiples if:

- You are between the ages of thirty-five and forty. Twinning peaks during these years, levels off at forty, and stops at forty-five.
- You are black. Blacks have the highest percentage of multiples (no one knows why), followed by Caucasians. Asians have the lowest rate of twinning of all races.
- You've been pregnant several times before.
- You've had one set of multiples before (a 10 percent greater chance for twins again, for instance).
- You've become pregnant within one month of stopping use of oral contraceptives. Researchers think this is due to the rebound effect of certain hormones that were suppressed by the pill.
- You took fertility drugs to become pregnant or became pregnant through *in vitro* fertilization. The drug called Clomid raises your chances of twinning 13 percent; the drug Perganol 20 to 40 percent. In the *in vitro* procedure, the surgeon

implants as many of the eggs harvested from your ovaries as were fertilized, saving only a few (if any) for later attempts at implantation.

- You have a female relative in the immediate family who has had fraternal twins. Yes, it's true. Twins do run in families. Twinning is a trait passed on by female descendants of mothers of twins.

A Good Time to Be Expecting Multiples

There has never been a better time in history to be pregnant with twins, triplets, quadruplets, or even quintuplets. Great advances in handling and treating multiple pregnancies and their complications are helping women stay pregnant longer. Early diagnosis, aggressive treatment of preterm labor, excellent nutrition, and delivery in facilities properly equipped to cope with the special problems of newborn multiples make a good outcome more likely than ever before. More and more women pregnant with multiples are making it close to or to term.

Getting as close as possible to term is key to a successful outcome in a multiple pregnancy, as prematurity is the primary factor in postbirth complications for twins, triplets, and higher multiples. The further a woman can progress into pregnancy, the higher the birth weights of her babies are likely to be (barring the complication called *intauterine growth retardation*—see Chapter 5—and the less likely they are to suffer from an inability to breathe properly (called *respiratory distress syndrome,* or RDS). If she can stay pregnant until the babies reach twenty-five hundred grams—about five pounds—their chances for survival become the same as if she had carried them each singly.

What Problems Might I Run Into?

A woman pregnant with multiples is five times more likely to have complications than if she were pregnant with only one fetus. By far the most common complications are premature rupture of membranes and premature labor and delivery. Up to 75 percent of all multiple pregnancies end before term (considered to be from the thirty-seventh to the fortieth week of gestation, depending on which medical text you read). This is due mostly to the inability of the uterus to hold the extra weight and volume of the pregnancy. In multiple pregnancy, the placentas (placenta, if identical twins) weigh more, there is more amniotic fluid, and there is more baby, taking up more room than with just one. Also, there is a growing body of evidence suggesting that the placentas of multiple pregnancies mature faster than those of singletons and that labor begins earlier as a result.

Here are the general rules on the length of gestation: Most twin pregnancies end at thirty-five to thirty-six weeks—about twenty to twenty-one days earlier than singletons. Triplets usually come into the world two weeks earlier than that; quadruplets two to three weeks sooner still.

Prematurity isn't the only potential problem. A woman pregnant with more than one baby also has a heightened risk of severe and extreme nausea and vomiting—called *hyperemesis gravidarum* (see Chapter 3). Although the exact causes are unknown, it is thought that the extra hormones necessary to sustain the early part of a multiple pregnancy make women more prone to vomit. Also, the uterus in a multiple pregnancy grows faster and much larger than with a singleton, crowding other internal organs and making nausea more likely.

Crowding of and pressure on the bladder in a multiple pregnancy also makes women more susceptible to urinary tract infection.

Because the fetuses need more iron than the mother can produce, anemia is common for mothers of multiples during the second and third trimester.

There is also an increased incidence of pregnancy-induced diabetes and hypoglycemia—low blood sugar (see Chapter 6, Gestational Diabetes).

Pregnancy-induced hypertensive disorders (high blood pressure and its complications) occur in up to 40 percent of all twin pregnancies, in up to 60 percent of the triplets (see Chapter 7, Hypertensive Disorders of Pregnancy).

And placental problems and difficulties with labor, delivery, and postdelivery are much more common than in singleton pregnancies. Placenta previa—a condition in which the placenta forms too low in the uterus (see Chapter 4)—is more common because there is more placenta covering more of the uterus in twin (and greater) pregnancies. The higher the number of fetuses, the more likely one (or more) placenta(s) may implant and grow unusually low in the uterus, creating the potential for serious maternal and fetal bleeding. Placental abruption—the premature separation of the placenta from the uterine wall—is more common during labor as well (see Chapter 9, Bleeding, Hemorrhage, and Placental Abruption).

The overextended uterus can also have trouble contracting properly during or just after labor. This is because the uterine walls are thinned from accommodating more than one fetus. During labor, weak contracting ability can lead to the need for or recommendations of a cesarean delivery. After birth, the same inability to contract well can prevent the uterus from sealing off the blood vessels opened up by the delivery of the placenta, causing hemorrhaging in the mother.

With all the potential for complications, it's important to keep in mind that no matter how complicated your pregnancy turns out to be, you still have an excellent chance of having healthy babies.

Lisa's is a typical success story. Her preeclampsia (a complication due to hypertension and its side effects) became so severe that her eyes swelled shut and her lungs filled with fluid. She was hospitalized for a month, and the babies were born prematurely, by cesarean. Her twins were ten weeks old when I talked to her about her experience, and they had already been home for over a month, normal and healthy. "I thought I had it really bad," Lisa said. "But after I saw these babies, I'd do it again if I had to. When they come out so sweet and cuddly and they're growing so well, it makes you real proud."

Cesareans and Multiple Pregnancies

Almost every medical authority recommends cesareans "liberally" with multiples. This is due in part to the size and fragility of multiples born prematurely. These infants tend not to react well to the rigors of vaginal birth. Also, in about half of all multiple pregnancies, one or more of the babies is positioned "improperly" for vaginal birth—that is, she would not come out head first. More fetal distress occurs in breech deliveries.

There is disagreement in the medical community about the need for a c-section when the first child presents herself head down, but the second does not. Some authorities believe that when this happens, it is safer for the babies to be taken by section. Other doctors feel that vaginal delivery works well, as long as they have everything prepared to shift right to surgical delivery if problems arise. The majority view seems to be to "play it safe" and do a c-section. If one or more of the babies is in a breech position, and you choose (with your doctor's agreement) to go with vaginal birth, you can expect a fair amount of medical intervention in the birth of the second child—a larger incision to widen the birth canal (episiotomy), possible internal manipulation of the second baby (which requires regional anesthesia for the mother) to help turn her to a better position for birth, and/or a forceps delivery.

Barring other complications, in almost all pregnancies in which both twins present themselves head down and close to term, the woman is encouraged to deliver vaginally. Conversely, in virtually every pregnancy in which the first twin is a breech, a cesarean is performed to prevent the twins from hurting each other during labor and delivery.

Also, most pregnancies in which the second twin is transverse—lying across the abdomen instead of up and down—are delivered by c-section.

How Can I Tell if I'm Carrying More Than One?

You may not be able to tell—especially early in your pregnancy. Until quite recently, up to 50 percent of all multiple pregnancies were not diagnosed as such until delivery! Some symptoms of multiple pregnancy mimic other pregnancy-related medical conditions.

But if you think you are in one or more of the "high-risk" categories for conceiving multiples, and you've had one or more of the following symptoms, it's time to discuss the possibility with your doctor:

- You are gaining weight more rapidly than you think you should be, but you're not overeating.
- You think you are bigger than you should be for the amount of time you've been pregnant (such as being ten weeks' pregnant and already "showing").
- You have dreams that you're pregnant with more than one baby.
- You can readily feel lots of small parts (hands, feet, and so on) or more than three large parts (heads, bottoms).
- You feel more fetal movement than you think you should for just one baby, or you feel more than one baby moving.

How Can the Doctor Tell?

If your doctor doesn't raise the possibility and you think you may be carrying twins (or more), talk to him about it. Ask him to check. The tests he'd do (a blood test and a sonogram) won't hurt you, so he should have no problem checking out your hunch. The doctor should have his own suspicions that you're carrying more than one baby, based on a combination of observations he'll make during routine exams and diagnostic testing.

For instance, every time you go to the office for a checkup, the doctor will feel your uterus to make sure it's growing at the right rate. There is an average rate of progression for every week of pregnancy. If the size of your uterus is four to eight weeks ahead of where it should be for the date you became pregnant, it's an obstetrical red flag that needs to be checked out.

After eight weeks of pregnancy, your baby's heart is audible with the aid of a special, sensitive microphone—called a *doptone*—that's placed on your belly. Each time you go to the office, your doctor or an assistant will listen to the heartbeat and let you listen to it, too. Hearing more than one fetal heart beating at a different rate is a dead giveaway that you're carrying multiples.

Another routine part of every prenatal visit is a weight check. Just as there is an average growth rate for your uterus, there is an average weight gain each week that is expected for all pregnant women. If you step on the scale and your weight has shot way up above the mean for your length of gestation, your doctor will start quizzing you about what and how much you're eating. If he's satisfied that you're not overeating or simply retaining water, he'll want to investigate further.

Most likely, he'll ask you to have a sonogram to determine if multiple gestation is the cause. In virtually every case, this ultrasound exam will successfully uncover the presence of multiple fetuses in the uterus—although it won't always catch the third or fourth fetus on the first go 'round.

Janet's triplets weren't all discovered until she was twenty-four weeks along. "At fourteen weeks, my doctor did a sonogram, and found only twins," she recalled. But Janet was sure she was having triplets. "I felt something on my lower left, but the sonogram didn't find it." At twenty-three weeks, Janet insisted on another sonogram. Sure enough, it was triplets, all of whom were born early, but are now healthy second graders. This is one reason doctors ask their patients to take repeat sonograms later in the pregnancy.

The doctor may also do a blood test to check the level of human placental lactogen (hPl) in your blood. HPl is produced by placental tissue, so women carrying twins have hPl levels that are much higher than for a singleton pregnancy.

How Am I Supposed to Feel? What's Normal?

"I wasn't comfortable," recounted Susan. "And I had pain in one hip that was really bad." Susan is a mother of triplets *and* quadruplets, all born at term with each baby weighing over five pounds. She had some swelling in her legs. "And sometimes it hurt just from the babies moving. You get to the point where you think about it before you move. It was hard to eat, but I did it anyway, because I knew that the babies really needed it."

Susan's litany of complaints were not due to complications. Hers were some of the *normal* aches and pains of plural pregnancy.

You may or may not experience Susan's difficulties. There is no one way you are *supposed* to feel when your multiple pregnancy is going right. But generally speaking, when you are carrying more than one baby, certain normal discomforts of pregnancy tend to increase. (See Chapter 2, When Pregnancy *Is* Perfect, for a discussion of the usual discomforts of a normal pregnancy.) For instance, you will probably be ravenously hungry, because your body is working so hard to nourish both you and the lives inside you. But it will be hard to eat so much more (from three hundred to six hundred calories per baby per day is recommended by most authorities) because your stomach will be compressed by your growing uterus.

Heartburn and nausea bother up to 60 percent of all pregnant women. In a plural pregnancy, these problems are even more likely to occur and with greater severity because of the extra hormones the mother's system creates to sustain the pregnancy and the larger size of the plurally pregnant uterus. This is normal for multiple gestation. Chapter 3 explains what happens to your digestive system as pregnancy progresses and why these discomforts are so common.

As your babies grow inside you, your uterus will grow and stretch much faster than it would for a singleton pregnancy. Your greater girth is likely to cause backaches, make it awkward for you to move around, and cause aches and pains in your lower belly, groin, and legs. You may feel extra pressure in your pelvis from the sheer weight of the uterus. Don't forget, toward the end, you'll be carrying at least twice the load that women pregnant with only one child must bear. All pregnant women can get varicose veins in their legs, hemorrhoids, and stretch marks. You can expect them, too—possibly in spades.

With multiples, from mid-pregnancy on, it is not unusual to feel short of breath as your uterus pushes up toward your diaphragm. Although uncomfortable, this is normal. It is also completely normal to feel very tired. Your body is working hard to do its job sustaining your pregnancy. The babies take a lot of nutrition and oxygen to grow. They also take a tremendous amount of iron from your body. It is not unusual for women in plural pregnancies to become anemic—and one of the side effects of anemia is tiredness.

How Do I Tell When Something Is *Not* Normal?

You may not be able to, especially if this is your first pregnancy. How are you supposed to know what feels right or wrong when you have no experience on which to base your evaluation? *If you have any ques-*

tion at all about whether something is wrong, call your doctor. That's part of what he's there for. He'd rather have you call and be able to tell you there's nothing to worry about than not have you call and have something go wrong.

It is particularly important for women with plural pregnancies to be aware of their bodies and what is happening inside them, since complications are more common with multiple gestations. Only you know what is normal for your body, pregnant or not. If you stay "in touch" with your body, you will become familiar with the way it reacts to being pregnant—like how much vaginal discharge is normal for you or whether you cramp up when you change position.

Here are the symptoms, which, if you have them, always warrant a call to the doctor:

- bleeding or gushing of fluid from the vagina (call, then go *directly* to the hospital)
- weight gain of more than two pounds per week
- sudden swelling (over the course of hours or a day or two) of the hands, feet, and/or face
- fever
- uncontrollable vomiting

Preterm Labor

The greatest danger to your babies is premature birth. With the uterus so stretched, it is often difficult to tell whether the pains you are having are labor or something else. What makes this even trickier is that preterm labor contractions are often painless. However, they tend to occur in a pattern. Chapter 8 fully explains preterm labor, why it happens, how to spot it, and what can be done about it. This is *must* reading for you. But, in short, here are the signs to look for:

- uterine contractions (a hard feeling over the entire surface of the uterus lasting from twenty seconds up to two minutes each) every fifteen minutes or closer
- menstrual-type cramps, especially if they are rhythmic or wavelike
- dull pain in the lower back, either constant or rhythmic, not relieved by a change of position
- pelvic pressure or a feeling of fullness in the pelvic area or back of the thighs
- persistent diarrhea

- intestinal cramps, with or without diarrhea
- vaginal discharge greater than is normal for you, or whose consistency or color changes (especially if the discharge is bloody)
- a general feeling that something is wrong, even if you don't know what it is

Some of these symptoms may be normal for your pregnancy. But if you have any of these symptoms, you need to lie down and check yourself for contractions, as explained in Chapter 8. If you have four or more contractions in one hour, **call your doctor** and **go to the labor and delivery room at the hospital.** Do not wait for his return call. Just go there.

YOURS IS A SPECIAL PREGNANCY: EXPECT—AND DEMAND—TO BE TREATED DIFFERENTLY.

Virtually every authority in the field recommends that women pregnant with multiples see doctors experienced in multiple pregnancies and that these women deliver in hospitals with level-3 neonatal intensive care units. These professionals and facilities are most capable of helping you get what you really want: full-term, healthy babies. And if—as 50 percent of all multiples are—yours are born prematurely, you will appreciate the expertise and special equipment that tertiary-care centers offer your newborns.

After interviewing several physicians, Pat chose an obstetrician who had delivered a number of multiples. "Thank God I chose the doctor and hospital I did," she told me. "I can almost guarantee you that if I had had anyone else in this area for my doctor, I wouldn't have done as well." Pat's triplets are three now, after a pregnancy that included premature labor and toxemia. Her doctor's skill helped her reach thirty-six weeks before giving birth to babies all weighing in over five pounds.

How do you find out your doctor's background on multiples or your hospital's ability to care for you and your children properly? Ask. Talk to your OB about it. Your multiple pregnancy requires, at a minimum, special attention and sensitivity to your progress, especially if you already have or have reason to anticipate complications.

It's a fair question to ask your doctor how many multiple pregnancies he has delivered. If he answers that the number is quite small (and in the case of triplets, quads, or greater, it's probable that your doctor has delivered one or none!) or he tells you he has little experience, you may want to consider switching to a physician with more experience in your type of situation. Also, if your practitioner has privileges only at a hospital without a level-3 neonatal intensive care nursery, you may want to consider seeing someone with privileges at such an institution.

Emotionally, switching doctors or hospitals in midstream is tough, to say the least. It's scary to leave a doctor you know and trust or a hospital with which you are already familiar. And by bringing up the issue, I am not suggesting that you should do so. But you should be aware that it is an issue to consider and think through carefully—one, hopefully, about which your own doctor will be open with you.

Once you've settled on an obstetrician to help you, you should expect a lot of scrutiny. What does that mean?

Well, to start, you will be going to visit your doctor frequently. Your obstetrician will ask to see you twice a month until your twenty-fifth to twenty-eighth week and weekly thereafter. When you are at the office, your blood levels will likely be monitored to check you for anemia and for gestational diabetes and other anomalies common to plural pregnancy.

You will have to take iron supplements to prevent or minimize anemia. This can cause constipation, so ask your doctor to recommend fiber supplements and/or stool softeners if you start having trouble moving your bowels.

Your doctor will also pay close attention to your weight gain and check you routinely for symptoms of toxemia—sudden swelling, protein in your urine, headaches, or visual disturbances.

Be prepared to eat more, and to gain more weight than you had anticipated—from forty to seventy pounds, depending on your doctor's bent. No matter how good your eating habits are, you'll have to learn what to eat (and what not to eat) to give your babies the best possible nutrition and opportunity for weight gain. Your doctor will give you nutritional counseling or will refer you to a nutritionist. The amounts and types of food you should be eating to both nourish yourself and give your babies the best chance to gain weight properly are different than if you carry a singleton.

Some physicians believe that an extra three hundred calories per day per baby is enough; others recommend at least double that. If your obstetrician does not have a written diet for you to follow, or does not have a nutritional counselor to refer you to, consult a nutritionist on your own. Your local hospital should be able to refer you to one. You can also get nutritional information from the twins/triplets support organizations listed at the end of this chapter.

Your doctor will recommend that you have several sonograms during the course of the pregnancy, to check the babies' growth rates and their position just prior to delivery. He may also want to test your blood and/or perform an amniocentesis to rule out fetal abnormalities. Amniocentesis near the end of the pregnancy (after thirty-one to thirty-two weeks) can tell the doctor whether your babies are ready to breathe on their own.

Normally, infants' lungs are not mature enough to avoid respiratory distress until thirty-six weeks' gestation. But many authorities believe that in multiple pregnancies or pregnancies in which there are complications, fetal lungs mature more quickly because of the stress on the babies. Thus many preemies from plural pregnancies breathe on their own much sooner than singletons born at the same week of gestation.

Besides amniocentesis, you can expect your doctor to order nonstress testing once or twice a week for you after you've reached thirty-two weeks of pregnancy. This test simply involves electronic monitors being placed on your belly to pick up the babies' heartbeats and any contractions you may be having. A strip of paper records fetal heartbeats and your contractions. From the readout, the doctor can tell whether your babies are still reacting well to being in your uterus.

Some doctors routinely put their plurally pregnant patients on bedrest from twenty-six to thirty-six weeks' gestation—considered the highest risk weeks for premature labor and delivery—on the theory that, by countering the effects of gravity and uterine weight on the cervix, being off one's feet betters the chances of going to term. To date, however, there are no universally accepted studies that prove that bedrest prevents preterm labor.

Once labor starts prematurely, though, bedrest, combined with other measures, such as contraction-stopping drugs (tocolytics) and hydration therapy, is effective in reducing or stopping contractions. And bedrest, especially when the woman rests on her left side, has been found to increase blood flow to the babies, which helps them to gain weight better.

Some OBs put their patients on home monitoring regardless of whether there is evidence that they're likely to go into premature labor. This involves spending some time (up to two hours or more) every day wearing an electronic monitor that records your uterine activity. The idea is to catch premature labor contractions before you actually go into hard labor.

Home monitoring requires your active participation. You have to strap the device on, follow directions, and report daily to the home-monitoring center nearest you (see Chapter 8). This can seem like a nuisance, especially when you are feeling no symptoms. But it can be a lifesaver. Literally.

"Monitoring wasn't available when I was pregnant," Marie said. "They told me I had the flu. Then they said I had a urinary tract infection. In fact, I was eight centimeters dilated. I lost both my babies, and I had no symptoms. I didn't feel any of those contractions," she said. "How nice it is to have that reassurance that now a monitor would pick my contractions up."

Another, more controversial prophylactic step is cerclage (stitching the cervix to prevent premature dilation and premature labor). Most recent medical literature recommends against such a step unless the woman has a history of incompetent cervix or has had previous cervical surgery that has clearly left her cervix in a weakened condition. These authorities say that cerclage, if done at all, should only be performed early in the pregnancy (up to eighteen weeks).

Mary Jo was a perfect candidate for cerclage. She had a history of previous miscarriages and cervical incompetence. Then, while taking fertility drugs, she became pregnant with sextuplets. One fetus miscarried in her sixth week. A sonogram to confirm the miscarriage diagnosed four remaining fetuses, with a possible fifth. Her OB decided to place a cerclage at thirteen weeks. "The thing that was most important to carry those babies was the cerclage," she told me. "I never would have gotten to thirty-two weeks without it." I spoke to her when the babies were eight months old. All five were doing beautifully.

But *cerclage is not for everybody*. If your doctor recommends this procedure to prolong your pregnancy, you should ask him to explain his reasoning. Cerclage is a surgical procedure and has risks associated with it, including the possibility of postsurgery infection (see Chapter 8). It may be that in your case, cerclage is absolutely the right move. But it needs to be discussed with you until all your questions about this measure have been answered.

There is one more suggestion that many doctors make to their plurally pregnant patients: They often advise that you quit working well before term. Again, the point of slowing down is keeping you pregnant until the babies are mature enough to survive outside the womb, and survive well. Some medical texts urge practitioners to require their patients to stop working by twenty-four weeks' gestation. My own obstetricians told me that I could expect to stop working at twenty-eight weeks and go on some rest schedule until I delivered.

What Happens if I Do Go into Labor Prematurely?

You will go to the hospital. How long you'll remain there depends on the stage of your labor when you arrive and whether it can successfully be stopped through intravenous hydration and/or tocolytic drugs. Most preterm labor, if caught early enough, *can* be stopped and the pregnancy prolonged until your babies are more mature. Frequently, it can be held off long enough to allow your babies to progress to the point that they'll breathe on their own after birth. Babies born as early as thirty-two weeks often breathe without any assistance at birth.

If your doctor can stabilize you—that is, get rid of your contractions, you may be able to go home. You may be told that you must rest in bed at all times, or you may be able to be up and around part of the time. Most likely, your doctor will require you to be on home monitoring with one of the several services available. You may need health care at home by a nurse practitioner and/or a social worker. For full discussions of preterm labor, prolonged bedrest, home monitoring, and what to expect when you're in the hospital, you should read chapters 8, 15, and 14.

Planning Ahead: Part of Your Job

No matter how complicated or easy your plural pregnancy is, you won't be fully doing your job unless you engage in a fair amount of preplanning—both for contingencies during your pregnancy and for after the kids come home.

After delivery, other stresses can take the place of the worries of getting to term. As a brochure from the support group TwinLine says: "Twins can be a hard happiness." You can make it so much easier by being well prepared.

This planning really isn't for your babies so much as it is for you. You know, if all goes well—as it does for the majority of plurally pregnant people—pretty soon you're going to have two or more little bundles to care for at home. It's at least double the work (and yes, double the joy) taking care of twins, triple for triplets, and so on. They may or may not have special needs, depending upon whether they are born prematurely or with other problems. The simple fact is that extra babies take extra planning.

One thing you should consider is what your physical condition is likely to be after you've given birth. If you've been on bedrest for weeks or months, you will need extra time to regain your strength, learn to walk properly again, and pick up stamina. There is nothing so enervating as lying in bed for a long time. And if you've had a cesarean, you will also be recuperating from major surgery. This takes weeks.

Adding to your energy problem will be lack of sleep. The feeding schedule of just one newborn is tiring for all new parents; the extra demands of twins, triplets, or more can be exhausting. A full night's rest is a luxury that you will not have for a minimum of several months, until the children mature enough to sleep through the night. Extreme sleep loss can be debilitating. So unless you carefully plan ways to ensure adequate rest—and this probably means getting in extra household help of some kind, night and/or day—your health, and thus the health of your children, can suffer.

You may feel depressed after the birth. Don't forget, you'll have extra hormones still running around in your body. The "baby blues" that many moms of singletons experience can be heightened for moms of multiples. So don't let sad or angry feelings surprise you too much right after the birth.

Your breasts are likely to be extra tender: You'll be producing a tremendous amount of milk. Adjusting to breastfeeding can be difficult. If you have questions or need help getting started or solving problems, call the La Leche League (LLL—listed in the Other Reading and Resources section of this book). The LLL will offer you support and can even recommend breastfeeding consultants who will come to your home and provide you with individualized, personal attention. Once you start breastfeeding, stick with it. The benefits to you and the babies will be well worth the trouble.

If your babies are in intensive care for prematurity, chances are you'll be leaving the hospital before they will. But you don't necessarily have to check out of the hospital in the usual three days (for vaginal delivery) or five days (for cesarean). If you ask your doctor, and if you can afford it, you may be able to stay an extra day or two, until you've better recovered your strength and are a bit more ready to enter into multiple parenting. Talk to your doctor about this possibility ahead of time.

Now is also the time for you to think about what kind of help you are going to have once you go home. Undoubtedly you will need some assistance, especially if you're anticipating bringing home more than two babies. Here are some of the other issues you should be considering and planning for as your pregnancy progresses:

- *Diapers*—disposable or cloth? If cloth, what diaper service will you use? (Some provide free or reduced-price service to moms of multiples.) Contract for it early.
- *Feeding*—do you plan to breastfeed, or bottle feed, or both? Read up on the pros and cons. Contact the La Leche

League. Research formulas. Buy bottles and the like ahead of time, or, if you can't bring yourself to do that, arrange for someone else to get what you need while you are in the hospital after the babies are born.

- *Baby equipment*—what else will you need? Where can you get it? Will you buy used or new? Do you want it in the house before you give birth? (Some women don't.)
- *Sleeping*—where are you going to put the babies? Cradles? Cribs?
- *Household chores*—who's going to do them? At first? As the babies grow? Can you afford household help? Do you have a relative or close friend who can assist you in the short term? The long term?

Of course, there are other questions to handle that are common to all pregnancies. But multiples make special demands of their parents.

But You Needn't Do It All Alone

Which is exactly why you should use every resource available to you. Support organizations can be of excellent assistance. Luckily, there are several to help you wade through the particular problems and pleasures of plural pregnancy and multiple child raising. These were started by women, who, like you, found themselves pregnant with multiples. The difference is that before these women had their pregnancy experiences, there were no resources for them to draw on.

I cannot urge you strongly enough to *use the services these groups have to offer*. The women involved in them know what you'll be going through. There's nothing like the example of others who have been through just what you have and who've come out on the other end smiling.

The two key groups that help women all across the United States are the Triplet Connection, and TWINLINE/Twin Services, both of which are based in California. The Triplet Connection is a not-for-profit informational and support network for women expecting (or who already have) triplets, quadruplets, and quintuplets or more. Begun seven years ago, the Triplet Connection has worked with over three thousand six hundred women who have given birth to larger multiples. Janet Bleyl, T-C's founder, had her triplets at twenty-nine weeks' gestation and "started the Triplet Connection because I wanted other women to get farther along in their pregnancies and do better than I did." She also wanted the Triplet Connection to help other prospective parents emotionally. "If you feel isolated with twins, you can imagine that being pregnant with three, four, or five babies will make you feel like the only one in the world.''

With the Triplet Connection, you'll quickly find out that you are *not* the only one in the world who's ever had your experience. The group offers a quarterly newsletter, plus information packets on multiple pregnancy and child care. T-C also offers support and "hot-line" consulting to women with questions or problems and will find plurally pregnant "buddies" for expectant mothers who want ongoing support and contact.

The group is guided by a medical board of advisors consisting of physicians who are at the top of the field. T-C does research on larger multiple pregnancy and sponsors bi-annual conventions where families with multiples can meet, exchange ideas, and get to know each other. Dues for joining the Triplet Connection are under twenty dollars. To get started, phone or write the group. Include your name, address, phone number, and due date. The address is:

The Triplet Connection
P.O. Box 99571
Stockton, California 95209
(209) 474-0885 or 474-3073

The other national organization is TWINLINE/Twin Services, a nonprofit agency founded in 1978 that provides professional health, education, and social services for families with or expecting twins, triplets, quadruplets, or more. The group maintains a TWINLINE "warmline" that provides telephone information, counseling, and referrals for families of twins and the professionals who work with them. Twin Services also publishes a variety of materials, including informational handouts, a quarterly newsletter, a survival kit for new families of twins, and other publications.

Membership fees are on a sliding scale, based on what you feel you can give. Services provided are free of charge. To join, send a self-addressed, stamped envelope with your name and address to:

TWINLINE/Twin Services
P.O. Box 10066
Berkeley, California 94709
(415) 524–0863

"I wish I had known about the support groups," Pam told me. "While I was pregnant with my twins, I had no one to talk to who had also had monoamniotic twins, and no one to tell me 'You can get through this.' I had nothing positive to go on and spent all this time lying there on my left side to think. Somehow I got through the months, though. And now that I have them, I know I'd never do it any different!''

You don't have to be in the dark, like Pam was. There are twin, triplet, and more support organizations equipped to answer virtually all your questions and get you started in the right direction. Use them. They exist only to help people like you. With a little planning, great health care, and a little luck, pretty soon you and your babies will be the talk of your town!

13

Cesarean Section

Technically, a cesarean section is not a complication of pregnancy; rather, it is an operation performed because of complications the mother experiences during pregnancy and/or labor. Then why am I devoting a whole chapter to c-sections? Because of the numbers.

Approximately one out of every four women who gives birth this year in the United States will do so by cesarean. In 1988—the last year for which statistics were available when this book went to press—out of 3,909,510 births, 965,649, or 24.7* percent, were delivered by cesarean section. Those numbers represent all pregnancies that resulted in births and include all those pregnancies that were picture perfect right up to delivery time.

What that one-in-four figure doesn't tell you is that for those of us whose pregnancies aren't perfect, the numbers are even higher, much higher. Having complications of pregnancy doubles or triples your odds of having a cesarean. For example, if you have placenta previa, you can virtually count on having a c-section. If you hemorrhage, you'll probably have a section. If the baby is premature, you have at least a 50 percent chance of giving birth surgically.

This chapter is here so that you can familiarize yourself with cesareans, what they entail, and what they're like from the woman's perspective. It's hard enough to go through a complicated pregnancy. You shouldn't have to enter the birth experience terrified because you don't know what's going to be done to you. The better you understand

*Source: National Center for Health Statistics

231

cesarean section, the easier it will be for you to tolerate if you must have one.

Just What Is a Cesarean Section?

A cesarean section is the delivery of a baby through an incision in the abdomen and uterus. Although it is done routinely throughout the United States, it is a serious abdominal operation that neither you nor your doctor should treat lightly. As with any surgery, c-sections carry certain risks, including accidents involving anesthesia, bleeding, and infection.

Still, it's important and reassuring for you to know the statistics on this method of delivery: The survival rate in the United States for this operation is greater than 99.9 percent. Those are pretty terrific odds. So, bottom line: Even though it is a major operation, there is every likelihood that you will recover, and recover fully.

It's Safe, But Not Risk-Free

There are, however, a couple of common complications that you ought to know about. The most frequent complication from this surgery is postsurgical infection of the incision or womb. You will also be at a slightly higher risk of postdelivery hemorrhage. And it does occasionally (though infrequently) happen that the bladder or urinary tract is damaged by the surgery. But these complications are the exception rather than the rule.

What you can reasonably expect as a result of the surgery is greater pain after the birth, a slower recovery, and a heavier reliance on pain medication than if you had delivered vaginally. Whereas most women giving birth vaginally leave the hospital within three days, c-section moms stay in the hospital from four or five days to one week. Breast-feeding can prove more difficult, because of the pain of the incision and because at first it will be harder for you to move around easily. Lifting and walking will also be tough for at least the first week. And you'll be more tired than a mom who's given birth vaginally.

"After my cesarean, I just wasn't myself for the first three weeks," Julia told me. "It was hard to do what I thought I ought to be doing. I was trying to do what I'd been told every new mom does—feeding my baby, changing her, bathing her. But my incision ached, and all I wanted to do was sleep. By the time a month was past, though, it all got much easier—except the lack of sleep. But that was because of the baby, not because of the surgery."

If you have a c-section, you'll find that the risks and discomforts are usually worth taking, because c-sections often improve the short- and long-term outlook for your baby. She is at less risk for birth trauma with a c-section. Also, if she is a breech baby, or has a placenta that formed too low in your uterus (placenta previa, see Chapter 4), she's much better off being born surgically.

And, as the pain of vaginal birth fades with time, so does the pain of a cesarean. I know that I'd do it again in a second if it meant ending up with a child as wonderful and delicious as mine.

Why Might I Need a C-Section?

The chances that you'll have to have a c-section are higher now than almost ever before. Over the past twenty years there has been a tremendous rise in the number of cesareans performed in the United States. In 1970, only 5.5 percent of all women giving birth did so by c-section. In 1988, that percentage had shot up to 24.7 percent.

Why the big rise? There are a number of reasons. For one thing, over 25 percent of all women having their first child are over the age of thirty. As a woman becomes older (not that any of us think of ourselves as such by thirty or thirty-five, but, obstetrically speaking, that's old) the numbers of and likelihood of complications she is apt to suffer go up. The more complications there are in a pregnancy, the more probable it is that cesarean section will be necessary.

Changes in obstetrics practice account for a majority of the increase in c-sections. For instance, today, nearly 86 percent of all breech presentations—that is, the baby enters the birth canal feet-, behind-, or knees-first, rather than head-first—are delivered by cesarean. Also, many babies who, years ago, would have been delivered by forceps, are now delivered by section because it is considered less dangerous to the fetus to do so. Plus, the electronic fetal monitor now allows physicians to follow every single heartbeat of the baby, so that problems and potential problems are easily spotted (although some studies now say that too many cesareans are performed based on these readings).

Doctors are increasingly concerned about avoiding lawsuits, too. Studies have shown that if there is a difficult vaginal delivery—if the baby has some distress, presents in a breech position, fails to come down into the pelvis within a certain period of time, and so on—many doctors will opt for the c-section to avoid the accusation later that they did not do everything possible to save or preserve the health of the child. The American College of Obstetricians and Gynecologists (ACOG) reported in the mid-1980s that nearly three-quarters of their members had had at least one lawsuit filed against them.

The Most Common Reasons for Having a Cesarean

You Had a Cesarean Last Time

Repeat c-sections account for 39 percent of all cesareans done in this country. Obviously, the old maxim "once a cesarean, always a cesarean" is still adhered to by many obstetricians, despite the fact that the ACOG recommends a trial of labor for almost all women who have had a previous cesarean. But despite ACOG's urging, the statistic on repeat c-sections has not changed significantly yet.

Failure to Progress

Failure to progress is defined as the failure of the cervix to continue to dilate, or failure of the baby to descend into position for passage through the cervix and vagina, during the active labor phase. It can be caused by inadequate or poorly coordinated uterine contractions, the position of the baby, or the failure of the baby to move into and engage in the pelvic cavity. There is no set time span that a woman must pass before this diagnosis is made, although it is usual for a doctor to allow at least eighteen to twenty-four hours of labor before intervening. Failure to progress accounts for 28 percent of all first cesareans.

Cephalopelvic Disproportion

This problem is really interchangeable with failure to progress. It is the inability of the part of the baby that would first pass through the pelvis (usually the head) to get through. This is caused either by the mother's pelvis being the wrong shape or size, or her soft tissues not expanding properly to accept passage of the baby. It can also occur when the baby is too big, when she is turned in such a way that she can't get through, or when her head isn't malleable enough to mold to the mom's pelvis and birth canal.

Although cephalopelvic disproportion is thought to occur in only 1 to 3 percent of all first pregnancies, cephalopelvic disproportion is listed, along with failure to progress, as the cause of cesarean birth 28 percent of the time in the United States. The term is used loosely to cover a range of conditions that prevent the baby from being born vaginally.

Claudie was one of that 1 to 3 percent who have true cephalopelvic disproportion. She was in labor for nearly twenty-four hours before her family practitioner brought in a consulting OB to try to figure out the problem. "He said, 'I think you could keep this up for the rest of the day, but that I'll have to take the baby eventually.' When it was over, the doctor who did the surgery said he thought it was good that we went with a section, because my pelvic bones were so thick that I couldn't deliver a baby any larger than a cyst through the pelvic outlet. I had never had an ultrasound. I had no prenatal testing that would have indicated that it was a problem, so it was a surprise, especially considering my build.''

FETAL DISTRESS

Ten percent of all c-sections are done as a result of fetal distress, a condition of the fetus that, if allowed to continue, could lead to permanent damage or death. It means that for some reason the baby has stopped receiving enough blood and oxygen. The baby's heartbeat becomes slowed, and, if deprived of oxygen for long enough, the baby will die or be permanently brain damaged. The trick is to diagnose the distress before it actually reaches this point.

Fetal distress is a diagnosis that is currently under debate in the medical community and often requires a real judgment call on the part of the obstetrician. This is because the electronic fetal monitor—a device that records the baby's heartbeat—makes possible detection of even the minutest deviation from the normal range. Some physicians feel that many cesareans are done too promptly—at the first sign of fetal distress—and unnecessarily.

Unless the heartbeat disappears altogether or is very slow, the doctor has another test he can easily perform to prove out his suspicion that something is wrong. Provided that the amniotic sac has already broken and the baby's head is in a position that can be easily reached through the vagina and cervix, the doctor can check the baby's condition by doing a fetal scalp blood sampling. For this he takes a tiny scraping of scalp tissue and blood from the baby's head, which is quickly analyzed by a technician for the amount of acid in the baby's blood. Too much acid signals fetal distress.

On the electronic monitor, if, after contractions, the baby's heartbeat is not in the 120 to 160 beat-per-minute range, or if the heart rate slows down in between contractions, the baby may be in distress. This usually happens in a pattern. A single dip in the monitor could be caused by many things and is probably transitory.

The doctor will try to improve the blood flow to the baby before doing anything as drastic as operating. That means he'll ask you to change your position to the left side. He may also ask you to breathe through an oxygen mask, so that the most oxygen possible reaches the baby. Most often, the condition that causes the blip(s) in the monitor is temporary, and the baby's *tracings*—the recording on paper of the heart rate—will improve. If they don't, and if the doctor feels that the baby is in real jeopardy, he'll tell you you need a c-section.

THE BABY IS BREECH

Over 85 percent of all babies who try to present themselves to the world feet- or behind-first are born by cesarean section, although these children account for only 7.3 percent of all cesarean deliveries. The baby's head is its largest body part, and the bones of the skull are movable, so that it molds to fit the mother's pelvis. When the baby comes down feet first, there is a danger that the feet, or other part that arrives in the pelvis outlet first, will get through, but that the mother's tissues won't stretch enough to accommodate the bigger parts of the fetus's body. The baby's head could get stuck, or the placenta detach before the baby's head is out, and the baby could asphyxiate. Or the baby could also have its head hyperextended during delivery causing damage to the spinal cord. Breech babies are taken by cesarean to prevent this from happening.

THE BABY IS TOO SMALL OR TOO LARGE TO HANDLE VAGINAL DELIVERY

Preemies and growth-retarded babies are very fragile and may not tolerate vaginal delivery or labor well. These infants are more prone than full-term, full-size babies to hypoxia—taking in too little oxygen—which can asphyxiate them or cause brain and nerve damage, and to physical damage during vaginal birth.

An extremely large baby might just not fit through the mother's pelvis or birth canal—as with some infants of diabetic mothers whose diabetes was poorly controlled during the pregnancy. These babies weigh more than nine pounds, are extremely chubby, and can cause injury to themselves and the birth canal. Delivery of these infants by cesarean as a routine matter is controversial, but it nonetheless is a reason for c-section in many places.

PLACENTA PREVIA

This is a condition in which the cervix is partially or totally covered by the placenta—that is, the placenta forms abnormally low in the uterus (see Chapter 4, Placenta Previa). Total placenta previa, where the placenta completely blocks the opening to the vagina, absolutely precludes vaginal delivery. Almost all forms of placenta previa create a serious danger of catastrophic hemorrhage for the mother, because as the cervix dilates, it shears away blood vessels between it and the placenta. This also causes loss of blood and oxygen for the baby and can permanently injure or kill her. Cesarean section, done before labor begins, usually takes care of the problem.

Multiple Pregnancy

Twins and higher multiples are often born by cesarean because of either their small size, their presentation, or their sheer number. Most multiple fetuses are smaller at term than their singleton counterparts, and they usually arrive significantly earlier than singletons (see Chapter 12, Multiple Pregnancy). Their prematurity or small size may make cesarean section a less traumatic birth method for them.

Sometimes the positioning of the babies inside you requires cesarean intervention. If the first twin is a breech, then the babies will always be taken by cesarean, for fear that their heads will lock together, causing asphyxiation.

And with higher multiples, there is a danger that one or more of the remaining babies' placentas will separate from the uterus, cutting off their blood supply and oxygen before it is their turn to be born. Also, the greatly overstretched uterus may have trouble contracting properly, hindering vaginal birth. Both factors weigh heavily in favor of cesarean.

Prolapsed Umbilical Cord

A prolapsed umbilical cord is an umbilical cord that falls under the fetus during labor and delivery. The cord may even fall through the open cervix, into the vagina, or out of the vaginal opening. This is a very serious birth complication, because the baby's downward journey causes her to press against the prolapsed cord during contractions or as she is delivered, and this compression cuts off her blood and oxygen supply coming from the placenta. If the condition is not reversed immediately, she can die.

Usually, as soon as a prolapsed cord is discovered, the doctor tries to move it up and out of the way by hand. If he does not succeed, an emergency c-section is performed to save the baby's life.

Diabetes, Gestational or Chronic

A woman who develops diabetes during pregnancy or who brings chronic diabetes into the pregnancy is at risk for blood sugar problems during labor. Controlling the mother's blood sugar level can be difficult during labor and, if it gets wildly out of control, can harm both her and the baby (see Chapter 6, Gestational Diabetes). As a result, doctors will often suggest a cesarean to avoid this and other potential birth-related complications.

PREGNANCY-INDUCED HYPERTENSION AND PREECLAMPSIA OR ECLAMPSIA

Doctors often deliver by cesarean when mothers have high blood pressure alone (hypertension), high blood pressure combined with swelling of the mother's tissues and protein in the urine (preeclampsia), or preeclampsia with seizures (eclampsia). These disorders increase the danger of premature separation of the placenta from the uterine wall (placental abruption), which can kill the baby. The hemorrhaging from abruption when the woman has a hypertensive disorder is also grave, because hypertensive women have less blood volume and go into shock from blood loss more readily than nonhypertensive women (see Chapter 7, Hypertensive Disorders of Pregnancy). Hypertensive women also may deliver prematurely, so there may be the added problem of a small or delicate fetus.

Delivery by cesarean in these instances may be safer than vaginal delivery, especially if the preeclampsia is severe. However, if her condition seems stable, and the cervix is partially effaced and soft, the trend today is to allow the mother a trial of labor for twenty-four to forty-eight hours, to see if she can deliver vaginally. If she does not deliver in this time, the doctor usually performs a cesarean.

GENITAL HERPES VIRUS

A woman who has an active outbreak of genital herpes, or has had one recently, is in danger of passing the virus on to the baby during a vaginal birth. A newborn is particularly susceptible to complications caused by herpes virus (see Chapter 11). Therefore, if active virus is present in the mother's genital tract, a cesarean is the only safe way to bring the baby into the world.

How Is a Cesarean Performed?

After you have been properly prepped and anesthetized, the doctor, with a surgical assistant, will make an incision in your abdomen. There are three techniques that he may use:

CLASSIC

The first, called the *classic* incision, is a vertical cut—that is, it runs up and down for several inches beginning just above your belly button. Classic incisions are no longer done much in the United States, because they have a higher rate of rupturing during the next pregnancy(ies). Women who have had classic incisions usually are not encouraged by their doctors to try vaginal birth the next time, for this reason.

LOW-SEGMENT, TRANSVERSE

The second incision is called a *low-segment, lower segment transverse,* or *bikini* cut—it runs horizontally, or from right to left, approximately where bikini panties would lie on your belly. The incision is several to seven inches long. In this country, the vast majority of operations are done as low-segment incisions. These have the best chance of healing without permanent damage to other internal organs, such as the bladder or the bowels. They also have much less chance of tearing or rupturing in subsequent pregnancies. They cause less blood loss and make an easier wound for the surgeon to sew together.

LOW-SEGMENT, VERTICAL

The third type of incision is a *low vertical* in which the cut is up and down, but below the navel. Low verticals can be done on the inside—that is, only up and down on the uterus, but bikini on the outside, so that the scarring is less unsightly.

Whatever kind of incision, the operation is done very carefully to avoid excessive bleeding and damage to surrounding tissues. The doctor cuts through each layer of tissue—first the skin, then the fat and muscle beneath, next the membranes (the peritoneum) that hold the bladder and bowels in place; then he moves the bladder aside and makes the final cut through the layers of the uterus.

Once the obstetrician reaches the uterus, he is even more careful about his work, so that he avoids cutting into the placenta or the baby as he enters the uterus. Once he has reached the inside of the womb, he gently ruptures the amniotic sac (if it is not broken already) and reaches inside for the baby. The baby's head is usually delivered first and her nose and throat suctioned out so that she can breathe easily. Then the baby's body slides through the opening. Afterward, the doctor reaches inside the uterus to detach and remove the placenta; he also wipes the inside of the uterus to remove any remnants of the pregnancy from the walls. The uterus may then be flushed with sterile saline solution for the same purpose.

As the baby's shoulders emerge from the womb, the surgical team puts oxytocin (a drug that stimulates contractions) into the mother's intravenous line, to help the uterus begin to contract to prepregnant size. The uterus has to contract tightly to seal off all the blood vessels that have been opened by the removal of the placenta. This is the same thing that happens during a vaginal delivery, but it is even more crucial in a cesarean section because of heightened chances of hemorrhage.

As carefully as the doctor has entered the body, he now begins to sew the uterus and all the overlying tissues back together. Each layer of tissue is sewn separately. This repair takes far longer than it did to get to and open the uterus, which takes approximately five to ten minutes. Suturing may take up to an hour and a half. The internal tissues are stitched with self-absorbing thread that will dissolve over time and be absorbed into the woman's system as healing progresses. The last layer—the skin—is sewn with thread that will later be removed by the doctor. Or, more and more commonly today, the skin is stapled together with plastic or metal staples. (I know staples sound ghoulish. But actually, many women I've spoken with say that the staples hurt less coming out, and bother less while they're in place, than regular thread stitches do.)

Are There Any Special Preparations?

Yes, there are several. If you come into the hospital knowing that you'll be having a c-section, you'll be instructed not to take anything by mouth for at least eight hours before the surgery. That means no eating and no drinking. The reason for this restriction is that anesthesia can make you nauseated, and if your stomach has food in it, you can aspirate—breathe in—your own vomit, which can give you pneumonia or cause you to asphyxiate.

If the c-section is an emergency, and you've had food within the past eight hours, the nurse will give you milk of magnesia or calcium citrate solution to drink, to lower the amount of acid in your stomach and diminish the possibility of acid getting into your lungs during the surgery. Most hospitals require their c-section patients to drink this mixture regardless of the length of time since eating.

The nurses or a lab technician will draw several blood samples from you to test and type your blood, just in case you need a transfusion during or after the surgery. These tests will also determine whether you are anemic or have any kind of infection.

Some hospitals still ask their patients to take enemas, to empty the bowels before surgery. I didn't have to have one, and most women no longer must. If you are told you must, it may be hospital policy. That shouldn't keep you from asking your doctor to forego that procedure (he can place an order specifying that you don't need one) if you really object to it.

If you don't already have one, the doctor or a nurse will insert an intravenous line (IV) into your hand or your arm, so that you can begin to receive the fluids that will replace the food you now will go without for the next forty-eight hours or so. The IV is also there in case you need a transfusion or fast-acting medication. You can ask that the line be placed in the hand or arm that you don't use for writing. It's going to be in place for two or more days, and you'll be up and moving around well before it's taken out, so it pays to have it inserted in the arm you use less. Once the line is in place, you'll start receiving fluids to hydrate and nourish you and the baby.

A nurse will also prepare your belly for the surgery by shaving it. She will remove the hair from an inch or two below the line of your pubic hair to a few inches above your belly button and from one hip bone to the other. This creates a clean area for the surgery.

URINARY IN-DWELLING CATHETERS

One other procedure you will undergo is the insertion of a catheter into your bladder. The catheter is a plastic tube with a balloonlike attachment that is pushed up the urethra (the natural outlet through which urine drains from the body) into the bladder; the balloon is inflated to make sure that the tube does not slip out. This procedure is necessary because you will have no bladder control during the surgery, or for at least twelve hours afterward. Urine drainage is important and crucial for the doctor and the medical staff to observe. It indicates whether your kidneys are functioning properly.

The placement of the catheter takes less than one minute. For some women, it is only mildly uncomfortable; for others, the pain is greater. I've had several surgeries in which I've had to have an in-dwelling catheter: They always hurt me—not extremely, but enough to make me wish I didn't have to know about them going in.

Many nurses and doctors prefer for the woman to have the catheter in place before she enters the operating room and before she receives anesthesia. As with any other routine operation, medical staffs at various hospitals have a regime that they like to follow; the catheterization before anesthesia is one of them. There is no real *medical* reason for this: It's simply easier for the staff—one less thing they have to do in the OR.

The nurse attending to me just before I was to go into the OR insisted that she put the catheter in beforehand. I refused. She told me that I'd be less embarrassed if she did it with fewer people looking on (there are a lot of people in the OR). I told her no. I had requested, and my OBs allowed me, to have the catheter put in place after I was anesthetized. It wasn't what the nurse on duty wanted, but it helped me feel more in control and more comfortable. Unless your c-section is a real emergency situation, you will have the opportunity to ask your OB to accommodate you in this small way if you wish.

CHILDBIRTH CLASSES AND BREATHING TECHNIQUES

Although the books on Lamaze and other breathing and relaxation techniques don't stress it, a woman undergoing a cesarean benefits tremendously from learning and practicing those methods of coping with stress and pain. It only makes sense: Major surgery is stressful, both emotionally and physically. Certainly its aftermath is painful. How better to get a handle on your fear and feel you have some degree of control over the pain than to be able to relax muscles and deal with physical discomfort?

The classes themselves, if you can attend them (that is, if you're not on bedrest and can go out of the house), will give you a forum to discuss your fears and ask questions. You'll find out that lots of your classmates worry about the same things that you do and that you are not an exception to any rule.

The breathing and relaxation exercises, if you learn and practice them until they're second-nature, will be enormously helpful to you before, during, and after your surgery. Using them before surgery will help you to stay calm and will make uncomfortable procedures, like catheterization, more tolerable. During surgery, you can do the deep breathing to focus your attention away from any discomfort you have and to control your natural anxiety. After surgery, they will again help you manage your pain; while breathing exercises can't eliminate pain, they will certainly help take the edge off it.

An added benefit: As one does the breathing with a coach (in my case, my husband), it also serves to keep you in close emotional contact with your loved one, at a time when it's easy to slip into feeling isolated and out of control.

My husband and I had a private instructor come to our house to teach us Lamaze. After I got to the hospital, I used those breathing and relaxation techniques fifty times if I used them once—especially the day of and during the surgery!

Can I Choose My Anesthesia?

You may or may not be able to choose the type of anesthesia you'll have, depending on whether the surgery is an emergency or is planned and whether your medical condition or the baby's allows a choice. Also, you have to be under the care of an obstetrician and anesthesiologist who are open to your participation in this decision. Most likely, your doctor and the anesthesiologist will recommend the type of anesthesia they feel is best suited to your unique situation. Most women abide by their suggestion.

Unless you are in a severe medical emergency, the anesthesiologist should come to your room or see you as you are being prepped for surgery, to explain what he'll be doing and how you will feel. If his explanation is not thorough enough to answer all your concerns, keep asking questions until you are satisfied. It is up to you to make sure you receive an adequate explanation of what the anesthesia entails, including its risks and aftereffects (if any). You will also sign a release form giving your permission for the surgery and stating that you understand what's going to happen to you and the risks involved.

Whether you are going to be awake or asleep during the surgery, you will most likely receive no or very little sedation before the event. Sedatives cross the placenta and can depress the baby's ability to breathe after birth. So, you'll probably enter the OR fully conscious and feeling everything, which can, of course, make you quite nervous. Now is a good time to practice Lamaze breathing to help you relax.

TYPES OF ANESTHESIA USED FOR CESAREAN SECTION

There are three main types of anesthesia used for cesarean sections today: the spinal block, the epidural, and general anesthesia. All three require the skills of an experienced anesthesiologist and, when done properly, pose minimal risk to mother and child.

The Epidural

The anesthetic most often used is the epidural. The epidural is an injection of anesthetic between the vertebrae, about one-third of the way up the spine, into a cavity called the *epidural space,* through which many nerves pass. The drug does not enter the spinal canal or the spinal fluid. The anesthesiologist can choose to use only one injection or can insert a very thin catheter into the space so that repeat dosages of the nerve-blocking drugs can be given as needed, including postoperatively for pain control.

First, the anesthesiologist will ask you to sit up, or lie on your side with your back curled into a C shape. This opens up the space between the vertebrae and gives him good access to the spot into which he has to inject. When you're in your last trimester, hunching over isn't always easy. Your belly gets in the way, but it's doable. You'll have to sit or lie completely still for the anesthesiologist to do his job, which may take up to five or ten minutes to accomplish.

"I was very nervous that I wouldn't be able to keep from moving when he put the needle in," Claudie told me. "I didn't see how they could do it, because I was contracting every minute and a quarter. I'd say, 'Here's one,' and all action would stop. The nurses would hold me until it was over, and then ten little busy bees were working on me again. They managed to do it within a minute, between contractions! And being awake for the birth was really great!"

Once the anesthesiologist finds the right spot, he'll inject you first with a local anesthetic (this stings a little, but it's far from awful). Once that takes hold (in a minute or two), he'll place a larger, hollow needle through your back into the epidural space. He'll inject a test dose of the anesthetic and then check to see whether the area he is working to numb begins to lose its feeling. If the injection takes, you'll then receive the full dosage. One shot is good for two to three hours, which is usually plenty long enough for the entire surgery. The anesthesiologist will tape the catheter in place, and the surgical team will help you lie on your back on the table. The full effect of the anesthesia is not complete for five to ten minutes.

The area that the epidural numbs is quite specific. You'll only be completely without sensation from a few inches below the incision line to a few inches above, although your legs will feel heavy, too.

The main disadvantages of the epidural include the fact that you may have a bad backache afterward, from the catheter. And epidurals sometimes are placed too far into the back and actually reach the spinal fluid. This can cause postoperative headaches, although very rarely. They are also occasionally not completely effective in preventing pain. Any manipulation above or below the line of numbness will hurt.

The Spinal

The spinal block—also called the subarachnoid block—places the anesthetizing agent directly into the spinal fluid. The needle penetrates to your spinal canal (thus the term, *spinal* anesthesia), which is deeper inside you than the epidural space. Only one dose is injected, so the amount of time you are numbed is finite (though enough for the surgery to be started and finished without your feeling pain). Unlike an epidural, a spinal numbs your entire pelvis and abdomen.

The anesthetic will be injected just as in the epidural; you'll have to either sit up and round your back into a C shape to open up the space between the bones, or lie on your side and assume a C position. First, the anesthesiologist will give you a local anesthetic in the area to be punctured. Then, he inserts a large, hollow needle into your back, in between your vertebrae, about a third of the way up your spine, and injects the anesthetic into your spinal fluid. The anesthetic is heavier than the spinal fluid, so the drug sits in the lower part of the spinal canal and blocks sensation only there.

One of the potential risks of spinal anesthesia is that it can lower your blood pressure too much, which will require the medical team to counteract that effect by rapidly infusing you with fluids and ephedrine, a drug that raises blood pressure. Your doctor could rule out this form of anesthesia if your baby is markedly premature or at risk, based on a concern that lowered blood pressure could deprive the baby of much-needed oxygen at a critical moment.

The other major drawback to spinals is that 10 percent of women who have them suffer severe headaches after the anesthetic wears off. The headaches, which can be excruciating, can last up to a week or more, although they usually get a bit better by the third postoperative day and are gone by the fifth day after surgery. No one is sure why the headaches happen, but one of the reigning theories is that they are caused by loss of spinal fluid at the puncture site. Then, when you sit up or stand, the lower volume of fluid irritates nerves in your system, causing severe headache.

Women once had no recourse but to suffer through the headaches. Today, there is an antidote that often works, called a *blood patch*. The doctor gives you a local anesthetic, then injects a few milliliters of your blood into an area just beside the spot where you received the spinal, and this seems to help.

Carrie had a spinal. "The anesthesiologist stood by my head and kept telling me what was happening, which was great because I had all these weird sensations. It felt like I couldn't breathe. I told him, 'I don't think I'm breathing.' He told me it just feels like that, but that yes, my lungs were fine. The bad part was really afterward," she said. "I had spinal headaches that lasted a week and a half or two weeks. They offered me that blood patch thing, but I couldn't face another needle in my back."

General Anesthesia

General anesthesia takes effect more rapidly than either spinal or epidural anesthesia. General anesthesia for cesarean delivery is usually limited to those cases in which the section is done as an emergency and quick access to the fetus is needed. It puts you to sleep and blocks most muscle movement in the body, including the lungs. With general anesthesia, you will be on a respirator that will breathe for you.

First, the anesthesiologist injects into the intravenous line one of several drugs that cause you to lose consciousness. Then, you receive a muscle relaxant in the same IV to help relax your throat muscles so that the respirator tube can be passed through your vocal cords and into your trachea (windpipe). The anesthesia is continued through aerosols that you inhale through the respirator.

The airway placed into your lungs after the general takes hold remains in place until you wake up. You can expect to feel throat discomfort upon waking. You won't be able to talk, and the tube will stay in place until the doctor is confident that you can breathe without the respirator. After the tube is removed, your throat will probably be sore, and your voice may be raspy for a day or two. Many women also complain of muscle stiffness and soreness all over the body the second day after general anesthesia.

The chief risk in general anesthesia is inhalation of vomit into the lungs while you are asleep. General anesthesia can make some women quite nauseated. And before or after the respirator tube is put into the airway, it's possible to aspirate some of the stomach contents. If that happens, you can come down with pneumonia and/or have lung tissue damaged by the stomach acid. There is also a risk of asphyxiation.

In addition, general anesthetics do cross the placenta to a certain degree and thus may depress the baby's ability to breathe at first and make her lethargic or have poor muscle tone. This disappears rather quickly after the birth, but is one of the reasons that doctors now tend to avoid general anesthesia unless it's an emergency.

Can My Husband (or Other Loved One) Stay with Me During the Operation?

That depends on the policy in place at your hospital and on whether you will be awake during the c-section. Most hospitals don't allow the husband to be present at a c-section in which the woman is unconscious. And, although more and more often, hospitals allow, and even encourage, husbands or a loved one to attend the cesarean birth, it is not yet a universal practice.

The hospital in which I delivered did not allow husbands in the OR. We questioned the policy. We were told that we could petition the hospital administrator to make an exception in our case, and my OBs would have backed up our request. But we weren't up to the challenge. One of my OBs stood in as my support person during the surgery.

If your hospital's policy forbids husbands in surgery, you should feel free to question the reasons. It's well-documented that having a loved one as a support person helps the woman emotionally and lowers her anxiety level. *And* there's no *medical* reason why the man should not be present in the OR.

You will probably get a better response from hospital administration if you are polite, use a rational approach, and maintain a calm tone of voice. The old adage that you catch more flies with honey than with vinegar applies here.

What Will Happen in the Operating Room?

What happens once you reach the operating room differs somewhat from hospital to hospital and depends upon whether yours is a cesarean that has been planned in advance or is an emergency. In general, unless either the baby or you are in immediate, grave danger, here's what you can expect:

THE ROOM

ORs are brightly lit places, full of chrome. They look antiseptic, and they are. The operating table in the center of the room is quite narrow (too narrow, you'll think, for you to stay balanced with your big belly). But you won't fall off. And there are all kinds of equipment lining the room—oxygen tanks, trays, sterilizing units for surgical tools, to name a few things.

PEOPLE

There will be more people than you would expect in the OR. At a minimum, you will see your obstetrician, his surgical assistant, two nurses assigned to help with you, plus one additional nurse to care for each baby as she is born. Also attending will be one pediatrician to care for each baby, and/or a neonatal specialist in case there are problems with the baby(ies). If the hospital allows husbands or other loved ones to be present during the surgery, your husband or another close friend will be there, too. And, of course, the anesthesiologist.

During the surgery, and before, all of them will wear surgical masks that cover their mouths and noses, to prevent you from being contaminated by germs during the operation.

FINAL PREPARATION

The first thing that will happen is that you'll be asked to slide from your bed or gurney onto the operating table. You may be able to do this under your own power, you may not. I've even heard of some women walking into the OR, but certainly that's not standard procedure.

Once you are up on the table, and before surgery starts, your belly has to be disinfected, so that no germs on your skin get into the incision and cause infection. A nurse will scrub your abdomen gently with a cold (so be ready . . .) detergent solution, then drape with sterile cloths the area to be cut. Some hospitals now use a sterile, gel-like film that is pressed onto and adheres to the abdomen instead of painting on the disinfectant. The doctor then cuts right through the gel as he makes the incision.

If you are having general anesthesia, this procedure will be done before you are anesthetized. If you are having a spinal or an epidural, most likely the scrubbing and draping will take place after you are numbed, since both epidurals and spinals require you to sit up or roll on your side to receive them, which would disturb the drapes.

If you chose not to have a catheter inserted before going to the operating room, now is when the nurse will insert it. Since the anesthesia (if it's a regional) will be taking hold, you shouldn't feel this at all.

Once you are anesthetized, the nurses will tie your legs down on the table. Try not to panic, even though being restrained this way may upset you. It's really for your own good: If they weren't tied down, your legs might slip off the table during the surgery. Also, the table may be tilted to the left, right, or slightly up during the operation, to give your uterus and the placenta (and therefore the baby) the best blood and oxygen supply possible. You'd fall off if you weren't secured! At least one of your arms (probably both) will also be tied down, either to your sides or out perpendicular to your body. This is to keep you from accidentally touching the surgical site or from flailing if you become nervous or excited.

Just before the surgery begins, a nurse will also hang a drape from a rod above your chest onto your chest or neck, so that your view of your belly is blocked off. This is so that you cannot see the surgery itself. In some hospitals, the nurse angles a mirror over your face so that you can see the baby coming out if you want. If your husband is in the room, he'll most likely be allowed to watch the whole thing from start to finish if he wants to. He may be able to take pictures and cut the umbilical cord. Both will depend on the condition of the baby at birth and hospital rules, which vary greatly on these points.

You may also be asked to breathe through an oxygen mask, to get the most oxygen to the baby during the surgery. The mask is usually a heavy rubber contraption that fits over your nose and mouth. The oxygen is supplied under pressure, so it is noisy, and you may feel like it's difficult to breathe it in. In fact, despite the feeling, the opposite is true: You'll be getting as much air as you can take into your lungs. The mask also can make it difficult for you to be heard when you talk. So, if you feel like people are ignoring you while the surgery goes on, just speak louder. They'll respond.

SURGERY BEGINS

If you are under a general, you'll feel nothing. Some women say that they were dimly aware of what was going on, but this is not common. If you have a regional, you will be wide awake, but you won't feel pain as the doctor makes the incision. You may feel some pressure from his hand as he moves through the layers, but you won't feel pain. That's the purpose of anesthesia.

The doctor will probably provide you with a sort of running commentary on what he's doing ("I'm making the incision now"; "You're going to feel some pressure for a moment"—things like that). Operating rooms can be noisy places. Some surgeons like music to be on; you may even be able to request it, although there's no guarantee that he'll oblige. People talk. I remember that when my doctor and the resident were sewing me up, they had a friendly argument about whose stitches were prettier!

Once the doctor cuts to the inside of your uterus, he's going to be pulling one side of the incision up or pushing it down so that he can reach inside you, take hold of the baby, and help her to be born. You will definitely feel some sensations then.

Every woman's experience of the physical sensations of the actual birth is different. Most epidurals only numb the part of the belly that is to be cut and several inches above and below the incision. At the least, you can count on feeling the tugging and stretching as the doctor reaches inside you, and as the baby comes out. If you're under a general, you'll feel nothing.

Every doctor I've ever spoken with about this says that the woman doesn't feel pain, just pressure. Many women I've spoken with (but not all) say that they definitely felt pain. I remember that it hurt, and that I said so, more than once while the operation was going on. But it certainly wasn't screaming pain, and it certainly was quite bearable. Remember, vaginal birth is no picnic; it hurts, too.

Once the Baby Is Born

If you know what to expect, and hold a positive attitude about the surgery, the actual birth will make the cesarean a strong positive event for you. Kate said that her second cesarean was a wonderful experience. She had been under general anesthesia the first time, but for the second one, she was awake. "When I was awake, I was excited—nervous, but excited. Everyone in the operating room except my husband knew it was going to be a boy. So that was thrilling. And the nurses, they were incredible—like a sorority cheerleading squad. They were just great!"

Here's what usually happens: As soon as the baby's head is delivered, you will be given oxytocin intravenously, to help get your uterus to contract and to cut off bleeding from the separation of the placenta from the uterine wall. Now the operating room becomes very busy. Someone will suction out the baby's mouth and nasal passages; someone else will get ready to carry the baby to the pediatrician, who is usually standing at the ready at the side of the room. Assuming all goes well, the baby will begin to cry vigorously. Someone will tell you the baby's sex (usually, they can't help shouting!), and that the baby is all right. You'll be laughing and crying all at once. Someone will bring the baby to you, so that you can see her. In some ORs, you can hold her for a while, or your husband can, before she is whisked off to the nursery for observation.

Once the baby is out, the operation isn't over. The doctor still has to remove the placenta, clear the uterus of all debris, and check you for damage before closing you up. Suturing the wound takes a fair amount of time, because each layer of tissue is sewn back together separately. After you're all stitched up, and the anesthesiologist is certain that your condition is stable, the surgical team will lift you onto a gurney and put the bars up to wheel you into the recovery room.

If your membranes were ruptured for more than six hours before the cesarean, your doctor may inject you with antibiotics to ward off infection. Studies have shown that up to 85 percent of all women whose water had been broken hours before their c-sections suffer some degree of infection during the recuperation period. Prophylactic antibiotics lower that rate to 20 percent or less.

The Recovery Room

The recovery room is where you go after surgery is complete. Each hospital's looks different. What they all have in common is that there is constant nursing there, to monitor your condition. Here is where the anesthesia wears off and where you will receive your first pain medication. You will most likely be in this room for several hours, until the medical staff is satisfied that your condition has stabilized and that you tolerated the surgery reasonably well. The nurses will check your heart rate and blood pressure four times an hour. They'll check to see the amount of urine your body passes through the catheter, which tells them how your kidneys are functioning. They will listen to your lungs to make sure they are not congested. They will ask you to cough and breathe deeply to clear your lungs. Your temperature will be taken, to make sure no infection is setting in. If you've lost a lot of blood during the operation, you may have a transfusion. (See Chapter 4 for a discussion of options for transfusion.)

The nurses will also check to see how much you are bleeding from your vagina (there is always some bleeding after the surgery) and check your abdomen to make sure that your uterus is tightly contracted. Whether one delivers vaginally or by c-section, it's very important that the uterus contract well, so that it clamps off the blood vessels opened by the removal of the placenta; if the uterus is not well-contracted, you can hemorrhage. Should your uterus not be firm and hard, you will be given more oxytocin to encourage it to contract.

It hurts having your stomach pushed around right after you've had major abdominal surgery. But you should be getting pain medication that takes the edge off everything (initially, the painkillers that are given are quite strong and almost knock you out); plus the nurse won't poke around your belly for long.

Once your vital signs are stable, the anesthesia has completely worn off, your uterus is returning to its prepregnancy size and firmness, and your kidneys are functioning normally, you'll be wheeled back to your room.

Pain Medication

Unless you are made of cast iron, you are going to need painkillers to get you through the first few days after surgery. The initial drugs that you receive are usually potent narcotics, which keep your discomfort manageable and encourage you to rest. The two most common of these are meperidine (Demerol) and morphine, and both are usually combined with an antinausea drug (nausea is a common side effect of the narcotics). Both morphine and meperidine are habit-forming and are given only for a brief period of days, to prevent the mother from suffering withdrawal symptoms.

Usually, the route of delivery for these drugs is injection into the buttocks. Their effect is only felt for three or four hours, and so repeat dosages are necessary. In some hospitals, although not all, a special device is now used to deliver tiny doses of the drug continuously via the IV line. The benefit of this machine is that it creates a steady level of pain control. You don't feel the effects of the drug wear off and take hold again, as you do with intramuscular injections. Some facilities even offer the woman the opportunity to control her own pain relief through this autodelivery system, allowing her to dial up or down (within limits) the dosage she receives.

"I was on a pump which meant I pushed a little button every time I felt I needed medication," said Liz. "It was kind of nice, and it worked out fine. I liked being able to control the amount of drugs I was getting."

Any narcotic given to relieve pain, including morphine and meperidine, gets into your breast milk in small amounts. Studies have shown that the quantity of the drugs in the milk does not affect the baby significantly. Being on these drugs will thus not keep you from breastfeeding if you desire to do so.

After you're able to ingest food again, you will be taken off the injected narcotics and will start taking pain relief medication by mouth. Your doctor will encourage you to take as little medicine as possible, since these drugs, too, get into your breast milk. The most popular pain reliever is acetaminophen (aspirin-free pain reliever, such as Tylenol), given alone or in combination with codeine, a narcotic. Acetaminophen and codeine each heighten the effect of the other, which is why they are prescribed in combination.

Will I Be Able to Breastfeed My Baby?

Yes, yes, and yes, unless your circumstances are unusual. As I just pointed out, even if you are on pain medication, your baby will not be harmed by your breast milk. Your milk is the perfect food for your baby: It transmits your immunities to her and may decrease the likelihood of allergy later in your child's life. And you can do it even though your incision hurts. The nurses will teach you how to find a comfortable position.

Breastfeeding isn't good only for the baby: The stimulation of your nipples by the baby's mouth helps your body release natural oxytocin, which in turn encourages your uterus to contract and return to its prepregnant size. Breastfeeding helps you to bond with your baby and may help you get past any negative feelings you may have about her birth.

Even if you can't breastfeed her directly (that is, if she's in the neonatal intensive care unit [NICU]), you can and should still pump your milk for the nursing staff to give her in the nursery. If this is the case, on the day after the surgery, the nurses will bring you a breast pump and show you how to express (push out) your milk. Providing your baby with breast milk this way will, at the very least, make you feel like you are caring for her at a time when you are not fully in control of what happens to her.

Of course, you are also free to choose not to breastfeed your baby. In that case, you should tell your doctor that this is your choice, and he will give you medication to stop you from producing milk.

At the back of this book, in the Other Reading and Resources section, several texts are listed that can help you better understand and begin the breastfeeding process.

Recuperating

What Happens Once I Get Back to My Room?

Mostly, you'll probably want to sleep. You may be in a fair amount of pain, despite the drugs. There's no easy way around that fact: You'll have just had major surgery, and the cut is still fresh. It's going to hurt. How much depends on your pain threshold, how extensive the surgery was, and your condition before the surgery.

"I don't know if it was just the great pain medication, or just the joy of finally having my baby," Carrie told me. "But I really did not have any pain at first. I was on such a cloud nine. I finally had my baby, and things were looking good. It did not really hurt until I started getting up to walk and stuff about sixteen hours after the surgery. Then it burned terribly."

I have yet to meet a woman who has told me that the first twenty-four hours after the surgery were a breeze. Still, it helps to remember a couple of things: You got a baby out of the deal, and the pain lessens with each passing hour. Really. I've had the surgery twice, and both times I was amazed at the difference between how I felt the first day, and how I felt after twenty-four, then forty-eight hours. And no matter how much it hurts: The pain is finite. You won't feel this way forever—not even for a whole week. Within two days you'll be eating again. In five days, you'll be out of the hospital and home in your own, comfortable bed.

"The first three days were the worst," said Liz. "It's hard to move side to side. Any little movement is a shooting pain. The second day, when my system was starting to work again, I had a lot of cramping and pain. And those nurses kept me walking, which was about the last thing I wanted to do. By the time I left the hospital, I could almost walk upright!''

But walking comes later. When you get back to your room on the gurney, the first significant task you have to accomplish is getting from the gurney onto your bed.

Nurses will come in and take your vital signs and your temperature at least once every four hours. If you're on continuous pain medication, you'll keep receiving small doses of the drug automatically for the first twenty-four hours. If your hospital doesn't offer that alternative, you'll get a shot every three to four hours for the pain. One aspect of that is tricky: The morphine or Demerol is injected into the buttocks or the rear section of the hips. It's difficult and painful to turn on your side just after the surgery. If you have the presence of mind, ask the nurses to alternate or rotate the location of each injection—these drugs, when placed repeatedly into the same site, can create painful lumps that can take up to several months to completely subside.

In addition to your vital signs, the nurses will also take blood samples from you on the first day after surgery, and maybe for several days after that, depending on your doctor's orders. The doctor will be looking to make sure that you are not losing blood internally, that your iron levels are going up, and that no infection is setting in.

And either the doctor or a nurse will check and clean your incision every day after the first twenty-four to forty-eight hours, to make sure it is healing correctly. The cleaning is usually not painful, but the antiseptic lotion is cold. Next they will change the dressing—which is usually just a couple of light, large, Band-Aid-type strips that are taped down. Don't be afraid to look at your scar. It will be both thinner and neater than you might imagine.

Until the third day after surgery, if you want to bathe, the nurse will give you a sponge bath. After the third or fourth day, you'll be able to take a shower. Depending upon the hospital, you'll be allowed to do this either alone or with a nurse standing in attendance or assisting you. If you don't feel steady enough on your feet, you can ask for a special chair to sit on in the shower. You may have to cover your wound with plastic and paper tape, to keep the stitches or staples and the cut itself from getting wet.

As your incision heals, you can expect it to feel sore, itchy, and tighter and tighter as the wound and tissues knit back together. Some women describe the sensation as a rubber band pulling tight.

At first—and in fact, for many women it takes weeks—you won't be able to stand up straight. This too is normal. Don't forget, your muscles have been cut, and until you are fully healed, they won't behave the way they used to. Your inability to stand erect will change your gait when you walk at first. It's usual to shuffle.

Also, don't forget that your body is undergoing the natural and normal reversion to its prepregnant condition, as well as healing from the surgery. Your pelvis will be starting to return to its normal size; your belly will be shrinking along with your uterus. This will also affect your gait and your balance.

Actually, you won't look much different from the women wandering the halls who had vaginal births. Most of them will have had episiotomies (an external incision from just behind the vagina toward the anus, made to widen the vaginal opening for birth and avoid jagged tearing of the tissue) so they will be moving "funny" too. You may still feel ungainly, but in a few weeks, you'll be walking tall and just the way you did before you became pregnant.

WALKING: THE ROAD TO RECOVERY

After you've been in your room for twelve hours or so, the nurses and/or your OB will come in and tell you that you need to start getting up and walking. You'll do this with assistance at first—at least twice during the first twenty-four hours. This may sound like absolute torture to you now—and you may not appreciate it much when it's suggested at the hospital—but it's really for your own good. Women who get up and walk soon after surgery recover faster, develop fewer respiratory problems, and lower their risk of blood clots.

At first, all you'll be asked to do is stand up. Maybe walk a few feet. On the second day, you'll walk to the bathroom, and maybe even into the hall, with assistance—that is, someone will help hold you up. Another reason it's crucial for you to get your "sea legs" back as soon as possible is that before long you'll be home with your baby, who will need holding and caring. Or, if your baby is in the intensive care nursery, you'll be wanting to see her, and you'll be making trips back and forth to the hospital. You've got to walk to do that.

GETTING YOUR BLADDER AND BOWEL FUNCTION BACK

Within twelve to twenty-four hours after the surgery, the urinary catheter will be removed. That means you'll have to get up and walk to the bathroom to pee—yet another reason to get out of bed early in the game. It may take you a while to get the hang of urinating again. One trick that sometimes helps is to spray warm water on your genitals, which helps you to relax the muscles that hold the urine back. Another relaxant can be placing your hand under warm, running water or into a cup of warm water. You can also sit in a warm sitz bath—again, to help you relax your muscles. And then there's the obvious: Leave the water running—the sound gives inspiration (if it works for two-year-olds, it'll work for you!). But, if all else fails, and at first you just can't pee, so that your bladder becomes uncomfortably full, the nurse can always reinsert a catheter to drain your bladder. Don't worry though, you'll get the knack of it again very soon, even if you have trouble the first time.

The same goes for bowel movements. You probably won't have one for the first forty-eight to seventy-two hours after the surgery. After all, you didn't eat for the eight to twelve hours before the surgery, and you won't take anything other than liquids by mouth for at least the first twenty-four hours afterward. Your system doesn't have much to let go of. At first, all you'll have is gas, which will be painful to pass, because it requires the use of the stomach muscles. If you are in severe pain from the gas, you can ask for medication, and even a tube that can be inserted into the rectum to allow gas to escape without your having to bear down.

When you finally feel like you have to move your bowels, it may be painful, and you may not have much success. This is normal. You should ask for stool softeners to take by mouth, and you can also take a rectal suppository that will help stimulate your system to eliminate. In addition, a small enema can help to loosen the stool and promote contractions. Once you've moved your bowels, the gas and pain in your intestines will pretty much disappear.

THE RETURN TO FOOD

By the way, as soon as you've started passing gas, that's when you get to start eating food again! In most cases, within the first twenty-four hours you'll be able to drink liquids. The next day, you'll move on to semi-solids, like Jell-O. Usually, by day three, you're on to real food, and you'll be able to eat what you like. Also, around the time that you begin eating solid food, the doctor will order the nurses to remove the IV from your arm.

The day of my c-section, my OB asked me what I wanted more than anything else once I could eat solids again. I had had gestational diabetes for the last six weeks of my pregnancy and had been on an extremely regimented diet. I told him that I wanted a Dove Bar, a chocolate, chocolate Dove Bar. On the afternoon of my third post-section day, he waltzed into the room grinning from ear to ear, dangling a brown paper bag from his hand. It was my Dove Bar: my first real, solid food. And it was heaven.

How Am I Likely to Feel Emotionally?

That depends on a number of factors, such as your physical and emotional state before you had the cesarean, the condition of the baby after she is born, and whether you believe—as too many women do— that having a c-section is a second-class way to become a mother.

It's important to remember that all women experience a broad range of emotions during the first few days after the baby is born. Wide mood swings are as common after birth as during pregnancy. Your hormones will be doing a tango inside you as your body shifts from its pregnant to its lactating state. "Baby blues"—from a little weepiness to severe depressions—are common to one degree or another for every new mother, not just the c-section mom. If your baby is well, you will also feel elated at the birth of your child, just like any other new mommy.

Some women who labored a long time before they had a section will feel very drained and may not want to have anything to do with the baby for the first few hours or even a couple of days. And, just having a c-section may make you resent your baby a little for taking away your "perfect birth" and making you scarred (by the way, within a year or two, the scar turns white and is almost invisible . . .). These feelings are not "unnatural," and they don't mean you'll be a lousy mother. You won't be the only woman ever to feel distant or resentful of her baby at first. It just means that you'll need to recoup a little before you can give everything to the new life you just brought into the world.

A very common emotional problem that c-section moms have is a feeling of inadequacy—that they "should have" been able to "do it right"—that is, have the baby vaginally. In fact, so many c-section moms feel bad about this and feel angry and cheated out of having a "normal" birth experience that many hospitals have c-section discussion groups for new mothers and couples who had a c-section. You should ask the nurses on your ward if such a group exits in your hospital and attend the sessions. They may help you.

Having any or all of these negative emotions doesn't mean you are crazy, or weird, or wicked. They are all in the spectrum of normal. They only become worrisome if, after a few weeks, you can't get rid of them. If you continue to have unpleasant thoughts about the baby, or can't shake a depression, seek professional help. With the right counselor, you'll quickly get back on track again.

One thing you should be prepared for: Well-intentioned but insensitive friends and relatives may continually offer their condolences that you had to have surgery to give birth or ask you for the gross details when you are not inclined to give them.

Marilyn found herself constantly bombarded with such questions and sympathies. She had two children by cesarean, the second after she attempted a vaginal birth after cesarean. "To tell you the truth, I was really getting pissed off at people who would say they're sorry for me for not having had a vaginal birth. I see c-sections as a positive birth experience." She says the following retort really worked for her: "Don't tell me you're sorry. I had a baby! I'm still a mom. Be proud for me. Be happy for me." You might try some variation of that statement to move people past their unthinking comments.

When Will I Feel 100 Percent Better?

Not for a while. How long it takes for you to recuperate fully depends on a number of factors: the shape you were in before you got pregnant, whether you are significantly overweight, how long you were bedridden before giving birth, if there were surgical complications, and how good a healer you are. In general, most women don't feel quite themselves for several weeks to two or three months.

In the early weeks, do not be surprised if you continue to have abdominal cramping and pain. You will tire easily at first. It may be difficult to walk any appreciable distance. It may also hurt to go up and down stairs; your doctor will probably forbid it, in fact, for the first week you are home, or longer. You will also not be allowed to lift anything other than the baby. You may have trouble turning from side to side while you're in bed, and it may be hard to roll from your back onto your side and sit up. Where you got all the pain medication injections may also hurt, and the lumps can take months to go away.

When Can I See My Baby?

As soon as you are ready if the baby is in the regular infant nursery. The nurses can bring her to you, and, although it may hurt your incision a bit, you can hold her, check out how many fingers and toes she has, dress her, undress her, just like any other new mother. Even if you are on pain medication, you should be able to nurse her if you have chosen to breastfeed (see above, Will I Be Able to Breastfeed My Baby?) Once you are able to walk far enough, you can also see the baby in the well-baby nursery, through the window, just like any other parent.

If your baby is in the NICU (neonatal intensive care unit), you'll be able to see her as soon as you are ready to make the trip. Where the NICU is in relation to the maternity floor differs from hospital to hospital. It may be right down the hall from you, or it may be quite a hike, even to another floor. If you can't walk there, you can usually go in with a wheelchair. Once you are inside, you'll have to don a paper gown and scrub your arms and hands with disinfectant.

When my son was in the NICU, for more than forty-eight hours I was not well enough to make the wheelchair ride to see him. The NICU nurses let my husband take instant photos of the baby for me to see, which he then taped to the wall beside my bed at my eye level. And although I couldn't see my son yet, I was already pumping my breast milk so it could be given to him by bottle.

Once I got down to the unit, the NICU nurses were great! They helped me to take Dylan out of his isolette and hold him, for as long as I liked. They showed me how to prop up his head (at six and a half weeks prematurity, he was like a Raggedy Andy doll, all flopping joints) and how to feed him his bottle. Once his sucking reflex grew strong enough, they even made a private little corner in the NICU for me to nurse him. And I could go in at any time of the day or night.

Going Home

It's important to arrange for assistance for the first weeks that you are at home. The usual interval that goes by before you can get out of the hospital after a section is five days. If your child has to stay behind in the intensive care unit or if you've been on bedrest for months and months like I was, your doctor may want you to stay an extra day or two. Up to eight days in all is not unusual. Undoubtedly, you'll be anxious to get home to familiar surroundings, especially if you were in the hospital for weeks before delivering. If you have other children at home, you'll be itchy to see them as well.

I can't counsel you to stay longer than you want to. But I will raise one point for you to consider: You're going to be caring for a newborn, and under the best of circumstances, this is a rigorous job. The baby won't be sleeping through the night; there will be diapers to change; and you'll have your own needs to meet, as well as those of your other children (if you have any). You'll still be weak and not up to 100 percent capacity for a while after you get home. You may want to take advantage of the 'round-the-clock care the hospital provides, to give yourself just a few hours more to build up your resources.

Make sure before you get out of the hospital that you arrange to get help in the house. Your main job in life for at least the first week after you get home is to heal and, if you are breastfeeding, to nourish your baby. If your husband can't take time off from work, import your mother. Or his mother. Your sister, an aunt, a cousin, or just friends.

If you can afford it, hire a nurse or a nanny to care for both you and the baby.

Your loved ones will want to help you. Let them. It makes them feel good, and you can use the assistance. If they call and ask what they can do, be specific. Ask for and expect help changing diapers, making meals, answering the phone, keeping visits from friends and relations brief. If a friend calls and offers to make dinner for you and your family one night and wants to know what you'd like to eat, don't be bashful—tell him. If another friend says she can take your toddler and five-year-old out for the day, let her. Ask others to run you over to the hospital for a couple of hours a day if your baby is still there and you need to see her. You have the rest of your life to pay back these favors one way or another.

Is It True: Once a Cesarean, Always a Cesarean?

It used to be, but not anymore. That was the case when almost all women received classic cesarean incisions—the vertical kind, which have a significant risk of rupturing during subsequent labor. Then, doctors did repeat c-sections on all their previously sectioned patients.

Nowadays, the ACOG recommends that women who have had one previous low-segment transverse c-section should be counseled to try vaginal birth for the next pregnancy. Such births are called VBACs— pronounced "vee-back"—and stand for vaginal birth after cesarean. Up to 80 percent of all women who have had one previous c-section can have a successful vaginal delivery the next time. Even women who have had more than one cesarean may be good candidates for a VBAC.

It has been found that VBACs are generally less dangerous than repeat cesareans and are probably better for the baby as well. The old fear that the uterus would rupture is now largely unfounded: Only one-half of one percent of women having a VBAC have scars that rupture partially or fully—less than for the repeat c-section rate!

If you do try VBAC, the hospital will require that your blood be typed and matched in case you need transfusion; electronic fetal monitoring and pressure monitoring of the inside of the uterus will be on standby; and an OR will be set up to do an emergency c-section if you need to have one. Don't let that daunt you. You have an excellent chance of delivering vaginally the next time.

A Final Word About Cesarean Sections

The final thing to remember about cesareans is that you are not a failure for not having a "normal" delivery. C-sections are neither unusual nor abnormal. And as long as the operation brings a child into life, it's a fine way to have a baby. As Marilyn said: "I wouldn't have cared if they had had to remove my head and turn me upside down to get that baby out. I'm still a mom, no matter how I delivered!"

14

What to Expect When You Go to the Hospital

When I first became pregnant, I didn't plan on spending any time to speak of in the hospital. I figured I'd go in for delivery, stay for three days, and bring home my happy, healthy baby. Just like on TV. I'd never known anyone who'd spent more than five days in the hospital after a birth—and that only for a c-section. I certainly wouldn't be having one of those! Why, with getting to know my baby, learning to breastfeed, and greeting all the visitors who'd be coming to see me, I'd barely have time to notice the hospital routine.

Well, as it turned out, I had more than ample time to observe and experience the daily ins and outs of hospital routine and pregnant patient care. I was in the hospital for a total of forty-two days. The first five, spent during my twenty-sixth week, were semi-planned: I had about half a week to prepare for my stay, during which my blood sugar would be brought under control and I would learn to inject myself with insulin. The last thirty-seven days were a complete surprise: My water broke at twenty-nine weeks and I went into labor. After an emergency ride to the hospital and a wild night in the labor and delivery suite, I took up residence on the obstetrics floor and didn't get out until seven days after I delivered by cesarean at thirty-three and a half weeks.

I learned a lot about hospital procedure during this time: Hospitals are creatures of routine. Everything from eating meals to giving urine samples is done on a schedule. It upsets the system when a patient asks for something that disrupts the normal flow of daily events.

I also learned that it is possible, within limits, to work with the staff and tailor your care to your own needs and rhythms. But in order to do that, you have to know how the system works. It took me a couple of weeks of trial and error before I understood what I could and could not expect and receive, if I asked. I'd like to pass on what I, and other women, have learned, so that you can be as comfortable as possible as soon as possible.

The Admissions Process

It all starts with being admitted—that is, checking in, letting the appropriate hospital personnel know you have arrived and are in need of medical attention, and giving them the information they need to keep track of you and bill you when you check out later. Where this takes place, how long it takes, and how it is accomplished depends upon whether your stay was planned or is the result of an emergency, whether or not you preregistered your insurance and medical history information earlier, and your condition when you arrive.

Bring Your Documentation with You

No matter when or under what conditions you go to the hospital, there is certain information about you and your family that the hospital is going to need. This usually involves filling out and signing a number of forms. If you are in the midst of a medical crisis, the staff will try to obtain this data as unobtrusively and appropriately as possible— most likely after the crisis is under control.

At a minimum you should bring with you a neatly typed or handwritten sheet with the following information on it:

- your full name
- your address
- your telephone number(s)
- your social security number
- any allergies you have
- pills or other medications you are taking (including vitamins)
- medical conditions you may have (such as kidney disease or heart problems)
- previous surgery you may have had (including cesareans)
- any other medical historical information you think may be important
- your next of kin's name (husband, partner, parent, and so on), address, and telephone number
- your medical insurance company's name(s), mailing address(es), phone number, caseworker's name (if you've been

assigned one), and your group number or policy number. (You'll also need the same information for your spouse if you are covered under his policy. If you have no insurance, include the name and number of a credit card or other information about how you intend to pay.)

- name and address of your house of worship if you wish to have your congregation notified of your admission.

Having these facts down on paper will make it easier for you or your loved one to get through the paperwork quickly, even if there are a lot of other distractions in the room. Once you've assembled the information, I recommend tucking copies of it in different items that you are likely to take with you if you have to leave for the hospital in a hurry—such as your purse, a prepacked suitcase (always a good idea), or your husband's wallet. Getting the information together ahead of time does you no good if you forget it!

FIND OUT IF YOU CAN PREREGISTER

To cut down on the red tape, some hospitals ask obstetricians to have their pregnant patients provide this information ahead of time. This is called *preregistration* or *preadmission.*

You send all the data in (including your expected delivery date) and sign all the forms early in the pregnancy. The hospital keeps this information on file. Then, if you do have to go in before term (or if you show up in labor at term), you tell the admissions clerk that you preregistered. She'll look up your file and ask you only a few questions.

If your doctor has not mentioned this option to you, now is a good time to look into it. One call to the hospital's admissions office will provide the answer. When you make the call, you can also ask whether the hospital will require any information from you other than the items listed above.

IF YOUR ADMISSION IS AN EMERGENCY

Early in your pregnancy, you should ask your doctor what part of the hospital you should go to if an emergency arises. Usually, the answer is to proceed to one of two places: the emergency room or the labor and delivery suite.

If you don't ask your doctor ahead of time, assume that you go to one of those two departments. *Don't* go to the admissions office! If you can, before you leave the house, make one quick phone call to your doctor. His office or paging service will pick up. Tell them that you are having an obstetrics emergency, how far along you are, *briefly* what the problem is, and that the doctor should meet you at the hospital. The service should then telephone the hospital to alert them to your arrival and will find your doctor and let him know you are on the way there, too.

Of the two choices—ER or labor and delivery suite—it is often preferable to walk or wheel into the latter as it is a specialized department in which all the staff are trained to deal with births and pregnancy-related problems. The nurses and physicians there should pretty much know what to do with you once you tell them what you think is going on. And your doctor may already be there, or he may have phoned ahead to tell the staff what he wants done with you initially. You are unlikely to have to wait more than a minute or two for treatment to start. And admissions formalities will most likely be dispensed with until your condition is stabilized.

The emergency room, on the other hand, specializes in critical care of all types, not just pregnancy-related crises. The ER may be crowded; the staff on call that day or night may not be very familiar with your particular condition; and, in very large facilities, you can get overlooked. **It is up to you not to let that happen.**

If there is a line, don't get on the end of it. You or your husband cut right to the front. This is particularly crucial if you are bleeding, are in preterm labor, or have hypertension—problems that can quickly get out of hand. Being a ''good girl'' and waiting patiently for the six people in front of you to be seen could jeopardize your baby's health. And you won't know how bad your situation is until you are examined. Another reason to be vocal: Some pregnancy complications—like preterm labor—are not readily apparent to anyone but you. If you don't tell the staff that this is an emergency, they just won't know.

Chances are you won't have to raise a ruckus to obtain speedy and proper treatment. But if you are told to wait in a chair along with a bunch of other people, or if you are placed in an examination cubicle and the nurse disappears for more than a minute or two, call out. *Insist* on being seen. Now.

Once treatment starts, the doctors and nurses will be working hard to assess your situation, stabilize you and the baby, and stop early contractions, if your condition warrants it. While they are doing this, there are a number of routine procedures that you are likely to undergo, regardless of your particular complication:

- You'll be asked to remove your street clothes, put on a hospital gown, and lie down on a hospital bed (lie on your left side—it increases flow of blood to the uterus and can help slow contractions).
- Someone will ask you a series of questions about how you

feel—things like whether you've had unusual vaginal discharge, cramps, bleeding, dizziness—to help them figure out what's going on with you.

- Someone will check your pulse, listen to your heart and lungs, take your blood pressure.
- Someone will take your temperature.
- You'll be monitored for contractions and possibly for fetal heartbeat.
- The nurse may also listen for the baby's heartbeat with a special microphone called a *doptone.*
- Many hospitals require you to have an intravenous line (IV) inserted to keep a vein open in case you need fluids or blood.
- You'll be asked for a urine specimen, or one will be taken from you with a catheter, to test for urinary infection and/or protein in the urine (if preeclampsia is suspected).
- A technician will draw several tubes of blood from your arm to type your blood and check you for anemia and infection (if you are diabetic, one sample will be tested to assess your blood sugar level).

Depending upon how far along you are, and how likely you are to deliver, the doctor may also:

- perform an amniocentesis (use a needle, inserted through your abdomen, to draw off a small amount of amniotic fluid) to assess the maturity of the baby's lungs.
- order an ultrasound to determine the fetus's true gestational age and condition.
- suggest (if the baby is under thirty-four weeks' gestation and he expects you to deliver within forty-eight hours) that you allow him to give you injections of corticosteroid drugs to speed up the baby's lung development.

In addition, you may be told to use a bedpan if you have to pee or move your bowels. You can ask whether your condition absolutely requires that you have no bathroom privileges, if you object to using a bedpan or are one of those people who just can't. Sometimes using a bedpan is hospital routine, rather than critical to your treatment. It's fair to ask.

On top of these procedures, you will also have whatever treatment is appropriate to stabilize your condition. The other chapters in this book describe in detail the likely treatment you would receive for a wide range of emergency complications.

Once your condition has stabilized, you will be moved to a room in either the maternity ward or the high-risk unit, or in some cases, sent home.

If Your Admission Is Planned

Of course you hope that, if you have to go to the hospital before you are due, it won't be under emergency conditions. There are several situations that may require a short, nonemergency hospital stay, such as bringing blood sugar under control with insulin therapy in gestational diabetes (see Chapter 6), or inserting a cerclage to strengthen an incompetent cervix (see Chapter 8). In these cases, you will usually be admitted to the hospital the same way that most nonpregnant patients sign in: through the admissions office.

When your doctor tells you that you will have to go to the hospital, ask him to explain what will happen when you get there. Ask him whether there is anything he can order or you can ask for upon your arrival that can help you remain comfortable or in compliance with your treatment. For example, if you are supposed to be on complete bedrest at home, you may be able to request a wheelchair or a gurney to meet you at the door. Or your condition may warrant expedited admissions (so you won't have to wait until your number is called to check in). If that is the case, your doctor should call the hospital before you get there to let the appropriate people know that you will be coming in and how he wishes your admission to be handled.

As you will have at least a day or two to get ready for your hospital stay, you will have time, if you have not already done so, to assemble pertinent medical and financial information. You can also call the hospital yourself and ask whether there is any particular time of day that the admissions office is less busy than others, so that you can go in when you are least likely to have to wait. Take advantage of the opportunity to prepare a little—it will save you time in admissions at a time when you will undoubtedly be a bit nervous and possibly physically uncomfortable.

There are a few items that you will find indispensable for a hospital stay. These include:

- one or more nightgowns
- a bathrobe and slippers
- socks
- hair clips, bobby pins, or whatever you use to keep your hair off your face
- several changes of underwear, including maternity and nursing bras

- a toilet kit, containing:

toothbrush	razor
toothpaste	shampoo
dental floss	conditioner
mouthwash	skin moisturizer
comb	deodorant
brush	

These are just the basics. Feel free to pack anything else you think you may want or need. And it's a good idea to prepack these and other items you think of, even if you're sure you'll never have to go to the hospital before term. Keep them in a bag that folds up (storage in your hospital room won't be expansive). By packing ahead of time, you guarantee that you won't forget essentials. If you try to pack during a crisis, I guarantee that you will.

The admissions office of a hospital is usually on the ground floor. If the location is not obvious when you walk in the door, ask at the information desk, which is usually a few yards inside the front door. Go right up to the admissions desk and make your presence known. Don't just sit down and expect somebody to notice you eventually, because that's exactly when they will—eventually. And that can be a couple of hours in a large metropolitan facility.

Explain that you are there to check in and that you are pregnant (if it's not obvious). If your doctor has given you special instructions, tell the desk person what these are. For instance, if you are to lie down while you wait your turn, say so, and ask where you should do it. If the answer is "Just sit over there; we'll be with you in a minute," insist, politely, that a place be found for you immediately. The vast majority of hospitals will honor your request promptly. But some are quite overcrowded and/or understaffed, and it will be the squeaky wheel in admitting that gets the grease. Speak up! If you don't get satisfaction, don't blow up at the desk attendant. She is most likely a volunteer or clerk. Ask politely but firmly to speak with the supervisor and deal directly with that person.

If the waiting room is crowded, you'll probably be assigned a number or your name will be put at the end of a list and you will be called in turn. Be ready with your information.

Every hospital's routine at admissions is somewhat different. Some admissions departments just do the paperwork; others also give you the initial physical and testing that all patients must go through upon arrival. In hospitals that do perform these common tests and exams as soon as you enter, this is generally what you can expect:

- A doctor or nurse will check your heart rate, blood pressure, and lungs and weigh you.
- Someone will take your temperature.
- You'll be asked to give a urine specimen.
- A technician will take one to several tubes of blood from your arm to type your blood and check you for anemia and infection.
- If you will be having general anesthesia, you may be asked to blow into a tube connected to a machine that checks your lung capacity.

The information that this brief examination reveals will be put into your chart and used as a basis for comparison during your treatment to make sure that your condition, whatever it is, remains stable or is improving.

The next stop will be your room.

What's a Hospital Room Like?

Rooms vary from one hospital to another, but have much in common. Things of beauty they are not—although at some facilities, the maternity wards are painted in pastels and have cheerful draperies and wall hangings.

Generally speaking, the rooms are small, square or rectangular in shape, and set up to be functional and easily cleaned. Furniture is sparse, usually limited to a bed, a bedside table, an adjustable tray table, and one or two guest chairs. Double these items and you get the picture of how a semi-private room is set up.

The beds in hospitals are no ordinary affairs. The head and foot can be raised or lowered by a hand crank or an electronic switch. And the height of the bed from the floor can be changed the same way. There are bars on each side of the bed that can be lowered, raised, and locked in place, to keep you from falling out. The mattress is usually pretty firm and covered with plastic-coated material. Pillows are made of hypoallergenic materials. Blankets are light.

On the wall at the head or side of each bed are a bunch of plugs and wires. These are there so that the staff can attach electronic equipment (such as a heart monitor or oxygen system). One of the wires or buttons is the nurses' call button—a gizmo that lights up a room number at the nurses' station so that you can call for help without having to shout. Often, the call button is attached to or hung on the bed via a flexible cable, so that you barely have to move to ring for a nurse.

Surrounding each bed is usually a heavy curtain hung from the ceiling that can be moved aside or pulled around the bed to provide you with some sense of privacy while you sleep, have visitors, or are examined. While these do create visual privacy, they provide absolutely no sound barrier.

If you have a single room, you may also have your own bathroom. Semi-private (that is, you get one roommate) and larger rooms either have one bathroom for all their occupants or have between rooms a bath that patients share. In some facilities, the patient must use a common bathroom down the hall.

If you want to watch TV in your room, you usually have to contract for it. The daily rental is nominal—a dollar or two a day. But you must specifically ask for it and usually pay for it separately as well. At some hospitals, VCRs are available for rental so that you can watch rented movies or cassettes from home (a great way to get to see your kids and for them to see you, if you can get someone to film you!).

Linens, soaps, towels, and the like are usually completely utilitarian. Don't expect anything better than plain bath soap, small towels, and unfitted sheets. The hospital isn't a place to expect to be pampered, even if you're pregnant. It's there to provide health care. Period.

SPECIAL REQUESTS

Hospitals all have strict schedules and routines. This doesn't mean, however, that you have absolutely no say in your daily treatment or your placement when you first arrive. Even if you come into the hospital on an emergency basis, it is possible to make certain requests, within reason, which the hospital staff will usually try to honor if they can.

Private vs. Semi-private Room

There are always many more semi-private or larger rooms than private ones. If you want a private room and can afford it, you'll have to ask for one at the time you're admitted. Otherwise, you'll be put in whatever semi-private space is available when you come in. You cannot reserve a room ahead of time, because the hospital has no way of predicting occupancy rates.

Please Don't Pair Me Up with a New Mom

Some women who are hospitalized for a complication of pregnancy find it difficult to be around mothers of full-term, healthy infants and their excited relatives. They find it painful to have roommates come and go up to three times a week and tough to deal with cooing newborns in the room when it's unclear whether their own child will be all right.

It's worth giving some thought to whether you might be upset if you had to have a new-mom roomie. If you feel that it would be more helpful to you emotionally to bunk with another woman with pregnancy complications or to be placed in with the general gynecology patients, find out who makes the decision on where to put you and talk to that person. Many hospitals today are sensitive to the emotional aspects of pregnancy complications and will try to honor your request. In fact, many of the larger facilities now have high-risk wings or units separate from the regular maternity floor.

I'd Like My Husband to Be Able to Stay Over with Me

In general, the maternity wards of hospitals try to cater as much as they can to their patients' wishes. If your room is a private room, even if the hospital policy is to send husbands home at the end of visiting hours, the floor nurses may just "overlook" his staying on. They may even provide a good cot or a recliner for his use. My husband stayed over in my room about half the time I was hospitalized. Some hospitals will even allow your other children to stay overnight (one at a time) on a cot or in a sleeping bag.

If you are in a semi-private room, the answer is likely to be no, your husband's presence might disturb your roommate. However, many hospitals will try to accommodate your request by providing a cot for your husband or loved one to nap on in another part of the floor. It certainly never hurts to ask.

Please Don't Use Me as a Teaching Patient

Some hospitals are teaching hospitals—they are affiliated with a medical school, and medical students receive training in the hospital, with real patients. This applies in obstetrics as well as any other department. Generally, a private patient—one who is sent to the hospital by her own physician—is seen only by her own OB and the residents whose job it is to work on the ward.

If a woman is a clinic patient, or has no doctor and just shows up at the ER or in labor and delivery, then she may very well have medical students studying her case. Medical students are under the supervision of the residents and department heads of the hospital. They may come in to the woman's room, ask her questions, examine her, draw blood (if it's required as part of her treatment), and so on.

It is your right to ask that you not be used as a patient on whose case medical students learn the ropes. Most hospitals will honor this request, if it is specifically made to the primary care physician or to the administration. It is true that the future doctors of America have to learn by doing. But if you don't want them to learn by doing to you, then say so.

What's the Daily Routine on the Hospital Floor?

Once you are settled in your room, your doctor will see you once or twice a day and tell the staff what special treatments you will be receiving. But your day-to-day care will largely be handled by the floor staff—the nurses, orderlies, and residents. These are the people with whom you will become most familiar and upon whom you will depend for your comfort. They all have a number of patients under their care—not just you—and they take care of them on a schedule.

Here, in general, is the drill you can anticipate:

The Morning

6:00–7:00 A.M.: The day shift arrives. A nurse or nurse's aide will take your temperature, check your blood pressure, and listen to your heart and lungs. She may also check for fetal heartbeats with a doptone monitor. You may be asked for a urine specimen. And if you have to have blood work drawn before you eat, it will be done now.

7:00–8:00 A.M.: An aide will deliver your breakfast, along with the day's menus, which you are expected to fill out and give back to her— probably when she comes by to pick up your tray in an hour or so.

7:30–10:00 A.M.: The resident or your doctor will drop by to see how you're doing, examine you, and tell you what, if any, tests you can expect that day.

8:00 A.M.–*12:00* P.M.: Room cleaning and linen change. If you have an IV that needs changing, it's usually done between these times.

9:00 A.M.–*12:00* P.M.: Aide brings you fresh water.

11:00 A.M.–*12:00* P.M.: Lunch. Nurse or aide checks your vital signs and listens to the baby's heartbeat. If you have to have blood work before eating, it will be done at this time.

The Afternoon

12–3:00 P.M.: Aide brings you fresh water and maybe a snack.

1:00–4:00 P.M.: Volunteers stop by and offer magazines or other reading material.

3:00–4:00 P.M.: Evening shift takes over.

4:00–5:00 P.M.: Dinner. If you have to have blood work before eating, it will be done at this time.

4:00–6:00 P.M.: Nurse or aide checks your vital signs and listens to the baby's heartbeat.

THE EVENING

6:00–8:00 P.M.: Aide brings you fresh water and maybe a snack.

6:00–9:00 P.M.: Room cleaning.

10:00–11:00 P.M.: Nurse or aide checks your vital signs and listens to the baby's heartbeat. If you have to have nighttime blood work done, it will happen now.

11:00–Midnight: Night shift takes over. If vitals have not been done before 11:00 P.M., the night nurse will check them now and listen to the baby's heartbeat.

Midnight–6:00 A.M.: Nurse may look in on you. If you have to have medication around the clock, you will be awakened to take it.

In addition to the usual routine, you may be visited by some of the following people up to once a day, or as infrequently as once every week or so:

- TV collection person
- hospital dietitian or nutritionist
- someone from hospital administration
- social worker
- medical students
- occupational therapist
- Candystriper
- volunteers

RELATING TO HOSPITAL STAFF

These people are going to be your lifeline. You will see them more than any other human beings during your stay. You would do well to try to cultivate their attention. Try hard not to alienate them. Even though you may be feeling rotten. Even though you hate being there.

These people have many responsibilities and may have over a dozen patients to care for every day. Whom do you think they're going to spend more time with, give the warmest smiles to, try to become a little personal with—the whining complainer, the hostile bitchy woman, or the one who tries to put on a good face and takes a positive attitude?

Am I telling you that you have to be a Girl Scout? No. I'm suggesting that you not take out your bad time on them. These are the people that you want in your corner, pulling for you and that baby of yours. If you're going to be in the hospital for a long time, you're going to come to crave every bit of positive attention you can get. Be courteous and warm to them and even the most surly orderly or nurse's aide will treat you with respect and a little kindness. And the really terrific nurses—and there are always several on the floor—will reciprocate your warmth in spades.

How Long and When Are Visiting Hours?

Visiting hours vary greatly from hospital to hospital. To find out what your hospital's rules on visitors are, you'll need to call and ask. In some hospitals, husbands are allowed to see you any time they wish. In others, husbands must adhere to the same hours as anyone else.

In many facilities, children are not allowed to visit at all, which can be a real problem for you if you're already a mom. You and your kids may be pretty desperate to see each other. You should find out if there is any way for you to see your little ones a couple of times a week (at least!) for short periods of time. If your children aren't allowed in your room, it can usually be arranged for you to see them in the patient lounge.

Tests and Procedures

Once you are on the hospital floor, the staff will have to monitor your condition daily. This means that you'll undergo a number of tests and procedures. Some of these are performed four or more times a day; others are done once or twice a week. Some hurt, some don't. Here's what you can expect on a daily basis:

- temperature and vital signs checked four to six times
- weight checked once
- baby's heartbeat monitored three to six times
- urine sample taken two to four times
- blood samples taken one to four times (if you are in for preterm labor, daily bloodwork might not be necessary)

Blood Tests: The Two-Stick Rule

It will seldom be your own obstetrician who draws your blood or places the intravenous line (IV), and medical personnel who perform these tasks may not all be experts in the needle department. The more relaxed you can be about getting your blood drawn or putting the IV in, the easier it will be for all concerned. I happen to have what nurses and doctors call *bad veins*—that is, they aren't big, tend not to sit in one place for the needle, and collapse when I get upset.

So when I was in the hospital to bring my gestational diabetes under control, I learned to adhere to what the residents called the *two-stick rule:* If someone is trying to put in an IV or take a sample of your blood, but they can't hit the mark after two tries, refuse to let them go for a third. Ask someone else to do it.

You can do so in such a way that you won't offend the person trying to do the blood work or the IV insertion. I often found that the person making the attempt seemed tremendously relieved to be asked to quit. They didn't like hurting me, and it was embarrassing for them to fail to "hit paydirt."

If your doctor anticipates having to order a lot of blood work on you over a period of days—as is always the case for gestational diabetes analysis—he may order the insertion of something called a *heparin lock,* also known as a *hep lock.* This is like an IV, but has no line attached to it. Its function is to keep a pathway to your vein open, so that each time you have to have blood drawn, the needle goes into the gizmo, not into you. It decreases your discomfort and makes it easier for the staff to do their work.

However, sometimes the hep lock doesn't work well, and then it may be back to sticking you each time a blood sample is needed. (I was in this category.) If the hep lock isn't used, over a period of days your arms might get fairly sore. In that case, you could ask the resident or nurse doing the drawing to use a *butterfly* needle, a smaller gauge needle, usually used on children or elderly people with delicate skin. Because it's smaller, I found it hurt less than the regular, larger needle. Not all hospital personnel are experienced with the butterfly, though, so it may be hard to find someone who can stick you with it.

Sometimes there is just no avoiding repeated pokes, but the two-stick rule should help you keep from feeling like a pincushion and your arms from looking like a battle zone.

In addition to the daily rituals involving scales, blood vials, and urine cups, there are other procedures that may be performed periodically, to check on the baby's well-being or your own:

- **Nonstress test**—NST—two to seven times a week. This is monitoring of the baby's heartbeat in relation to your uterine activity. A special microphone allows the baby's reactions to be transcribed on a paper strip, which also notes when uterine activity occurred. The final readout can be evaluated by a doctor or technician and provides valuable information on whether your baby is thriving inside you.

- **Contraction stress test**—CST—one to seven times a week. This is the same test as the NST, but it records the baby's reactions to uterine contractions you self-induce through stimulation of your nipples or mild contractions induced by an injection of the natural hormone oxytocin.
- **Electrocardiogram**—EKG—one or more times during your stay. Your heart pattern will be electronically monitored and recorded. This is done for hypertensives and women on tocolytics to make sure that their hearts continue to function normally.
- **Ultrasound**—also called a *sonogram*—one or more times per week. Using ultrasonic soundwaves, an image of the baby in the uterus is transmitted to a video monitor. This test can measure fetal growth or its slowdown, along with amniotic fluid volume. It can also reveal certain gross physical abnormalities and may be used to confirm fetal death.
- **Amniocentesis**—one or more times during your stay. A hollow needle is inserted through your abdomen and the uterine wall into the amniotic sac, where a sample of amniotic fluid is withdrawn. An examination of the fluid determines fetal lung maturity.

GETTING SOME REST

The truth is, you probably won't be able to rest very well. Your room has no lock on it, people are constantly rushing by in the hall and talking outside your door—sometimes even in the middle of the night—and hospital staffers will come into your room a minimum of ten times a day. Your roomie may be a whole other kettle of fish. She may be a talker or a moaner, or she may have a constant stream of relatives parading through the room.

If you find that this routine becomes stressful for you and you are exhausted but can't get more than a catnap, talk to your doctor. You can ask him to order that you not be disturbed for a number of hours, so that you can catch up on sleep. But be prepared to put a sign on your door if he gives you permission to forgo a set of vitals or afternoon bloodwork; such a change of routine may not register quickly with the staff. In fact, you may need to have your husband or friend "stand guard" to prevent people such as volunteers and clean-up crews from inadvertently disturbing you.

A noisy roommate requires different tactics. If she turns up her TV or radio too loud, ask her politely to turn it down or to use the earpiece that usually comes with the set these days. Most will understand your need for rest and will try their best to keep their activities and the noise level to a minimum. But you can't expect her to sit still as a stone, take no visitors, and stop living because you need your rest.

To minimize the amount of noise you hear, especially at night, try using earplugs. They really did the trick for me. Also, get someone to bring in a personal stereo with headphones, so you can listen to soothing music while you drift off to sleep.

Is Hospital Food as Bad as They Say It Is?

At the risk of alienating every hospital dietitian in the country: Yes, it is. It's not that all hospital chefs are bad cooks. They're not. It's not that the dietitians who plan the menus don't do a good job. They do. The problem is that hospital kitchens have to buy in bulk and on a budget, and bulk-bought items are often of the canned or bottled variety. It's hard to create a delicate sauce from such raw materials, especially when you're cooking hundreds of meals a day. And even if the food looked great and tasted even better when it left the kitchen, it still has to go into a warming cart for delivery to the patient. The crispest vegetable and crustiest roll succumb to limpness when they spend half an hour or more being steam-heated while waiting to be served.

What can you do about this? The answer is BYOF—bring your own food—*if,* and *only if,* you are not on a restricted diet, *and if* your doctor tells you it's okay to deviate from hospital-provided fare. Get your loved ones to bring in take-out once in a while. Ask them to bring you fresh fruit and other little snacks that you can keep in your bedside table. Most hospital rooms don't come equipped with a refrigerator, so you probably won't be able to keep things like dairy products or meats on hand. But don't let that keep you from sending friends out for daily portions of your favorite foods—*if both your medical condition and your doctor will allow this.*

Other Ways to Make Your Stay More Pleasant

No one enjoys being hospitalized, not even for the birth of a healthy, full-term baby. While the hospital provides quality care for you and your baby, staying there doesn't have a whole lot to recommend it. Especially when it comes to creature comforts.

So, do you sit there, miserable and forlorn? *NO!* You can make your hospital room much more pleasant and homey by bringing in every creature comfort you can think of. You are allowed to do this, and it will really lift your spirits. Here are some ideas:

- Bring your own pillows from your own bed—big and small (boudoir pillows add a nice touch and can be placed under sore spots or under your right hip to help you lie on the left side). Put pillowcases from home on them—your favorite pattern. You can send out the cases with your spouse or partner for periodic laundering.
- Have your husband or a friend buy an "egg crate" mattress pad (a thick, foam rubber pad that has peaks and valleys resembling an egg carton) to make the bed more comfortable.
- Take your silkiest, softest, prettiest nightgowns along. There may be some days (if you are bleeding or leaking amniotic fluid) that you'll appreciate the hospital-provided gowns. But most of the time, you'll want to wear your own clothes.
- Don't confine yourself to nighties, either. You can also wear stretch pants and tops, a housedress, or pajamas. Getting out of your bed clothes can really give your mood a boost.
- Also, take your favorite bathrobe. Who cares if it's all worn in and tattered at the bottom? If you love it, bring it!
- Got a favorite pair of slippers or socks? Don't forget them! You'll be doing at least a little walking, and you'll want warm, clean feet.
- Have someone bring you an inexpensive cut-glass water pitcher and drinking glass for your bedside.
- Take your makeup (if you wear any) and some funky earrings to wear during the day.
- If you have long hair, bring along some favorite hair clips and your curlers and hair dryer. Even if you're on total bedrest, you can still get your hair washed—nurses are skilled at giving in-bed hair washes!
- Bring nail polish and nail files.
- Bring perfume and scented soaps to bathe with.
- Take along some framed pictures of family for your nightstand or windowsill.
- Bring a string or mesh bag that you can hang on the bedrails; it will make it easier for you to reach magazines and handiwork.

If friends or family ask what they can do for you, or bring to you, don't be shy. Tell them, and be specific. Most will be all too glad to oblige you.

The idea is, the less impersonal and unpleasant you can make your temporary living quarters, the less imprisoned and the more in control of your situation you will feel.

How Is Being Hospitalized with Complications Likely to Make Me Feel?

You can expect to have a wide range of strong emotions, especially if the stay drags on for weeks or months. Nobody enjoys being in the hospital. It's a stressful rather than restful environment. For a pregnant woman whose pregnancy is in trouble, it can be doubly so. Most women experience a heightened emotionality while they are pregnant. It comes with the territory. The stresses of a hospital stay add to this. So, whatever your emotional state, it's going to be understandable under the circumstances.

For instance, nobody should blame you if you are angry at having to be cooped up in bed in a strange place with a stranger for a roommate, no privacy, and, possibly, a bedpan for restroom facilities. It is common and normal to feel angry at being so restricted. You may even periodically hate everyone who can be up and leading a normal life (I especially detested pretty, thin women with small breasts). If you get a little testy when the technician comes to take the fourth tube of blood for the day, you needn't berate yourself for not being an angel. In fact, given the circumstances, we'd have to wonder about you if you didn't exhibit some signs of edginess from time to time. You don't have to pretend things are fine, because they are not!

As you're there because there's a problem with your pregnancy, it's reasonable to assume that you'll be worried and anxious about the baby's safety and maybe even your own. The knowledge that you're in the best place to be if anything goes wrong probably won't be enough to quell all your unsettled feelings. On the flip side, you may also find it comforting to know that you are in good hands. Feeling alternating emotions of anxiety and comfort is normal.

One of the most universal feelings when you're in the hospital for even a couple of days is *boredom*. Lying in bed all day *is* boring, let's face it. Chapter 15, Bedrest: Keeping Yourself from Going Bonkers, should help you cope. It applies to hospital stays as well as home rest. When you finish this chapter, you should read that one.

You may also get depressed or simply be sad. You may cry at the smallest provocation. It's important to remember that feeling blue "for no reason" happens to everyone. All pregnant women get a little weepy from time to time. But you're in the hospital. You probably miss your family—your children especially, if you already have any—your normal routine, your own bed. In other words, no one can blame you for feeling sad or sorry for yourself now and again as you go through this experience. So don't add to your own misery by beating yourself up about it.

As your stay wears on, you'll also find that the littlest niceties make you happy. A new hair clip, a bunch of new flowers, a thoughtful card from a friend can really make your day. And when you have tests run and the results are good, you'll feel great. There's nothing more heartening than hearing your doctor say, "The untrasound shows that the baby is gaining weight and growing nicely." If such things make you giggle insanely, don't give it a second thought. Feeling emotional extremes is natural for you right now.

Remember, the entire spectrum of emotions *is normal,* and you can expect to have most of them while you are hospitalized. Problems arise when you can't lift yourself out of your negative feelings, despite a desire to do so. If you find that you have persistent dark thoughts that you cannot shake, if you can't put your fears aside even though you want to, or if you just cannot stop crying no matter what you do, it's time to consider reaching out for counseling. This is not a defeat or abnormal. Lots of women become overwhelmed by their negative experiences during a tough pregnancy.

If this happens to you while you're hospitalized, let the staff help you. Ask to see the hospital social worker or staff psychologist. The hospital should be able to provide you with a professional who understands your predicament and who can help you work through your feelings.

How Friends and Relatives May React to You

You may want to just "talk it out" with family, friends, or your husband. Often, if you are feeling lousy, friends and relatives can really boost your spirits. But just as often, you may have the sense that they'd rather not hear about how it really is for you. They change the topic to the weather, current events, their Aunt Martha's pet pig—or just cut the visit short. This can hurt your feelings and make you feel uncared for.

It's usually not that they don't love or care about you: They are probably having trouble coping with their own feelings about finding you in this fix. Their normal image of you is of the vital, active woman you've always been (and will be once again after this is over!). But when they see you in the hospital, you're supine and tired, and they can't make you all better. For some people, this is too much to deal with. So they withdraw.

Now it's not your job to make them comfortable with your condition. You've got enough on your hands keeping yourself together. But you may want to hold off on "having it out" with them until you're back on your feet after giving birth. You can always save your thoughts and feelings about their behavior to discuss with them at a later time. Clearing the air when you have the internal wherewithal to listen to their emotional "stuff" about your pregnancy can help you get your friendship back on track.

LACK OF CONTROL

When you're in the hospital, especially for a long stay, it's easy to feel like everything is out of control. Your body is playing nasty tricks on you, and you can't will it to stop. You're being poked and prodded and looked at half-naked by strangers who don't even make appointments ahead of time. And the people you want to see most—your friends, your family—sometimes can't get in to see you at all because of hospital visiting hours. Of course you feel out of control!

But you don't have to keep feeling that way. By becoming actively interested in the medical care you are receiving, you can regain a feeling of control and personal dignity. It may be hard for you to do this at first, since you'll also be feeling grateful that the medical staff is taking good care of you and is helping to prolong your pregnancy and win you a good outcome. To feel in control, you must speak up if you have questions and fears or if something someone is doing to you is causing you pain.

Medical personnel do the tests and procedures that you now have to undergo so often that they can become desensitized to the individual. You have the power to make sure this doesn't happen to you. Even though it may not feel like it, this is still *your* body. You have every right to see to it that you and it are treated with the gentleness and respect you deserve.

How do you do this? Ask questions. Calmly, politely, in a friendly tone of voice: What is each procedure for? How is it done? Will it hurt? Tell your doctor, nurses, and residents that knowing what's going on is important to you.

Request that your doctor, the residents, and the nurses inform you ahead of time if you are to have blood work or other testing done. Tell them that if a test or examination will be painful, you want the person performing it to let you know before they do the part that hurts. Ask about test results. Ask what the results mean for you and the baby. Ask the nurse what your temperature or blood pressure is when she takes it. Engage your caregivers in conversation about your condition and the routine things they're doing for or to you.

This is called taking an active role in your care. Your queries will help you understand what's going on with you, what the doctors are considering for your treatment, and what effect those treatments will have on you physically. It's fair to ask your doctor about treatment options and whether there's any less invasive or uncomfortable way for him to find out what he needs to know.

Your doctor should welcome your interest in your treatment and treat your questions, no matter how small, with respect. If he does not, call him on it. He should know that a well-informed and involved patient is a better patient. You are more likely to comply with treatment, even if it is unpleasant or painful, if you know why and how it's being done.

Remember Why You're in the Hospital

Finally, keep your eyes on the prize. You're in the hospital because you want to do everything you possibly can to have a healthy baby. All the bad things about being in the hospital are temporary. The lack of privacy, the needle sticks—all the testing will be finished soon. No matter how long you're in the hospital, and I know it can feel like forever, this experience is going to be over. With the skill of your doctor and the hospital staff and a little luck, eventually you'll be taking home a happy, healthy baby!

15

Bedrest: Keeping Yourself from Going Bonkers

When I was ordered to bed in my third week of pregnancy, the only other woman I'd ever heard of who had to spend her whole pregnancy in bed was Sophia Loren. I had seen a made-for-TV movie of her life that pictured her, gorgeous, beatific, dressed in satin in a magnificent, luxurious room, patiently and happily gestating away. She made bedrest look like fun.

What the movie didn't tell me was that by the third day in bed, I'd be bored to tears and terrified that I would lose my twins. It was impossible to comprehend the coming total change in my and my husband's routines. I was a real doer: I had a demanding job that often took up ten to fourteen hours of my day; I had an active social life; I worked out three to five times a week.

But a few words from my doctor changed all my doing to don'ts. Go to bed, be as quiet as you can, until you've stopped bleeding for at least forty-eight hours. Don't get out of bed except to go to the bathroom. No, you should not even stand up long enough to make yourself a cup of tea. Don't lift anything heavier than a paper plate with food on it that *someone else* prepares for you in advance. No sitting up straight, not even to eat. Call your office and tell them you won't be coming to work for the foreseeable future. Oh, yeah, and no sex.

Once I figured out that this prescription of inactivity was going to be a long-term proposition, I was devastated. I was left with the telephone, the television, a radio, and twenty-four hours a day to fill with activities that could only be done in bed, without moving around. It meant nearly total dependency on my husband. Up until then we had always pretty evenly divided the household chores: Now he had to do my half, too, plus take care of me. I was worried about him. How would he do all that, keep up with his job and his other activities, his friends. . . . Could our relationship survive the stress? Would my babies make it? Would I lose my job? Would my friends and family really understand? Would I go stark, raving mad?

I didn't know it at the time, but those questions represent the normal, natural worries that any woman confined to bedrest may have. (If you are sent to bed when you also have one or more children to take care of, the fears compound: Will my kids understand? Am I hurting them by staying in bed? Who's going to take care of them? How can my husband do the housework, and his job, and take care of the kids and me?)

Why Do I Have to Go to Bed?

Bedrest is the treatment of choice for a surprising number of pregnancy complications. For instance, bedrest is the best therapy for premature labor. Bedrest alone—that is, without drugs—stops premature labor in up to 50 percent of all cases. Bedrest in combination with tocolytics (drugs that stop contractions) stops premature labor in 80 percent of all cases, making it a highly successful treatment.

Bedrest can be essential in stopping premature effacement (shortening) and dilation of the cervix—a key cause of premature birth—by taking the increasing weight of the growing baby and uterus off the cervix. This is particularly important for women who in the past have lost pregnancies because of a weak cervix and who now have a cerclage (a surgical procedure that sews the cervix closed to help hold the pregnancy).

Bedrest is also considered the best treatment for intrauterine growth retardation (IUGR)—when the baby is small for gestational age and is not receiving as much nutrition from the mother as she should. Why? Because the less blood and oxygen the mother needs to use, the more the baby receives, thus encouraging growth.

Bedrest can be crucial in treating placenta previa—a condition in which the placenta covers all or part of the cervix and the woman is in danger of bleeding or placental separation from the uterine wall. And bedrest is important in encouraging water loss in pregnancies complicated by hypertensive problems.

And though still not universally accepted within the obstetrical community, bedrest is often prescribed for women pregnant with multiples. The theory here is that the extra weight such women carry is more likely to cause premature labor when they are upright than when they are supine. Lying down lessens the downward pull of gravity.

In short, this "medicine" usually works for a broad range of problems, which means that it helps you get to term or close enough to term that your baby can survive outside the womb without serious problems. That is, when you take the doctor's prescription and follow the directions faithfully.

But I Don't Feel Sick . . .

"I hear women say that all the time: 'If I just looked sick or sounded sick, then I wouldn't want to get up.' For active people, bedrest is really tough to try to implement," said Marie, a social worker and mother of two who spent both of her successful pregnancies on bedrest from fourteen weeks on.

Most women whose doctors order them to bed don't really feel sick. Unless you are bleeding, there may be nothing tangible externally to remind you that your pregnancy is or could be in jeopardy. Even if you are bleeding, you are probably not in pain. And that makes it hard to stay in bed once you get there.

That's the bottom line about bedrest: It's very hard work. Your doctor most likely hasn't told you that. He probably hasn't referred you to a support group for bedresters or told you that physical, psychological, and occupational therapy is available and appropriate for women in your situation. He almost certainly hasn't offered you advice on how to break it to your boss that you will have to stop working.

These omissions are not purposeful. Your OB is concerned with getting under control the underlying medical problem that requires bedrest as treatment. He was probably not trained to look at bedrest as anything other than a prescription for what ails you. It is only very recently that the medical community has begun to consider the physical and psychological effects of bedrest.

And that's a shame. As anyone who has been through a long stint of bedrest knows: The more information you have about what to expect, and the more support that you can arrange for yourself, the better your experience is going to be. Also, the more positive you feel about what you're doing, the more likely you are to stick with it and not cheat.

And cheating—getting up to vacuum those dust bunnies in the corner, sneaking out to the deli because it's such a gorgeous day and how can you stay inside—is always a strong temptation. It's difficult to believe that a walk to the corner can be dangerous. But giving in to temptation can be the difference between a good outcome for your pregnancy and an outcome you'd rather not think about.

Keeping Your Eyes on the Prize:
A Healthy, Full-Term Baby

If it hasn't hit you yet, it will soon. You're going to be giving up an awful lot during the next weeks or months. Although it doesn't feel like one, this is a choice you are making. You can always get out of bed and resume a normal schedule. But if you do, you'll be taking a calculated risk that could hurt you and your baby.

So it's important to keep straight in your head *why* you are choosing to comply with the bedrest. "Remember," says Patricia, a mother of three healthy girls, all of whom were born after twenty to twenty-four weeks of bedrest, "you're working for a goal here, and if you can just mark off time, and if all goes well, you'll end up with a good result—a healthy, full-term baby." It sounds so obvious, but it bears repeating because there will be times during your confinement that you're going to forget it. Your goal is a live, normal infant.

And staying in bed will be as much as you can possibly do to insure that outcome. If you are the kind of person who prefers to prepare for the worst as opposed to the best, then know this: By being religious about staying in bed exactly as much as your doctors tells you to, if your pregnancy doesn't end up well, you will have the comfort of knowing that you did everything in your power to protect and nurture your child. Luckily for both optimists and pessimists, bedrest usually ends up well.

The Best of Times, the Worst of Times . . .

What's it like? Well, at its worst, bedrest is incredibly stressful, for you, for your family, and for your friends. For you, lying still all day is boring. When it's not boring, it's frustrating. It's likely to do a number on your self-image. It's going to make you feel helpless. Your muscles will ache from the inactivity. Your work and the rest of your social life will feel like they're going to hell in a handbasket. Your partner, unless he's up for beatification, is likely to get cranky and distant at times and may be overwhelmed by the extra responsibilities that now fall to him. Your friends will be interested in helping you at first, but then they'll get on with their lives and you'll feel lonely and abandoned. Some of them may not be able to cope with your inactivity; most of them won't be able to really empathize with your problem.

At its best, bedrest is a time for reflection that most of us never have the luxury to spend. It creates a stronger relationship between you and your husband and a stronger family unit if you already have young ones at home. And you will get to know your baby in ways that women who remain active during pregnancy never do. Small moments in life will seem magnified and wondrous. You will have a terrific feeling of accomplishment. It will change your life.

How Long Am I in For?

That depends. The duration and strictness of bedrest prescribed for the various complications of pregnancy is different for every woman. For the first thirteen weeks of my confinement, I bled almost daily. I could get up and sit on the couch in a semi-reclining position, and I always had bathroom privileges. After that, I was in bed for intrauterine growth retardation (IUGR). For that, most of the time, I was supposed to be supine and get up only to use the toilet.

Some women are more restricted than I was and are told to be on complete bedrest, including having to use a bedpan. Other women just have to "put their feet up" for several hours a day and can continue to work at least part-time. Most bedrest regimes, no matter what their level, involve stopping work if you work at an office outside the home.

Even if you are on total bedrest, once your baby has reached the stage (about thirty-six weeks) where the lungs are mature, your doctor may tell you that you can get up and move around more. That's because once the baby's lungs reach maturity, she will be able to survive outside the womb. Even if you immediately go into labor, the baby should be okay.

What's Going to Happen to My Body?

If you've read Chapter 2, When Pregnancy *Is* Perfect, you already know that under normal circumstances, pregnancy causes profound, progressive changes in the body. (If you haven't read Chapter 2, you should.)

When you go on pregnancy bedrest, your body will still make these changes, and you will still feel these effects. But the bedrest will cause other changes as well. You can expect to lose some muscle tone from the lack of exercise, especially in your legs, abdomen, and back. You will feel tired more often and will tire more easily. You will also feel stiff when you get out of bed and may have body aches the rest of the time. You may even find it painful to walk, since lying constantly in bed with legs relaxed can cause tightening of the Achilles tendon.

If you are on total bedrest, with no exercise allowed, it's going to be impossible to avoid these problems. And most of them will follow you for some time after you give birth. You will recover quickly, though, especially if you embark on a reasonable exercise regime as soon as your doctor gives the okay to do so.

IF YOU GET PERMISSION TO EXERCISE IN BED

If you are allowed to do any exercise at all, while you are resting, you should regularly and religiously. The following exercise regime was developed by a team of doctors, occupational and physical therapists at the Albert Einstein Medical Center for a study on the effects of physical and occupational therapy on sixty pregnant women confined to bedrest for at least one week.* The women's complications were much like yours: Some had premature labor and/or preterm premature rupture of membranes; others had PIH (pregnancy-induced hypertension), bleeding, incompetent cervix, or were pregnant with multiples.

The physical therapy portion of the program (the twenty-four exercises that follow) began on the third to fourth day of hospitalization and was performed three times each day, under medical supervision. **MEDICAL SUPERVISION IS VERY IMPORTANT WHEN UNDERTAKING ANY PHYSICAL EXERCISE PROGRAM WHEN ON PREGNANCY BEDREST.** The exercises were designed to help prevent the muscle weakness, limit the loss of range of motion, prevent lung congestion, minimize the effects of bedrest on the heart, and help the woman maintain sufficient tone to be able to walk without assistance after delivering (as women who don't spend their pregnancies in bed do). Each woman was tested after each exercise session to make sure her heart rate and blood pressure did not go too high; the fetal heart rate and number of contractions per hour were also measured following exercise.

What this should tell you is that **YOU MUST NOT DO THESE OR ANY OTHER EXERCISES WITHOUT THE KNOWLEDGE AND CONSENT OF YOUR OBSTETRICIAN. CONSULT WITH YOUR OBSTETRICIAN TO MAKE SURE IT IS SAFE FOR YOU TO EXERCISE. EVERY BEDRESTER'S CONDITION IS UNIQUE, AND YOU MAY REQUIRE MODIFICATIONS IN THIS REGIMEN TO MAKE IT SAFE FOR YOU AND YOUR BABY** (doing all exercises tilted slightly to your left side so as not to compress the major veins that lie under the uterus, for instance). **LET YOUR PHYSICIAN SET THE NUMBER OF REPETITIONS FOR EACH EXERCISE. DO NOT DECIDE FOR YOURSELF HOW MANY OF EACH IS SAFE. THEN, IF YOU RECEIVE PERMISSION TO EXERCISE, DO ONLY THE NUMBER OF REPETITIONS OF EACH EXERCISE THAT YOUR DOCTOR SPECIFIES.**

*Sherry Blumenthal, M.D., principal investigator; Ellen Kolodner, M.S., O.T.R./L, F.A.O.T.A., co-principal investigator; Mary McLaughlin, P.T.; Caryn Johnson, O.T.R./L., research coordinator.

Also, ask your OB specifically how to record your heart rate and check for contractions (see Chapter 8, Preterm Labor and Premature Rupture of Membranes, for information on how to self-monitor).

Remember, you are on bedrest to keep you pregnant as long as possible. Don't undo all your good work toward this ultimate goal by being overzealous or second-guessing the professionals on your exercises. You're only trying to maintain reasonable body tone and overall good health here, not win a marathon! If you follow doctor's orders, these exercises may go far in helping you maintain muscle tone and the strength you will need in preparation for labor and your recovery after the baby is born.

These are the exercises:

1. DEEP BREATHING
Purpose: to clear lungs and relax
Position: lying on your back or sitting up
Action: A. inhale through your nose
            B. exhale through your mouth
             • Never hold your breath while exerting energy!

2. PELVIC TILTS
Purpose: to maintain abdominal tone and pelvic mobility
Position: lying on your back
Action: A. arch your lower back
            B. while exhaling, flatten small of your back into the bed

3. KEGELS
Purpose: to maintain pelvic floor muscle tone
Position: lying on your back
Action: A. use your imagination to pretend you are on an elevator going up. As the elevator ascends, exhale as you draw the muscles of the perineum up slowly until they are completely contracted, stopping at each "floor" for two to three seconds
            B. inhale and slowly allow the muscles to relax fully, again stopping at each "floor," while imagining that the elevator is returning to the ground floor

4. GLUTEAL SETS
Purpose: to maintain buttock muscle strength
Position: lying on your back with knees slightly bent
Action: A. exhaling, tighten buttock muscles together
            B. hold for two to three seconds
            C. inhale as you relax the muscles

5. LEG ROLLS

Purpose: to maintain range of motion in hip joints and muscular strength

Position: lying on your back with your knees straight, toes and kneecaps pointing straight up toward the ceiling

Action: A. rotate both legs outward at the hip by keeping knees straight and turning toes and kneecaps outward

          B. rotate both legs in at the hip by rolling your kneecaps and toes toward each other (pigeon-toed)

6. ANKLE PUMPS

Purpose: to stretch calf muscles, promote return of blood from the legs to the heart, and maintain range of motion in the ankle

Position: lying on your back with your legs elevated on a pillow

Action: A. inhaling, and without lifting your leg off the pillow, flex toes and entire foot up, toward your head, holding for two to three seconds

          B. exhaling, push the ball of your foot downward and while pointing your toes (as if you're stepping on a gas pedal of a car), again, holding for two to three seconds

7. HEEL RAISES

Purpose: to maintain strength of calf muscles

Position: lying on your back, knees bent and legs together, feet flat on the bed

Action: A. keeping your toes on the bed, exhale and raise your heels off the bed

          B. inhale as your return your heels to the bed and flatten your feet against the mattress

8. KNEE EXTENSION

Purpose: to maintain strength of your thigh muscles

Position: lying on your back with a firm pillow or large towel roll under your knees so that your knees are gently flexed and supported

Action: A. exhaling, and keeping upper leg pressed against the pillow or towel roll, slowly raise one foot up until knee is straight (leg no longer flexed)

          B. inhale and slowly lower heel to the bed

9. HEEL SLIDES

Purpose: to maintain strength and range of motion at hips and knees

Position: lying on your back, knees bent, heels flat on mattress

Action: A. inhaling, keeping one knee bent, and never taking the heel off the mattress, slowly slide the other leg down until it is straight and flat against the bed

         B. exhaling, slide the straight leg back up to the bent position, never taking heel off the mattress

         C. repeat with the opposite leg

10. QUAD SETS

Purpose: to maintain strength in the thigh muscles

Position: lying on your back in a comfortable position, keeping one leg straight and the other bent

Action: A. exhaling, tighten the thigh muscles in the straight leg (your kneecap will move up slightly toward your hip), holding for three to four seconds as you inhale, then exhale again

         B. repeat with other leg

11. LEG LIFTS

Purpose: to maintain strength of the hip muscles

Position: lying on your side with your lower leg bent for balance, upper leg in a straight line with the trunk of your body, head resting on lower arm, other arm bent to steady you. Don't let your hips roll forward (use a pillow under your abdomen to steady yourself if necessary)

Action: A. exhaling, raise upper leg up toward ceiling four to six inches (leg should remain straight and your side flat against the mattress)

         B. inhaling, slowly lower your leg

         C. repeat with other leg

      Note: If this exercise is too difficult for you, or if your doctor prefers for you not to do it, ask him if it is all right to do the exercise while lying on your back. In this version, keeping both legs straight and pressed against the mattress, slowly slide one leg out to the side, keeping knees and toes pointing straight upward (like you're making angels in the snow)

12. ARM RAISES

    Purpose: to maintain strength and range of motion in the shoulders

    Position: lying on your back, arms at your sides

    Action: A. exhaling, and keeping elbows locked, raise one arm off the bed and over your head

             B. inhaling, return the arm to the starting position

             C. repeat with other arm

13. CHICKEN WINGS

    Purpose: to maintain range of motion in shoulder joint

    Position: lying on your back with your hands clasped under your head, elbows pointing up (arms hugging the sides of your head)

    Action: A. exhaling, press elbows back against the bed

             B. inhaling, return to the starting position

14. UP AND OUT ARM RAISES

    Purpose: to maintain strength and range of motion in the arms

    Position: lying on your back with left hand on right hip with your hand in a loose fist

    Action: A. slowly move your arm up and out above your head in a sweeping motion toward your left side, while opening your hand and spreading your fingers

             B. slowly return your hand and arm to the starting position, ending with left hand in a loose fist on your right hip

             C. repeat with other arm (right hand on left hip for starting position)

15. UP AND IN ARM RAISES

    Purpose: to maintain strength and range of motion in the arms

    Position: lying on your back, left arm on bed perpendicular to your body, hand open, palm down

    Action: A. slowly turn your palm up, closing your hand while you sweep the arm up and in across your chest toward your right ear

             B. slowly return to the starting position

             C. repeat with the right arm (right arm perpendicular to the body, hand open, palm down, for starting position)

16. SHOULDER SHRUGS

Purpose: to relax and strengthen neck and shoulder muscles
Position: lying on your back, arms relaxed at your side
Action: A. exhaling, shrug your shoulders as high as possible up toward your ears
           B. inhaling, relax and slowly lower your shoulders

17. SHOULDER BLADE SQUEEZE

Purpose: to strengthen the muscles between your shoulder blades and improve posture
Position: lying on your back, chin tucked against your chest, arms relaxed
Action: A. exhaling, and keeping your chin tucked, pull your shoulders back against the bed, pulling your shoulder blades together (try to bring your elbows in close to your side)
           B. inhaling, relax and return to the starting position

18. ELBOW BENDS

Purpose: to strengthen the upper arm muscles
Position: lying on your back, left hand touching the right shoulder so that left elbow is bent
Action: A. exhaling, raise your left hand toward the ceiling until the elbow is straight
           B. inhaling, return to the starting position
           C. repeat with opposite arm (right hand touching the left shoulder for the starting position)

19. WRIST CIRCLES

Purpose: to maintain strength and range of motion in the wrist and forearm
Position: lying on your back, hands held comfortably in front of you
Action: A. rotate your wrist in a large circle in a clockwise direction
           B. move wrist up, down, left, then right

20. HAND PUMPS

Purpose: to maintain strength, range of motion, and circulation of the hand
Position: hand bent back slightly at wrist
Action: A. curl your fingers up, starting at the tips, until you make a fist
           B. uncurl your fingers completely, straightening and spreading them out

21. CHIN TUCKS

Purpose: to maintain range of motion in your neck, decrease stiffness and improve posture

Position: lying on your back with a pillow under your head

Action: A. without tipping your head back, lift your chin straight up toward the ceiling

B. pull chin back and tuck it in as much as you can (make a double chin)

22. CHIN RAISES

Purpose: to maintain range of motion and prevent pain and stiffness in the neck

Position: lying on your back with the head of the bed slightly elevated, place a pillow behind the shoulders to allow your head to bend back

Action: A. exhaling, tilt your head backward, raising your eyes and face toward the ceiling

B. inhaling, slowly return to the starting position

23. NECK DIAGONALS

Purpose: to maintain strength and range of motion of the neck

Position: lying on your back, chin tucked in (make a double chin)

Action: A. tilt your chin down toward the right shoulder

B. exhaling, raise your chin up and over your left shoulder

C. repeat in the other direction

24. NECK CIRCLES

Purpose: to maintain strength and range of motion in the neck

Position: lying on your back, head of the bed slightly elevated and shoulders supported by pillows so that they are pushed forward

Action: A. bring your right ear toward your right shoulder

B. roll your head backward with your eyes facing the ceiling

C. roll your head around to the left, bringing your left ear toward your left shoulder

D. roll your head forward until your chin touches your chest

E. repeat in the opposite direction

The Psychology of Bedrest

If you're feeling sad, worried, panicked, depressed, angry, even euphoric about being on pregnancy bedrest, you're in excellent company. Every woman who has to spend part or all of her pregnancy in bed feels just like you do right now at some point before, during, or after her confinement. We'd have to wonder about you if you didn't have a strong reaction to it. After all, you're being asked to put all your normal activities and most of your needs on hold, to limit yourself to a small physical space, and generally to turn your entire life upside down—all for the sake of this tiny person you've never met. Your perfect pregnancy—the one we're brought up to believe every woman gets to experience—has now become that other thing you read about in magazines. You are now in the high-*risk* category. Everyone, from your obstetrician to your own mother, is behaving differently toward you.

And most likely, even though they are trying, not one of them is being tremendously helpful in the coping-with-it department. It's likely that you don't know anyone else who's been on bedrest for her pregnancy, so you have absolutely no idea whether what you're feeling is usual, or whether you're going to get through it.

I can assure you that yes, you will get through it. What you're feeling, whatever that feeling is, is natural under the circumstances.

You'll have to trust us experienced bedresters on this one. There is no definitive body of scientific or academic research to back us up. Only three of the twenty leading medical obstetrics texts discuss bedrest and its implications; only one of these even mentions the psychological impact of having to rest in bed during pregnancy.

But there are a number of psychologists who now specialize in treating women with complicated pregnancies. Their insights, plus the first-hand experiences of the thousands of us who must spend our pregnancies in bed each year, make it clear that there are certain issues and feelings common to all pregnant bedresters.

The very first feelings that most pregnant women have in response to the news that they have to spend some or all of their pregnancy in bed are shock, disbelief, and denial. It takes awhile for the information to really sink in—days, sometimes a couple of weeks.

You may have prepared for your stint of bedrest like a trooper, organizing your life to meet the situation. You've kept your spirits up, or at least attempted to. Everyone says you're being so brave. Then all of a sudden you find yourself crying "for no reason" or simply feeling blue. It hits you that you're in bed for the long haul. And you feel miserable. But then just as suddenly, you feel chipper again.

You can expect these mood swings to continue on and off for your whole pregnancy. They are particularly likely around the time that each medical event in the pregnancy takes place. You may be "up" on the day you get to go out to the doctor's office, but "down" and frightened when you have another bout of whatever it is that needs bedrest to fix. This is natural. Remember, even women with "uneventful" pregnancies have mood changes.

One of the key issues that you are likely to struggle with around this time, especially in the beginning of your bedrest period, is the common ambivalance that all mothers-to-be have about pregnancy. When a pregnancy becomes high-risk, these feelings tend to get blown up.

You may also feel that you are to blame somehow for the pregnancy complication that's forcing you to bed. You can't find a logical reason for the problem, and usually, your doctor doesn't know why it's happening, either. In that case, it's easy to make it your own fault, as a means of trying to understand it and explain it. But while it is common to blame yourself, you must understand that in reality, *it isn't your fault*. What is happening to you falls into that these-things-sometimes-happen category. It's not a satisfying explanation, but often it's the only one there is. You shouldn't blame yourself for something over which you have no control.

Which raises another big issue. Loss of control. At some point, all your volition in life will seem to have disappeared. Your body is out of control, and it will be easy to feel "done to." The doctors and nurses *do* things *to* you—take your blood, monitor you for contractions, send you home to stay in bed.

On top of that, you won't be able to participate the way you are used to. Your family or friends will constantly be *doing for* you—making your meals, doing your shopping, cleaning your house, and so on. You, the woman who can do whatever she pleases in life, are now limited by what and when others can do for you. It's terribly frustrating, and it happens to all bedresters.

For Mary, this was the most difficult aspect of being on bedrest. "I'm used to being a giver," she told me. "I'm a mother and a wife. I'm active in job and career and used to being part of things. I had the hardest time putting my whole life on hold. I felt angry about not being able to participate in life. I was at the mercy of everybody around me. My husband was really great, and so was my family. But enough is enough. You have to ask somebody for everything! I really had a problem with that."

It made Mary feel guilty, like it does most of us. So many people are doing so much for you and you can't reciprocate in kind. You'll feel that that's not right. You'll feel selfish and unworthy of the attention.

These feelings are normal, but they are not the reality. The fact is that by staying in bed, you are protecting and nourishing your unborn child. There is no more selfless act of giving to your child than complying with bedrest during pregnancy. It is an act of pure love and commitment to the life you have inside you. It's an incredibly adult act, one that most people, when told about your situation later, will tell you they could never have done themselves.

That won't necessarily help you feel better about the fact that you cannot reciprocate for all the help you've been getting right now. Paige, who had to spend months in bed while carrying three of her four children, knows this problem all too well. "It's hard to rely on friends," she told me, "because the problem is chronic. You have to ask and ask and ask, and you feel like you'll never be able to give back what you've taken."

What Paige and many bedresters find helpful is to realize that rarely can you reciprocate on a one-for-one, give-and-take basis during a high-risk pregnancy. Instead, think of it in a more universal sense. There's an opportunity to give back many times over in your lifetime. You'll help others later in similar, or other, situations.

It may also help you to remember that most people find it easier to give than to receive. You'll find that it actually helps your friends and loved ones feel better about what has happened to you if you allow them to do something concrete to assist you. In many ways, they feel out of control too, because they can't make you better.

You will also be dealing with other feelings that relate to your self-image, how you see yourself and your role in the world. For example, if you are a professional person, a lot of what makes you feel good about you may be tied up in your work—doing a good job, achieving, performing. When you're pregnant and on bedrest, unless you can do most of your work over the phone, a fax, a Dictaphone, or on a computer, continuing to work is quite difficult. Your doctor may even tell you working from bed is not a good idea because the stress of your job may counteract the benefits of resting.

Plus, you may normally be an extremely active person—one who works out a lot or spends a lot of time doing physical things outdoors. Now you aren't even allowed to pick up a half-gallon of milk.

Then there is how you see yourself as a woman. As women, we are all brought up believing the fiction that pregnancy is easy, that everyone can do it without much effort. We all should be able to carry a fetus to term, working the whole time, and with no complaints. When your pregnancy doesn't proceed that way you feel like your body has betrayed you. You may even feel failed as a woman.

But you have not "failed" at anything. Your baby is still alive and is growing every day. Your staying in bed is making this so. The truth is that having a complicated pregnancy is more normal than you think. One out of five women (some physicians say one of every three) have some kind of complication of pregnancy.

The other major emotion you're likely to experience during this difficult period is fear. It will run the gamut from simple nervousness, to feeling really anxious, to sheer terror. Most of the fear is focused on the potential for losing the baby.

For Marie, the hardest part of it was "being scared to death that the baby was going to die. I was doing all these things to keep the pregnancy going, and it still might not work out."

The fear is cyclical and will ebb and flow depending on how you feel you're doing each day. We tend to fear what we don't understand. Communicating with your doctor is one way to help yourself keep on top of the fear. Get as much information from him about your condition as you can, and ask him specific questions about what you can do to affect positively the way your pregnancy turns out. Read the chapters of this book that describe your complication(s) so you can understand the mechanics of what is going on inside you (see also the Other Reading and Resources section). And take reassurance in the fact that by complying with bedrest and your physician's other instructions, you will be doing everything you can to make things turn out well.

Even so, don't be surprised when you find yourself simply angry about it all. At some point during your confinement, you can expect to feel angry at your baby (for keeping you in bed), your husband (for getting you into bed in the first place), your doctor (for not just fixing the problem), and everyone else you can think of. You may not think so now, but they will all survive your wrath.

Getting Practical: What You Can Do to Help Yourself

It is important for you to take an active interest in your care during bedrest, not only to counteract your fear, but also to deal with your other emotions as well. If you act helpless, you'll feel helpless. As soon as you can, start planning for your own care. Commit to a goal of getting all the way to term without another hitch, and then plan for every contingency you can think of.

DETERMINE HOW INACTIVE YOU MUST BE

Start by quizzing your doctor thoroughly about exactly what you can and cannot do. The questionnaire on the opposite page, compiled by Lennette Moses of Intensive Caring Unlimited, a Philadelphia/ Southern New Jersey parent support group, covers just about every contingency. You should make sure that you ask these questions of your doctor as soon as possible, and again if your medical condition changes.

WHAT IS BEDREST?

The term "bedrest" is a familiar one to mothers experiencing high-risk pregnancies, but they are often confused about the exact parameters of their limitations. Variabilities depend on each mother, the extent of her complications and even on the physician himself. This chart has been developed in an attempt to help mothers and their OB/GYNs mutually define needs in specific situations. Since variables change during each individual pregnancy, you may wish to make several copies of this chart, to be completed at various stages of your pregnancy.

Date   Date

What Can I Do Right Now?
1. Activity Level
Maintain a normal activity level __
Slightly decrease activity level   __
Greatly decrease activity level   —

2. Working Outside the Home
Maintain my full-time job   —
Work part-time (how many
hours?)   —
Work in my home (how
many hours?)   —
Stop work completely   —
Why: _____

3. Working Inside the Home
Continue doing all housework   —
Decrease housework including:
Heavy lifting (laundry,
moving furniture, etc.)   —
Preparing meals (standing on
feet for a prolonged period
of time)   —
Vigorous scrubbing   —
Other: _____
Why: _____

4. Child Care
Care for other children as usual __
No lifting children   —
Have another caretaker watch
an active toddler   —

Have permanent caretaker for
children   —
Why: _____

5. Mobility
Continue normal mobility   —
Limit mobility (sit down
frequently)   —
Lie down each day (how
many hours?)   —
Recline all day (propped up)   —
Lie down flat all day (on side?) __
May walk stairs (how many
times a day?)   —
Stairs forbidden   —
Take a shower/wash hair   —
Eat lying down? Sitting up?
Sitting at table?   —
Why: _____

6. Driving
May drive a car   —
May be a passenger in a car
(frequently?)   —
May not ride in a car, except to
doctor   —
Why: _____

7. Bathroom Privileges
May use bathroom normally   —
Should actively avoid
constipation   —
May not use bathroom (use
bedpan)   —
Why: _____

Date   **Date**

8. Sexual Relations
May continue normal sexual
  relations   ___
Should limit relations
  (maximum times a month?)   ___
Should avoid intercourse   ___
Should avoid all types of
  relations which stimulate
  female orgasm   ___
Should abstain from sexual
  relations   ___
Why: _____

9. Maintenance of Pregnancy
Should monitor fetal activity
  ___ hours each day by hand,
  counting movements   ___
Should drink wine each day
  (When? How much?)   ___
Should abstain from all alcohol ___
Should limit cigarette smoking
  (no. per day?)   ___
Should stop smoking cigarettes   ___
Should monitor fetus by
  electronic home monitor
  ___ hours daily   ___
Should take (drug) _____
  ___ times daily, dosage: _____
  Reason: _____
Should take (drug) _____
  ___ times daily, dosage: _____
  Reason: _____
Should follow these dietary rules:
Plenty of: Protein, vegetables,
  fruits, calcium,
  other: _____
Avoid: Excess salt, excess
  fats, junk food, spicy foods,
  other: _____
Approximate number of calories
  a day: _____

What Might I Expect in the Future?
1. Decrease in Activity Level   ___
2. Limitations on Work
   Stop working completely   ___
3. Decrease Housework   ___

4. Need for childcare helper   ___
5. Need to recline in bed   ___
   Need to stay in bed
   (total bedrest)   ___
6. Limit driving   ___
   Stop driving   ___
7. Limit sexual relations   ___
   Abstain from sexual relations ___
8. Need to self-monitor fetal
   activity   ___
9. Need to use a home monitor ___
10. Need to take labor-inhibiting
    drugs   ___
11. Need to have a cervical stitch
    put in   ___
12. Need to stay in hospital for
    some period of time   ___
13. Need to have amniocentesis ___
14. Need to have sonograms/
    ultrasounds   ___
15. Need to visit OB/GYN more
    frequently than normal   ___
16. Need to visit a High-Risk
    specialist   ___
17. Need to have Alpha-fetal
    Protein Levels done   ___
18. Need to have blood sugar
    screening   ___
19. Need to have a Non-Stress
    Test   ___
20. Need to have a Stress Test   ___

**If Problems Arise and I Go into
Premature Labor . . .**
1. When should I contact my
   OB/GYN?   ___
2. Where will I be hospitalized? ___
3. Where might I be transferred? ___
4. Name of OB/GYN at other
   hospital?
5. Where would my baby be
   hospitalized?   ___
6. Could my husband be present
   at delivery?   ___
7. Is there a possibility of a
   cesarean?   ___

Date   **Date**

HOSPITAL BEDREST

1. **What position do I have to be in?**
   Trendelenberg (head lowered) ___
   On side (left or right?) ___

2. **Do I have to use a bedpan?** ___

3. **Can I reach for things, or should I use a reacher?** ___

4. **Personal hygiene**
   Can I take a shower? ___
   Can I take a bath? ___
   Do I have to take a bed sponge bath? ___
   Can I get out of bed to wash my hair? ___

5. **Mobility**
   Can I walk the halls? ___
   Can I walk in my room? ___
   Can I sit in the chair in my room? ___
   Can I take a wheelchair to the lobby? ___
   Can I take a wheelchair to the nursery? ___

Can I take a wheelchair to hospital support group meetings? (If applicable) ___

6. **Visitors**
   When can my husband visit? ___
   (If you do not have a husband):
   Can I have another friend or relative visit at the times husbands are normally permitted to visit? ___
   Who can visit? When _____
   Can my children visit? When? ___
   How many people can visit at a time? ___
   If I am admitted to the labor room, who can visit? _____
   Who can be present in the delivery room? _____

7. **Consults**
   If appropriate, may I see:
   a physical therapist ___
   an occupational therapist ___
   a neonatologist (about fetal development and/or a typical preemie) ___
   a social worker ___
   an opthalmologist ___
   a dermatologist ___

8. **Other directions:**

This chart was developed by Intensive Caring Unlimited, a Philadelphia/Southern New Jersey parent support group. Copies may be made without permission. Please address questions and comments to: Lennette Moses, ICU, 910 Bent Lane, Philadelphia, PA 19118.

Give Notice at Work

If the need to go on bedrest is immediate, and you are a working person, you'll have to inform your boss that you won't be coming to work for a while, and you'll probably have to do it over the phone. If you have some time to plan, you'll be able to sit down with your supervisor ahead of time and explain the situation, and you should. Help your company by giving them as much lead time before you leave as possible.

Before you call or meet with your boss, consider that you may have to let your supervisor know where your unfinished files or other projects are located in your office. Think about whom you can suggest to cover for you during your absence in the short term and in the long run. Write down everything you want to talk about beforehand. Otherwise you'll tend to forget details.

Find Out About Company Maternity and Disability Leave Policy

Your company may have its own policy on maternity leave that includes some coverage for disability before the baby is born. Ask your direct supervisor about this, or check with your personnel department. Many larger firms treat pregnancy disability the same as any other medical disability and will continue full pay for some period, followed by partial pay for the duration. In some cases, you may be able to continue working from home and remain on full pay until the baby is born. It is more than worth your while to check into this—and to try to negotiate some form of pay continuation if your firm has no set policy that it follows.

Find Out About Medical Insurance Coverage

As soon as you found out you were pregnant, you probably looked into your medical insurance to see what your coverage provides for pregnancy. But you probably did not explore what your coverage would be if you were disabled by the pregnancy. Now is the time to check into it.

Unfortunately, insurers generally are not terrific about reimbursements or coverage for such bedrest-related items as in-home helpers, home-monitoring devices that detect preterm contractions, and in-home IV hookups. You will have to be prepared to fight for yourself when it comes to getting reimbursement in many cases. Insurers seem to need to be convinced that reimbursing seventy-five dollars a day for a mother's helper who performs the services you really require (someone to fix meals, take care of the kids, tidy the house, do the shopping) is more cost-effective than paying five hundred dollars a day for in-hospital supervision.

But in fairness, there are a few companies that do provide at least a modicum of coverage. Some companies will cover in-home, non-nursing care—but only if you've spent at least five days in the hospital first. Others will cover such care only if the helper is "supervised" by a registered nurse. The visiting nurse associations in most metropolitan areas provide such a service. If your obstetrician will cooperate with the insurance company and act as your advocate, you'll have a better chance of having your costs covered at least partially.

ARRANGE FOR CHILD CARE

If you have children, arranging for their care is one of the most stressful aspects of bedrest. You'll be out of commission for some time, and you will worry constantly about their well-being if you don't make firm arrangements for them. This is also important for the children. Having a mommy who can no longer do the things that they are used to will upset them. Providing reliability through other adults (even if you have to string together ten friends to take care of it all) will help your kids to continue to feel secure. So start thinking immediately about the changes in care-taking arrangements that your bedrest will necessitate.

If you are your family's primary caregiver, someone will have to take over for you almost fully. Someone else will have to get them up in the morning, make their meals, take them to and pick them up from day care or school or watch them at your house, take them to playdates and lessons, bathe and feed and put them to bed. You will want to keep their schedules as close to normal as possible while you are on bedrest. If you have a husband or helpmate, you have at least some built-in assistance; if you don't, now is the time to call your closest relative or friends and tell them you have an emergency. If you have the money to do it, hire an au pair or other full-time child care worker.

This does not mean that you will or should give up all your responsibility for or contact with the kids. There are lots of quiet activities that you can still do together. Drawing, painting, watching TV, reading books, sewing, playing with dolls or playing games, listening to the radio, and just talking to each other are some of the many pastimes suitable for bedresting moms and their kids. Make one or more of these part of your daily regimen and their daily schedule. Consistent, loving contact with your children while you are on bedrest is essential for them—and for you.

Of course, your kids are going to demand an explanation for why you can't get out of bed (or off the couch) to play with them. They will want to know why Mommy is "sick." Tell them the truth: Mommy isn't sick, but she has to stay in bed to help the baby inside her grow and stay well and be strong. Mommy won't always be in bed, just until the baby is born. You will probably have to repeat this message often.

As long as you are straight with them, and keep communicating your love for them through your words, your touch, and your activities, your children will suffer no permanent psychological harm from your bedrest. Remember, children are extremely adaptable. They will probably cope with your bedrest better than you will.

ARRANGE FOR YOUR OWN CARE

In your rush to take care of everyone and everything else important to you, *don't forget to take care of yourself.* That means making sure that you have someone to prepare your meals and make them readily accessible to you and keep you supplied with magazines, books, newspapers, and things to do. It also means thinking about and arranging to have those items and comforts around your bed that will make your life as easy as possible. Lying around in bed twenty-four hours a day is boring and stressful. There will be times when, no matter what you do, you'll feel like you are going out of your mind. But the more you plan ahead and the more organized you are about your activities, the less maddening staying in bed will be.

SETTING UP YOUR ROOM

The questionnaire on page 299 will help you define your exact limitations, and you can then begin planning around them. Set up your room so that you have at least the following within arm's reach:

- telephone and telephone book
- radio
- remote control for the TV
- pad of paper and pens, pencils
- box of tissues
- pitcher of beverage and glass
- your essential toiletries
- prescription medicines
- magazines, newspapers, books
- knitting, crocheting, embroidery, and the like

Also have ready your slippers, a robe, and an extra nightie if you decide to stay in bedclothes. Or have a change of clothes at the edge of the bed, so you can stay fresh all day if you want.

If you have no kitchen privileges and no one at your beck and call to bring you refreshments, keep a cooler or small refrigerator near the bed, stocked with snacks and liquids. Make sure it's at least at waist level, so you won't have to bend down for it.

A Word About Working from Bed

If you are one of the lucky few who have jobs that can be continued from bed, you may have a tough time finding ways to set yourself up comfortably. As a reporter, I kept writing stories from bed by using a laptop computer, a modem, and the telephone. But the computer became unwieldy once my belly got big. I have since learned that you can buy or rent hydraulic platforms to attach to everything from your phone and fax to your computer. Once installed (you may have to bolt it to the wall), the unit is operable with one hand and can assume numerous positions, so that even if you are lying on your side, you could work a keyboard. Absent one of these, you can purchase or rent a hospital-type bedside stand that rolls under your bed and swings up over the mattress. It has a height adjustment so you can compensate for your big belly, and you can push it out of the way with one hand when you're tired of working or need to get up.

You needn't be computer-literate to work from home. You can dictate documents and send the tapes to the office via a courier service. You can even handwrite or type reports and then fax them to the office. And you don't have to own these devices. Almost every city has an office-equipment rental store that will outfit you with whatever you need.

There's a lot of room for creativity if your company is willing to support your desire to work from home. One woman I spoke to had a life-size photo of herself propped in her chair at the weekly office managers' meeting and then participated in each conference via speakerphone.

CREATE A SCHEDULE AND STICK TO IT

Setting up a daily routine for yourself is a key way to counteract the feelings of helplessness and listlessness that are the natural consequence of spending weeks in bed. It doesn't really matter what your regimen is, as long as you keep it consistent. At the least (if you are allowed), you should awake at a regular time, bathe, dress, or change your gown, and take meals at consistent hours of the day. If you are a makeup wearer, put some on each day, even if no one is going to see you.

Plan your other activities to give you some constancy, too. Setting a schedule for yourself gives you daily markers against which to measure off time and creates stability. So if you have favorite TV shows, note when they are and watch them. Don't leave the TV on all day just for background noise or it will lose its usefulness as a separate activity. Listen to music instead. Set specific times aside for phone calls, letter writing, reading articles or books. If you've never taken up hand crafts, now's a good time to learn to knit, crochet, or do needlework. (I did needlepoint throughout my confinement. I haven't done it since, but it helped pass a couple of hours of every day.) Arrange regular visiting times for certain friends or family members.

Everyone has a different way to keep herself busy while she's in bed. Be creative and do what you think will work for you. To get you started, here are some ideas from women who have been in your position and made it through to the end:

> "I would set up special evenings for 'dates' with my husband. He'd bring home a different kind of take-out dinner every time, and sit in bed with me for a dinner 'out.' Then we'd watch a rented movie and eat popcorn." —Joan.

> "Get someone to teach you relaxation techniques, so you can feel like you are in control."—Caryn

> "I often worked out a schedule that the children could count on, like watching *Sesame Street* together. We did puzzles, memory books of photos, and we read together."—Paige

> "Two of the things that really helped me were that Peter brought all the prisms up that I had in the house, so I had rainbows in the room all day long. He also got me fresh flowers every week throughout my whole pregnancy. It didn't cost very much, and it really helped me."—Lennette

> "I couldn't do fine motor things because I was on ritodrine to stop contractions and it made my hands shake. But I had my husband bring me dresser drawers, and I'd rearrange each one. I got the baby's room ready by having my husband do the laundry and bring it to me. I'd read the kids stories. I did a lot of writing. A friend of mine in Germany was also on bedrest, so we wrote to each other a lot."—Lori

> "I got dressed, whether I could be up or not. I earned those maternity clothes, so I was going to wear them."—Patricia

> "I kept a journal, and that helped me."—Marie

"We were house hunting when I was sent to bed. So I had my husband bring home pictures of each house he saw. Then, every time we saw a house I liked, I'd decorate it. I'd draw floor plans."

—Shelley

Use Emotional Support Groups or Counselors

This is no time for you to be a martyr. You're going to want a lot of support and comforting, and it's a mistake to expect your loved ones or friends to provide it all. They can't. They're going to be quite busy taking care of your physical needs and tending to their own feelings.

"You need to know the people that you can talk to," says Patricia, a former bedrester who started and runs a bedrest support group called High Risk Moms, Inc., in Naperville, Illinois. "There are a lot of people who don't understand what you're going through, and they unintentionally say things that hurt you because you're in a raw state emotionally." Also, it's a fact that after a while, most people get tired of hearing how scared or rotten you feel. That doesn't mean you should stop talking about how bedrest is for you. You just need to find an appropriate outlet for your feelings.

No one understands how you are feeling better than another bedrester. There are an increasing number of bedrester support groups that you can turn to at no cost. And you can always turn to a psychologist or other licensed counselor who is trained and whose job it is to help you through this difficult time. Talk to your obstetrician about getting trained professional support, if he doesn't offer that information to you. Be firm about asking for a referral. If he doesn't have one handy, request that he make inquiries.

Bedrest Support Groups

The following groups are some of the best organized and most stable bedrest support groups in the United States. The list is not comprehensive, since more support groups spring up all the time. If none of the groups described below has a branch in your area, ask your obstetrician if he knows of any bedrest support groups. If he doesn't know of one, ask him if he can introduce you to another one of his patients who is on bedrest, or, failing that, one of his colleague's patients on bedrest. I can almost guarantee you that you're not the only woman in your town on pregnancy bedrest.

Also, check with your local hospitals' maternity wards and ask if they sponsor a pregnancy bedrest outreach program or discussion group. If you turn up nothing, call one of the groups listed below.

They will try their best to find someone for you to talk with, even if it has to be long-distance. Or, at the very least, they will talk to you and send you material to help you start a group of your own. Now there's something that will keep you occupied while you rest!

INTENSIVE CARING UNLIMITED
910 BENT LANE
PHILADELPHIA, PA. 19118

This group will try to match bedresters up with each other in the greater Philadelphia and southern New Jersey areas. ICU is a parent support organization to share information and resources with parents and professionals who care for children who are premature, high-risk, or have special problems, parents who are experiencing a high-risk pregnancy or who have lost a child. They also publish a bi-monthly newsletter that includes information on pregnancy bedrest and maintain a resource list of other parent support organizations and services. For referrals in Greater Philadelphia and surrounding counties, subscription information or resources, telephone: (215) 328–3128. For referrals in Southern New Jersey, call: (609) 799-2059

THE CONFINEMENT LINE
C/O Childbirth Education Association
P.O. Box 1609
Springfield, Va. 22151
(703) 941-7183

A resource and referral service and support network for women confined to bed in the Washington, D.C., area. They will find you a bedrest buddy and check in on you from time to time to see how you are doing. Supported by the March of Dimes, they publish a newsletter on bedrest, a checklist of questions for you to ask your doctor and a "Yellow Pages" of services in the D.C. area for homebound women. They are also compiling a how-to manual for starting your own "confinement line."

HIGH RISK MOMS, INC.
P.O. Box 4013
NAPERVILLE, IL 60567-4013
(708) 357-5048

A tax-exempt support group that maintains a telephone network for moms on bedrest in the greater Chicago area. They will connect you with other women who are currently on bedrest, plus check in with you at least twice a month to see how you are doing. They also hold monthly support meetings for women who have completed bedrest.

PARENT CARE, INC.
101½ SOUTH UNION STREET
ALEXANDRIA, VA 22314
(703) 836-4678

This is a national organization that supports the establishment and maintenance of parent support groups in neonatal intensive care units. The national headquarters does not provide services for bedresters. However, a number of state and local chapters do. Parent Care, Inc., can tell you whether the groups in your area offer bedrest support.

VERY IMPORTANT PREGNANCY PROGRAM (VIP)
HEALTHDYNE PERINATAL SERVICES
P.O. Box 11085
ROCKFORD, IL 61126
(800) 999-2416
(800) 779-7676 (Ask-a-Nurse)

A program co-sponsored by HealthDyne Perinatal Services—one of the several companies in the country that provide home-monitoring equipment for premature labor—and Rockford Memorial Hospital. VIP is a volunteer complement to the services offered by the company. Among its other services, the program will pair both hospitalized and at-home high-risk moms who want a telephone buddy who has previously experienced similar problems. VIP publishes a bimonthly newsletter and will send it to anyone who calls or writes with a request. They will also assist women who want to start local support groups of their own.

PREPARING FOR CHILDBIRTH

When I had been in bed for twenty-two weeks, my husband and I hired a private Lamaze instructor who came to the house once a week. Pam was great. She was kind and funny, and she just happened to be a nurse at the hospital where I planned to deliver. Practicing my breathing and relaxation exercises a few times a day gave me something new to do when I really needed it.

We hadn't quite completed our course when my water broke and I went into labor at twenty-nine weeks. Over the last five and a half weeks of my pregnancy, in bed, in the hospital, I must have used those

Lamaze techniques at least fifty times. They helped me control my fear during my cesarean and helped reduce the pain after the surgery, too.

You may find it difficult to focus on the birth of your child right now. You have medical complications, and you may choose not to attach yourself too strongly to the notion of a positive outcome. One way or another, though, it's a fact that you are going to give birth. Whether you expect to deliver vaginally at term, prematurely, or by cesarean, you should focus some attention on the process and prepare for it. What you learn from books or a childbirth instructor will serve you well no matter what happens.

Listed in the Other Reading and Resources section of this book are several suggested books on childbirth preparation. I urge you to read at least one of them and to practice the breathing and relaxation techniques it describes (if your condition and physician allow it).

Ideally, you should read several texts, and go to group classes. But if you are in my situation, then hire a private instructor to come to your home and give you lessons on ways to get through labor and birth with as much awareness and as little pain as possible.

A Final Word About Pregnancy Bedrest

Having to go to bed to maintain your pregnancy is at once one of the most benign treatments for your unborn child and, outside of long-term hospitalization or surgery, the most radical treatment for you. It is a difficult prescription to take, and getting through prolonged bedrest successfully will take great effort on your part. Your life as you've known it will change radically for the next few weeks or months and will require adjustments by your loved ones as well as you.

Once your healthy baby is born, you won't regret a single minute of having been in bed. A bedrester named Sarah states the bottom line: "When I look back on it, the two and a half months I spent on bedrest was a small price to pay to have Kyle. In the two years we've had him, he's more than paid me back for my confinement."

16

For the Fathers: What Happens to You When Pregnancy Isn't Perfect?

"For every woman with a complicated pregnancy, there's a man out there somewhere who is affected, too." That's how Ron began the story of *his* complicated pregnancy and the subsequent death of his son shortly after birth. It took Ron and Barbara over a year to conceive, and once she was pregnant, Barbara began having bleeding problems. She was placed on partial bedrest and, at fourteen weeks, was given a cerclage (a stitch through the cervix to help it stay closed). In the fourth month Barbara quit working and rested even more, but bouts of bleeding continued off and on.

"While all this was going on," Ron told me, "I felt helpless. There wasn't anything I could do about Barbara's condition." And Ron was frustrated that his wife wasn't able to give him complete information about her condition: "She would go for a checkup herself, and then I would ask her, 'Well what did he say?' She'd answer, 'I don't know. The doctor said a lot of medical things, and I don't remember.' So I took to calling the doctor myself. It would have driven me nuts not to know what was going on.

"At home, I did everything. I wouldn't let Barbara do anything. I did all the housework. And I carried on at my job. I was exhausted, but I was just so excited about the baby. I wallpapered the whole damn house. It didn't really sink in how severe the problems were in the pregnancy.

"On December tenth, around the twenty-eighth week, Barbara started to bleed noticeably. So at one in the morning, I took her to the hospital—the oldest obstetrics hospital in the country. A resident did an ultrasound. Basically nobody told me anything, except that my wife had an abrupted placenta. I didn't realize how grave that was. That was on a Saturday night. I went away that night figuring everything was under control. Sunday I visited her. Monday I had to go back to the office, but I got a call from the doctor, who said we have to take the baby tonight. So I go dashing down there, and my son is delivered.''

The baby was born twelve weeks prematurely. He had severe respiratory distress syndrome, bleeding in the brain, and numerous other problems. Sixteen days later, the baby died.

''And that whole time, from the beginning of the pregnancy until well after the baby died, no one, not even my own mother, asked me how I was doing! It felt like I had been excommunicated from the world. And when anybody asked, it was always, 'How's Barbara?' Nobody ever said 'How are you? How do you feel?' The message is that number one, a man's not supposed to show any emotion. Number two, not only is he not supposed to show it, he's not supposed to have it. How's Barbara?! She was a disaster!

''There's nothing established to ask the guy how he's doing. I don't know why. I guess because it's not on anybody's agenda. The father's like the forgotten person in a complicated pregnancy—even more so if the baby dies. It's like you don't really exist.''

TRADITIONALLY, MEN ARE LEFT ON THEIR OWN WHEN THEIR PARTNER'S PREGNANCY ISN'T PERFECT.

There are no books, in medical or lay terms, that address the man's side of the bargain. Hardly any psychologists or social workers specialize in counseling the male partner of a complicated pregnancy. And there are pitifully few organizations to which you can turn for a little support or even a reality check on whether what you're going through is normal under the circumstances.

We all know that your wife has gotten a raw deal with her pregnancy. What everyone, maybe even including your wife, forgets is that you've been dealt a lousy hand, too. Not many, if any, people will stop and acknowledge your rotten luck during your wife's complications. Even though you'll probably get a healthy baby when all this is over, it's okay to call a spade a spade: What you are going through, or may go through if problems have just started, stinks, plain and simple.

What Changes Can I Expect in My Own Routine?

If your partner has just been diagnosed with complications, you may not have had time yet to think about what those complications will mean for you. But you are definitely in for some changes in routine. There are certain common responses and stages you'll be likely to go through as your wife's pregnancy moves forward.

MORE RESPONSIBILITIES

To begin, you can expect to have to take on much more responsibility than you already have, particularly if your wife is confined to total bedrest. This is true even if you normally share the household chores fifty-fifty. It will now fall to you to do not only your own chores, but hers as well. You'll also need to do all the shopping and other out-of-house errands that she may usually do.

In the house, the doctor may forbid her to do even the lightest of housework. She may not be allowed out of bed except to use the bathroom. You may have to help her in and out of bed. You may have to cook her meals and yours.

If you have other children, most child care, except for quiet activities that can be done in bed with Mom, will be yours until after the delivery. That means dressing, washing, and feeding them, taking them to lessons and other outdoor activities, putting them to bed at night, and calming their natural fears about their mom's condition.

You will be the most constant tangible link your wife has with the outside world. She's going to want your attention when you get home from work or when you have a break in the household routine. She'll be lonely for company and probably pretty starved for news of the outside world.

If she's in bed, she's bored to tears, angry at the loss of her perfect pregnancy. She may be depressed, demanding, any number of widely ranging emotions, which change like quicksilver from day to day. She's terrified she'll lose her child. She's frightened that something awful and permanent may happen to her. She hates being made helpless by her body and her circumstances. She feels like she let you down, like she's stuck you with the burden of her ''imperfection.''

And it may not be easy for you to deal with her moods. ''I never really knew what the tone would be like when I came home,'' said Mike, whose wife Marie spent virtually her entire pregnancy on bed-rest each time she was pregnant. ''Did Marie have a good day? Were there concerns about the day, physically? I didn't know from one day to the next what to expect. Having to deal with that was the most difficult thing for me.''

"In a lot of families, these changes happen overnight," says Ann Paciulli, a coordinator of volunteers to support women on bedrest. "The man assumes the child care, shopping, cooking, laundering. He's busier than he's ever been in his life. He doesn't have time to himself to relax, or to feel."

Your Sex Life Will Change

"When you're dealing with a complicated pregnancy, your sex life as you knew it is often one of the first things to go," says Sharon N. Covington, one of the few clinical social workers who counsels the male side of complicated pregnancy.

Many pregnancy complications require the woman to refrain from intercourse or orgasm. For instance, a woman experiencing preterm labor cannot afford the contractions caused by orgasm, since these may set off stronger contractions that can cause changes in the cervix, which in turn may lead to premature birth. In another case, a woman with placenta previa may be told not to have intercourse or orgasm because it might provoke serious bleeding.

You, of course, can still function normally, and while your physical needs may stay the same, your wife's may not. She may feel too frightened that her own arousal will somehow bring about injury to the baby, or she may not be up to participating sexually with you in other ways. You may not be willing to ask her to help take care of your needs when she is not allowed to let you reciprocate; or she may be willing and able, but *you* may worry that somehow sex could injure her or the baby.

When you can't have sex or make love with your partner, it can remove the most important way you have of experiencing intimacy and closeness with her. You both might feel frustrated or angry at the situation. And it's not unusual for some of this to translate into strained feelings between the two of you.

If this happens, it may help you to remember that this is a temporary situation. Once your partner gives birth and recovers from the pregnancy and delivery, both of you will be able to resume a more satisfying sexual relationship.

It will also help if you can talk about your feelings with your wife and listen to how she's feeling about the intimate part of your relationship. You can remind each other that sexual expression can take many forms. You needn't have intercourse, and she does not have to have an orgasm for you to have fun with each other.

And something else to keep in mind is that you can love each other without *making* love. As difficult as it may be at this time, try to find a way to put a little romance into your relationship. For instance, even if your partner cannot get out of bed, you can still plan and share a candlelight dinner, or rent a videotape for the VCR, make some popcorn, and cuddle up for a "night at the movies." You can send her flowers, bring her balloons, give her a beautiful nightie—anything to express your love for her. Believe me, she will appreciate these little things, because chances are she's not feeling her most attractive or lovable.

How Do I Fit into the Doctor/Patient Relationship?

"I felt like I was an outsider," said Mike. "The woman and her doctor develop a real strong bond between each other. Marie came to be dependent on that relationship. And not just on the doctor, but also the nurses. As a spouse, I really had a hard time feeling like I was part of that communication. Marie was real good about sharing what she knew, so I didn't feel that I was lacking information. But the doctor/patient relationship kind of made it feel like we had 'another man' between us. It wasn't until after the birth that I finally felt like I had my wife back."

Mike's sentiments are common. As the pregnancy progresses, especially if there are ongoing problems, your wife will develop a special relationship with her obstetrician. She has to: Your wife is counting on her doctor to get her through the pregnancy with a good outcome. She will be relying on his advice, talking with him frequently. She may need to believe in him completely in order to feel safe and maintain some degree of calm about her situation.

You may feel like there's not much room for you in this. After all, the doctor's main relationship is with your wife and the life inside her. He is most concerned with her physical well-being and that of the child. He's not likely to come to you with information about your wife's condition; you'll have to go to him.

And when the man does try to take an active role, some doctors don't welcome the additional input and questions. In fact, some doctors—although one hopes not many—will not even talk to the husband about his wife's condition unless the wife signs a release form specifying that he can have the information. And the doctor needn't be a man for you to feel like the odd person out.

But there are also a great many obstetricians that welcome the man's participation. My OBs made my husband feel included at every office visit. Sometimes, especially when I was in the hospital with preterm labor and preterm premature rupture of my membranes, my doctors gave more complete information to my husband than they did to me! Ideally, your wife's doctor should treat you as an ally and an indispensable part of the whole process.

You Are Your Partner's Advocate

You *are* an indispensable part of the whole process, whether you are made to feel that way or not. There are going to be times when you'll be called upon to be your wife's advocate. And you'll need to be prepared.

The most important part of that preparation is being informed. "You should know as much as or more than your wife does and be aware that there may be many instances when you have to act as your wife's advocate," said Aaron, whose wife was hospitalized in the middle of the night when her water broke in her sixth month. "If you end up in a situation such as mine, and your wife is gravely ill and has complications, being as equipped as possible to be her advocate will give you the best chance to feel like you're in control of the situation, and that you're doing the best job for her and your child. It's too late to read the books once you go into the hospital.

"Depending on what the complication is, and my wife had quite a few of them, there may be times when she is just not able to consider what the ramifications are of the treatments that the doctor is discussing for her condition."

Aaron felt that he didn't know enough to do the best by his wife when her complicated pregnancy reached this crisis. "My wife was given mag sulfate," a contraction-stopping drug. "We were at the hospital for an emergency and they said it would stop the contractions, but I didn't understand completely what the drug was. When my wife had a terrible reaction to it, we'd only been in labor and delivery for about half an hour, so I was still just going along with whatever the doctor was saying. My wife had an intense reaction to the drug; she became almost hysterical. And she's lying there asking me to tell them to stop it. So I did.

"At that point, either I represented her or she wasn't going to get her way because she was too upset to make demands that would be paid attention to. They were treating her like an object—in a caring manner, but they were doing their job and they were just not going to pay attention to her, so I forced them to stop. If I had understood better why they were using the drug, what it was for, and how long this really awful reaction my wife was having would last, I would have instead helped her get through it for the sake of the baby. If I had been better informed, I would have been a better advocate. And I could have explained it to her."

The mag sulfate was only one of the decisions Aaron was called upon to make. "The first night we were in the hospital, there were all sorts of choices to be made, including whether we should let the contractions go on and allow the baby to be born that night, or stop them with the drugs. It was our decision to make. That's a real surprise when it happens.

"That's the level of advocacy that I'm talking about. There are those kinds of decisions that you will be expected to take part in. And if you're not ready, you'll feel like an ass. You'll feel incompetent. And you'll feel like there's nothing you can do. And at that point, being your wife's advocate is all you *can* do."

Being the Best Advocate You Can Be

Educate Yourself

How do you go about equipping yourself to be your wife's best advocate? You're going to have to do some reading and ask a lot of questions. The idea is to become as well-versed as possible in your wife's condition. There are several ways to do that.

Gregg educated himself by computer when he found out his wife was carrying twins with a rare complication. "I searched out all the medical information I could find. I found an on-line database with data on this complication. I got the statistics so that I could make decisions and understand. You know, doctors don't tell you everything, and sometimes they don't know everything. It wasn't very hard to become—at least statistically—as knowledgeable as they were."

Michael used a hands-on approach during his wife's triplet pregnancy. "I got involved pretty much. Whenever my wife went to the hospital, I went with her. Whenever I felt something wasn't right, I said so. I was looking at every aspect like that. I wanted to find out what was going on for sure. I didn't want guesswork. I was all demands. I think it really helped. If you don't ask, you just don't know. I asked a lot. And I got a lot of answers. I was happy about that. You have to know what's going on."

Jim, whose wife had hypertension, read portions of all the books his wife read. "At least that way, I knew what to expect," he said.

And you can do reading on your own. You may want or need to know more about certain issues than your wife does. For example, your wife might not be prepared to read about pregnancy loss. But you may want to know what options you'll have available to you if the worst should happen, so that you can help guide the two of you through it.

As a start, I encourage you to read the other chapters in this book

that pertain to your wife's problem(s), including the chapters on cesarean section and pregnancy loss. Even if your wife doesn't read these,
you'll be able to explain things to her at the appropriate times. It will
give her a sense of security knowing that she can turn to you for
information. You will also feel better able to handle discussions with
medical personnel, and you'll feel more in control generally.

View Yourself as a Full Participant

Your wife may be the one with the baby in the belly, but these are
your problems, too. You need to know as much as you can about the
situation. I encourage you to participate in the whole treatment process. Go to each office visit if you can; certainly accompany your partner to the hospital if humanly possible. When you do go, ask questions.
And go with the attitude that the doctor and other medical staff should
view you as an integral part of the pregnancy. Jump into the conversation when you have comments or questions. Speak up, even if you
perceive that your presence makes the health care provider uncomfortable. You have as much a right to be fully informed as your wife.

Dealing with Hospital Personnel

Part of your advocacy role will involve assuring that your wife gets
the kind of care you want to see her receive, especially at the hospital.
Hospitals thrive on routine. But it is possible, within limits, to work
with the staff to help tailor your wife's care more to her own needs
and rhythms. In order to do that, you have to know how the system
works. Chapter 14, What to Expect When You Go to the Hospital,
will give you a good idea of what it will be like for her there.

Once you understand what the routine is at your wife's hospital,
you'll want to start trying to make sure that she doesn't become just
one more body that the staff attends to. Here's where the old saying
that you catch more flies with honey than with vinegar applies.

"I had quite a few talks with nursing staff, humoring them, strok-
ing them, if you will, so they'd be more responsible, so they'd give my
wife some special attention that they might not give someone else, even
though she might be demanding or unpleasant because of what she
was going through," said John. "I wanted them to take care of Maureen just as if I was in the room. I was hoping that they would be an
extension of me when I wasn't there—to take care of her the way I
would."

Sometimes your efforts will be well rewarded; other times they
won't. I was in the hospital for a month before I delivered, and then
another week after that recovering from my c-section. My husband

struck up a friendly relationship with one of the night nurses, who later looked the other way every time he stayed over in my room. Eventually, she even brought him a cot to use, so he wouldn't have to sleep on the floor. I got friendly with her, too. She'd come and keep me company sometimes, in between floor rounds on the nights my husband couldn't be with me. Her personal interest in what happened to me made my prolonged hospital stay easier. And I have my husband to thank for that.

Sometimes being your wife's advocate at the hospital will mean interceding to help her retain her dignity or sense of privacy. For instance, there are no locks on the door to the room. Hospital personnel think nothing of walking in on your wife while she's changing her clothes or using the toilet. Something as minor as your "standing guard" while she slips into a clean nightgown can make her day better.

John arranged with the nurses on the floor that they would clean out his wife's bathroom more often than the twice-a-day schedule called for, "so that she felt more at home and comfortable. For my wife, that little nicety made the difference in her being able to tolerate being hospitalized for weeks."

And being an advocate may also mean suggesting ways of coping to your wife. One man I spoke with said that when the doctors came into his wife's room, they were so hurried that she would get flustered and not remember what she wanted to ask them. He helped her get into the habit of writing down her questions when she thought of them, so that she had a list to refer to each time a doctor paid a visit.

What Am I Going to Feel?

It is inevitable that you will have strong feelings about what's going on, similar to those that your partner will express to you about herself. You, like she, probably won't like them much. But have them you will. There is no "right" way for you to deal with your situation. Every man has his own way of handling the stress and fear that are part and parcel of the complicated pregnancy experience.

Some of the feelings that are most common among men in a similar situation are discussed below:

Anger and Frustration

It is normal and natural for you to feel angry and frustrated. Anger at the situation, at the doctor for not being able to make your wife better, at friends and family who may not understand what you're going through and don't even ask—and, anger at your wife. Almost all men experience it at one point or another in the pregnancy.

Some of that anger may not seem rational to you. "I kept sort of yelling at myself," said Jerry, whose wife spent several months on bedrest. "I felt so furious at her. And I kept saying to myself: How can you be angry with her, in her condition? She didn't do this on purpose! It was very confusing, and I didn't want to fly off the handle at her. She had enough trouble already. So I just stuffed it."

Your wife's behavior toward you while she's confined to bed may anger you from time to time. While you are turning all of your attention outward and doing doing doing for her, your wife will be turning her attention inward. It's almost impossible for her not to when she's fighting to keep her baby safe inside her. And her self-absorption may sometimes make her unaware of all that you are doing for her. She may act uninterested in your daily activities, while at the same time demanding that you listen to everything she did or thought that day. Her behavior, while understandable given what she's going through, may make you feel unappreciated—which is bound to engender some negative thoughts and feelings.

"We fought some about that kind of stuff," Mike said. "There were times where we didn't understand each other. While Marie was on bedrest, we fought more than we normally would. I didn't have the patience to always be the supporter she needed me to be. Sometimes we didn't really appreciate what the other one was going through, even though we tried."

"I think everyone has at least one fight," Judy, who was on bedrest for most of her pregnancy, told me. "It was hard for me to listen to my husband's frustrations and anger, but when I could, it really cleared the air."

You're also likely to feel angry at hospital personnel, especially when you don't like how they're treating your wife (and there will be times when you won't like it). If your wife is hospitalized, there may be procedures she will have to undergo that cause her physical pain or discomfort. You won't be able to prevent these, and that frustration can make you mad. "When the staff did something that would hurt my wife," said Michael, "I'd really get teed off."

POWERLESSNESS AND HELPLESSNESS

"It was the worst nine months of my life," said Bill, whose wife had bleeding and hypertensive disorders during pregnancy. "It was difficult from the very beginning. I felt helpless, and there was nothing I could do about it. It made me so mad!"

Helplessness in the face of the situation is part of what creates the anger and frustration. It can be a real challenge to the way you normally operate in the world. Most likely you think of yourself as someone able to influence outcomes, to make your life what you want it to be. In your relationship with your wife and children (if you already have some), you may see your role as that of provider and protector. Under normal circumstances, if you see someone or something hurting your loved ones, you'll take action.

But this is a situation that, no matter what you do, you can't fix. You can't make your wife's complications go away. You can't ensure your baby's health. And because of the uncertainty involved in what will happen next, you can't even anticipate your own schedule the way you're used to. It can seem as if there's nothing left within your control.

FEAR

"I was so afraid," Bill told me. "I lived with a feeling of dread most of the time. I just lived with it. I talked to a friend or two about it. But mostly, I just lived in it."

Every man has to live with the fear, at some level. You might classify it as feeling worried, or nervous, or as Michael termed it, feeling "high-strung." Whatever you call it, fear will be a component of your journey through a complicated pregnancy.

It's natural to worry or be scared. You don't know whether your baby will be all right. You worry that your wife won't be okay. You'll worry that the one time you have to stay late at work or leave your wife alone while you're out, something will happen and you won't be there. You'll worry that you'll fly off the handle at an inappropriate time or that you just won't be able to handle the whole situation.

SADNESS AND DISAPPOINTMENT

You may also find yourself feeling down or depressed. Think about it: It's not just your wife's perfect pregnancy that has just turned into a bout with Murphy's Law; it's yours, too. It's a colossal disappointment for both of you. The baby may not seem quite real to you yet, but you probably have had thoughts about what this time would have been like for you—taking your wife shopping for baby things, helping to plan the room. Maybe you were anticipating showing off your wife's big belly or looking forward to having sex without using birth control.

Now, instead, you're shuttling back and forth to doctors or the hospital. You won't be able to take that last romantic vacation alone, just the two of you.

You may not think so, but the loss of the "perfect pregnancy" you'd imagined—that you'd counted on—*is* a real loss. And it doesn't matter that you'll still probably have a healthy baby at the end of this time. It's the loss of the ideal pregnant time that hurts.

ISOLATION

Most likely you won't have many external resources available to you to help you sort out the emotions that a complicated pregnancy brings up. This can make you feel isolated and reinforce your belief that the best way to deal with it is to just keep pushing ahead with your responsibilities.

"Psychologically, for me, it was a real time of isolation," said Stephen. "Complications don't happen during visiting hours or times of the day when you can get in touch with someone else about how you're feeling while your wife is being examined or is in the OR. You're by yourself. That's how it was for me. It was so isolating. I felt like a soldier, just waiting for the next conflict."

Having any of these feelings and more is a "normal" response to the severe stress that complicated pregnancies bring into your relationships and your life.

DON'T BE SURPRISED IF YOUR SITUATION AND FEELINGS AFFECT YOUR PERFORMANCE.

It is also normal for what you are going through to have a negative impact on your ability to concentrate at work or in your other pursuits.

"I kept going to work. I had to," said George, whose wife was hospitalized for over three months with a series of complications. "We were trying to preserve my vacation time and four weeks' leave for after the baby came. So I showed up every day; I mean, my body did. But productivity-wise? I was nowhere close to normal."

WORK AND TIME-OFF POLICIES

Although George's company didn't give him extra time off while his wife was hospitalized, it didn't penalize him for his lessened output either. Most good employers will, if asked (and may even offer without prompting), do what they can to accommodate your needs during this difficult time. Some will provide paid time off; some will dock pay; still others will offer a combination of paid and unpaid leave.

Now is a good time to inquire about your company's policy,

and if it is not favorable, to petition your management for an exemption in your case. It never hurts to make the request: The worst thing they'll say is no.

Of course, how each man deals with his work situation will vary. You may want and/or need to keep working because it offers you an emotional and physical break from the problems at home (or hospital). You may not be able to afford taking time off. Or you may feel compelled to drop everything, if you can arrange it, to be with your wife and family. There is no "right" choice. You should do what feels right to you and your wife under your unique circumstances.

Aaron started a leave of absence when his wife first went to the hospital. "I was very lucky that my supervisor allowed me to do that, because my wife hadn't delivered yet," he said. "In fact, she didn't deliver for another five and a half weeks. So I was already using my paternity leave before the baby even arrived. That was stressful.

"If I knew another man who was in the situation that I was, I'd tell him: Overcome what normal reticence you have in your business life, whatever that may be, and explain the situation to your superior. I think people are always comfortable providing time off if someone has died in the family, and that's understood. This situation is like that: You'll find that people understand when your wife is ill, even though it's not a disease. They will understand, or they should if there's not something wrong with them.

"For me, the reality was that there are very few instances in life where it would be more important for me to be with my wife, and I needed for my employer to understand that. And they did."

Some Coping Strategies

There *are* ways to deal with what is happening to you and your partner. This discussion of strategies certainly can't change your situation, but it may help you get to the end of the pregnancy and beyond without feeling like a total wreck.

DON'T JUST "TOUGH IT OUT"

"I didn't look for any support systems. I usually just handled my problems alone. I just lived with them."—Bill

"Emotionally . . . boy. I just kept going. I don't really have a true friend that I turned to to share my feelings with."—Mike

"I didn't seek out anyone."—Aaron

When faced with a pregnancy crisis, this is how most men respond. In our society it's customary to view men as "strong" when they are unemotional, and this is what many men believe is expected of them. Ron's example is typical: He felt that somehow, he "wasn't supposed to cry. I was supposed to be the strong one."

Even when a sympathetic ear is offered, many men say that they would turn away the opportunity to let off steam or share their feelings. For instance, one man I spoke to said that in retrospect, "If somebody had approached me while I was going through it and tried to get me to open up, I would have pretended to be strong enough not to do it."

Handling emotions by holding them in and just getting on with it works to a certain extent: At least you get things done. But you're still left with the emotional baggage that will leave you feeling rotten somewhere down the line, with a permanent distaste for the entire experience. From a mental-health standpoint, it's better to look for outlets for the natural and normal emotions that you are going to be experiencing in the days, weeks, and months ahead. There are numbers of ways to do this.

TALK IT OUT

This means emotional support. You tell how you feel, and the listener just listens and offers some sense of understanding.

You may be surprised at how little you need to make you feel better. A few thoughtful words, an acknowledgment that it must be very hard for you, can give you the support you need to go on with a tough day. It won't take your feelings away, but it will help you to deal with them in a healthier manner.

When looking for people to talk it out with, be aware that not every person you know or to whom you are referred will be a good and sympathetic listener. If you run up against platitudes or attempts to make you "behave like a man," look to someone else for support. Here are some suggestions of where to turn:

- friends or colleagues you feel may be good listeners
- your clergyman
- your partner (she's probably not as fragile as you might think; and sharing your feelings can also help the two of you feel closer during this period of stress)
- another man who has had or is going through a similar experience (if you don't know anyone, ask your wife's OB or the hospital social worker to give you a name and telephone number; you may feel very awkward about doing this, but if you overcome your reticence, you may find that it helps)

- a professional counselor (again, if you don't know one, ask for assistance at the hospital; talking to a therapist or social worker doesn't mean you're admitting you're nuts, or that you have to make a long-term commitment. Just one or two sessions may make the difference between your being miserable and being able to tolerate the situation)
- family members who have the patience and are good listeners

TAKE TIME OUT FOR YOURSELF

You're probably going to be busier in the next few weeks or months than at any other time in your life. And the temptation may be to give up all of your normal outside activities because you don't think you could focus on them. But it's important for your sanity and health that each week you squeeze in some time during which you *do* focus on something that's pleasurable. When you give yourself some breathing space in this way, you'll find you have more of yourself to give to your partner and other children. And you won't end up resenting the situation quite as much. Some suggestions:

- schedule lunch or drinks with a friend
- go to a movie or play
- find a way to jog or work out for an hour several times each week
- take an hour or two for yourself to pursue a sport or a hobby, or just spend time relaxing

You may argue that doing these things is impossible because you can't leave your wife or kids alone. Then don't leave them alone! Arrange for someone you trust to stay with her/them during the couple of hours of well-deserved R&R.

GET HELP WITH CARETAKING RESPONSIBILITIES

Now is no time for you to be a martyr. You're going to be doing enough as it is. Getting help with logistical things does more than just take some of the burden off you. It clears some time for you to spend with your wife (and kids, if you have them). There will be few, if any, times in your life when your support and presence will be more important to your wife. And your need to be with her may be so powerful that it will feel instinctual. Here are three ways to free up some of your time:

Enlist Your Partner's Help

Discuss your responsibilities with your wife, and ask her what she feels she can take on. If she's bedridden, she can still use the phone, pay bills, and so on. In fact, remaining intellectually active and involved in household planning will help her feel useful and like less of a burden. Among other things, she can make shopping lists, fold laundry, arrange for the children to visit neighbors and for friends to come sit with her if she is not supposed to be alone.

Allow Friends and Family to Help

Friends and family will want to assist you. Let them. Be specific about your needs. It will make those people who are close to you feel useful at a time when they desperately want to help. Friends and relations can keep your wife company while you go out, bring over meals, take the kids out, pick up necessities for you when they're out shopping, and take your wife to doctor's appointments. It is no sign of weakness to accept assistance. It's just good sense!

Hire Household Help if You Can Afford It

If you are lucky enough to be able to afford it, hire a housekeeper or housecleaner to help with the extra tasks. While I was bedridden, we hired a cleaning person to clean the house once every other week. It saved my husband hours of work that he was really too busy to do.

Although housecleaning is a service you must pay for yourself, you may be able to obtain reimbursement from your insurer for personal care services provided by nurse's aides, visiting nurses, home health care workers, or social workers who visit your home. Check with the medical insurance companies for both you and your wife on rules and restrictions for coverage.

Loss of Privacy

"Support people were really welcome, but they were also a source of frustration," Mike told me. "When you let them in, you give up control of your house—what you're going to eat, what they've done to take care of your wife. I appreciated them, but I didn't like people being there all the time. I like the privacy of my home, and I didn't get that back until after the baby was born and my wife was home for a while."

As Mike discovered, there is a trade-off you have to make when you accept logistical help: You give up some of your privacy when they take over part of the burden of running the house. If you find your ability to feel and act hospitable wearing thin—and there may be occasions when you do—it may help you to take a step back for a moment and remember that these people are here to help. You want them to treat your wife—and you—well. So you don't want to alienate them.

At the same time, you needn't give up complete control of your home to your helpers. You should feel free to tell your caregivers— politely but firmly—when you need and want privacy. Try to set up your physical space so that it is possible for you to get some private time for yourself, even when caregivers are present. And encourage your wife to do likewise.

GOOD COMMUNICATION IS KEY.

In any crisis situation, tensions build between people. With complicated pregnancies, it's a given that tempers will flare occasionally and that you will get on each other's nerves. Unless you work at keeping the lines of communication open during the coming months, you may find yourselves squabbling more frequently, resenting each other, and/or growing distant, when what you really wish for most is to support each other.

For your part, it may help you to remember that it's your wife's body, not her mind, that is malfunctioning. Even if her condition is delicate, she probably will still be able to listen to your thoughts and fears—even your negative ones. Try to be open with her. Push yourself to share your thoughts with her. It will help you cut through your isolation, and hers, too.

There will be times when it may not be easy for her to listen to some of your feelings, and there may be times when you legitimately believe that your wife won't be able to deal with some of the thoughts you are having. In that case, save those thoughts to share with a friend or a counselor.

Conversely, there may be days when it will drive you crazy to listen one more time to how bad, sad, or scared your partner feels. Those are feelings that, if you want your wife to continue to count on you for support, you had best keep to yourself and handle elsewhere. This is one more place where you will be called upon to be a little more selfless than you may normally be.

"I think in order to understand how your wife is feeling," Aaron told me, "you have to get it that she had the same kind of fantasy, the same ideal, that you did going into this pregnancy. But it's even harder for her, because she's the one who's not living the fantasy that she had expected. And, boy, can it make her cranky! I tried to keep that in mind most of the time. That she'd gotten a really rotten deal. That we both had.

"But I was the one who could still go out of the house; while I was at my job, I was leading a normal life. I just tried to keep in mind that this was something that was going on inside of her, and it was with her day and night. I wasn't always able to do that, but I thought that my whole job was to be supportive. I figured there weren't going to be many other situations in our entire married life where I'd have to be that uncritical of her and just be behind her one hundred percent. But this was one of them. She got enough crap and platitudes about stuffing her emotions from everyone else—family and friends. Because they can't handle it after a while and they just want her to stop talking about it. If you become like that, where's your wife going to turn? It really is one of those times that you really have to be what she needs you to be."

This Too Shall Pass

"It's almost like being in a war," said Gregg. "It's so long and stressful." When you're caught up in the daily stress and crises that complicated pregnancies can bring, it can be terribly hard to remember that this is a temporary situation. Eventually (much sooner than it feels) you're going to be new parents. And as time passes after that, these few months will become a dimly recalled bad patch of time. That's all. Just a fuzzy memory.

"When the boys were born, whatever was balled up inside me totally vanished. It was like a whole new beginning. I feel so lucky. My sons are doing really good."—Michael

"It was worth it. But I wasn't so sure while it was going on. I'm glad now, though."—Bill

"Our relationship got better, and I got stronger, and our relationship got stronger because of it. It's a crisis, and if you survive it, make it through together, you feel better prepared to handle the next one when it comes along."—Mike

Remember, the time, caring, and nurturing you are investing now, combined with great medical care and a little luck, will soon bring your healthy baby into the world. Handling a crisis the best way we know how makes us grow. And no matter how tough it is now, when it's over, you'll be glad you did it, and did it right.

OTHER READING AND RESOURCES

HIGH-RISK PREGNANCY

Brewer, Gail S. *The VIP Program: A Personal Approach to the Art and Science of Having a Baby.* Emmaus, PA: Rodale Press, Inc., 1988.

Hales, Dianne, and Timothy R.B. Johnson, MD. *Intensive Caring: New Hope for High Risk Pregnancy.* New York: Crown Publishers, Inc., 1990.

Harrison, Helen. *The Premature Baby Book.* New York: St. Martin's Press, 1983.

Semchyshyn, Stefan, MD, and Carol Colman. *How to Prevent Miscarriage and Other Crises of Pregnancy.* New York: Macmillan Publishing Co., 1989.

CHILDBIRTH PREPARATION

Bing, Elisabeth. *Six Practical Lessons for an Easier Childbirth.* New York: Bantam Books, 1977.

Cogan, Rosemary, and Suzanne Logan. *Lamaze for the Joy of It.* Garden City Park, NY: Avery Publishing Group, Inc., 1984.

Dick-Read, Grantly. *Childbirth Without Fear: The Original Approach to Natural Childbirth.* New York: Harper & Row, 1987.

Lamaze, Fernand. *Painless Childbirth: The Lamaze Method.* Rev. ed. Chicago: Contemporary Books, 1987.

Novak, Janice. *Enhancing Lamaze Techniques.* Los Angeles: Price Stern Sloan, Inc., 1988.

WHEN PREGNANCY IS PERFECT

Eisenberg, Arlene, Heidi Eisenberg Murkoff, and Sandi Eisenberg Hathaway, RN, BSN. *What to Expect When You're Expecting.* New York: Workman Publishing, 1988.

Flanagan, Geraldine Lux. *The First Nine Months of Life.* New York: Simon and Schuster, 1962.

Junor, Penny. *What Every Woman Needs to Know: Facts and Fears About Pregnancy, Childbirth and Womanhood.* North Pomfret, VT: Century Hutchinson, David and Charles, Inc., 1989.

Samuels, Mike, MD, and Nancy Samuels. *The Well Pregnancy Book.* New York: Summit Books, 1986.

Simkin, Penny, RPT, Janet Whalley, RN, BSN, Ann Kepler, RN, MN. *Pregnancy, Childbirth and the Newborn: A Complete Guide for Expectant Parents.* Deephaven, MN: Meadowbrook, Inc., 1984.

Subak-Sharpe, Genell J., MS, ed. *The Columbia University College of Physicians and Surgeons Complete Guide to Pregnancy.* New York: Crown Publishers, Inc., 1988.

Verilli, George E., MD, FACOG, and Anne Marie Muesser, Ed.D. *While Waiting: Prenatal Guide Book.* New York: St. Martin's Press, 1987.

GESTATIONAL DIABETES

Brudnell, J. M. *Diabetic Pregnancy.* Dallas: Churchill, 1989.

Chahul. *Diabetes and Pregnancy.* Stoneham, MA: Butterworth Publishing, 1988.

Folkman, Jane, and Hugo J. Holleroth. *A Guide for Women with Diabetes Who Are Pregnant or Plan To Be.* Boston: Joslin Diabetes Foundation.

HYPERTENSIVE DISORDERS OF PREGNANCY

Rubin, P. C., ed. *Hypertension in Pregnancy: Handbook of Hypertension,* Vol. 10. New York: Elsevier Science Publishing Co., Inc., 1988.

PRETERM LABOR AND
PREMATURE RUPTURE OF MEMBRANES

Katz, Michael, MD, Pamela Gill, RN, Judith Turiel, RN. *Preventing Preterm Birth: A Parent's Guide.* San Francisco: Health Publishing Co., 1988.

Robertson, Patricia Anne, MD, and Peggy Henning Berlin, PhD. *The Premature Labor Handbook: Successfully Sustaining Your High-Risk Pregnancy.* New York: Doubleday & Co., Inc., 1986.

Semchyshyn, Stefan, MD, and Carol Colman. *How to Prevent Miscarriage and Other Crises of Pregnancy.* New York: Macmillan Publishing Co., 1989.

PREGNANCY LOSS: WHEN THE WORST HAPPENS

Borg, Susan, and Judith Lasker. *When Pregnancy Fails.* Toronto: Bantam Books, 1981.

Cohen, Marion D. *Ambitious Sort of Grief: Pregnancy and Neo-Natal Loss.* Las Colinas, TX: Liberal Press, 1986.

Fritsch, Julie, with Sherokee Ilse. *The Anguish of Loss.* Long Lake, MN: Wintergreen Press, 1985.*

Ilse, Sherokee. *Empty Arms: Coping with Miscarriage, Stillbirth and Infant Death.* Maple Plain, MN.: Wintergreen Press, 1990*

Ilse, Sherokee, and Linda Hammer. *Miscarriage: A Shattered Dream.* Long Lake, MN: Wintergreen Press, 1985.*

Lachelin, G. C. *Miscarriage: The Facts.* New York: Oxford Univ. Press, 1986.

Limbo, Rana K., and Sara Rich Wheeler. *When a Baby Dies: A Handbook for Healing and Helping.* LaCrosse, WI: Resolve Through Sharing, 1986.

Morrow, Judith Gordon, and Nancy Gordon DeHamer. *Good Mourning: Help and Understanding in Time of Pregnancy Loss.* Dallas: Word Publishing, 1989.

Panuthos, Claudia, and Catherine Romero. *Ended Beginnings: Healing Childbearing Losses.* New York: Warner Books, 1986.

Pizer, Hank, and Christine O'Brien Palinski. *Coping with Miscarriage: Why It Happens and How to Deal with Its Impact on Your Family.* New York: New American Library, 1980.

Resources:

Burial Cradles: Bay Memorials, Thomas Zerbel, Funeral Director, 321 South 15th Street, Escanaba, MI 49829, (906) 786-2609

Centering Corp., P.O. Box 3367, Omaha, NE 68103-0367 (for a catalog)

National Center for Education in Maternal and Child Health (NCEMCH), 38th and R Streets, NW, Washington, D.C., 20057, (202) 625-8400 (a guide to resources in perinatal bereavement)

National Center for the Prevention of SIDS: (800) 638-7437

National Funeral Directors' Association: (414) 541-2500

National SIDS Foundation, 2 Metro Plaza, 8240 Professional Place, Landover, MD 20785, (319) 322-4870

Parent Care, Inc., 101½ South Union Street, Alexandria, VA 22314-3323

Perinatal Bereavement Team, Women's College Hospital, 76 Grenville St., Toronto, Ontario, M5S 1B2 Canada

MULTIPLE PREGNANCY

Alexander, Terry Pink. *Make Room for Twins: A Complete Guide to Pregnancy, Delivery and the Childhood Years.* Toronto: Bantam Books, 1987.

Clegg, Averil, and Anne Woolet. *Twins: From Conception to Five Years.* New York: Ballantine Books, 1988.

Novotny, Pamela P. *The Joy of Twins: Having, Raising and Loving Babies Who Arrive in Groups.* New York: Crown Publishing, 1988.

Resources:

Center for the Study of Multiple Birth; mail-order publications, medical referrals: 333 E. Superior St., 476, Chicago, IL 60611, (312) 266-9093

*Publications written by and/or in association with Sherokee Ilse are available from: Wintergreen Press, 3630 Eileen St., Maple Plain, MN 55389, (612) 476-1303

Doubletalk (quarterly newsletter about twins); P.O. Box 412, Amelia, OH 45102, (513) 753-7117

International Society for Twin Studies; organization of scientists involved in a wide variety of twin research: c/o The Mendel Institute, Piazza Aleno, 5, 00161 Rome, Italy

International Twins Association; support, social events for adult twins, annual Labor Day twin convention: P.O. Box 9157, Denver, CO 80209

Moonflower Birthing Supply, P.O. Box 128, Louisville, CO 80027, (800) 747-8996

National Organization of Mothers of Twins Clubs; referrals to local clubs, info. on starting a club: Lois Gallmeyer, 12404 Princess Jeanne NE, Albuquerque, NM 87112, (505) 275-0955

Parents of Multiple Births Assn. of Canada (POMBA); mail-order publications, Canadian club referrals: P.O. Box 2200, Lethbridge, Alberta, Canada, T1J 4K7, (403) 328-9165

Supertwin Statistician; information and statistics about multiples from around the world: "Miss Helen" Kirk, P.O. Box 254, Galveston, TX 77553, (409) 762-4792

Twins Foundation; newsletter, support for adult twins: P.O. Box 9487, Providence, RI 02940, (401) 274-TWIN (8946)

Twins Magazine (bimonthly), P.O. Box 12045, Overland Park, KS 66212, (913) 722-1090 or (800) 821-5533

CESAREAN SECTION

Cohen, Marion D. *A Flower Garden: All About It, Pregnancy, Cesarean Birth and . . . .* Las Colinas, TX: Liberal Press, 1987.

Donovan, Bonnie. *The Cesarean Birth Experience: A Practical, Comprehensive and Reassuring Guide for Parents and Professionals.* New York: Beacon Press, 1986.

Hausknecht, Richard, MD, and Jean Rattner Heilman. *Having a Cesarean Baby.* New York: Dutton, 1982.

Rosen, Mortimer, MD, and Lillian Thomas. *The Cesarean Myth: Choosing the Best Way to Have Your Baby.* New York: Penguin Books, 1989.

Royall, Nicki. *You Don't Need to Have a Repeat Cesarean.* Hollywood: Fell Publishers, 1983.

Shearer, Beth, and Aleta F. Cane. *Frankly Speaking: A Book for Cesarean Parents.* Washington, D.C.: Abbe Publishing Association, 1989.

BEDREST

Johnston, Susan H., M.S.W. and Deborah A. Kraut, M.Ed. *Pregnancy Bedrest: A Guide for the Pregnant Woman and Her Family.* New York: Henry Holt and Company, 1990.

BIBLIOGRAPHY

Texts and Treatises:

Benson, Ralph C., MD. *Handbook of Obstetrics and Gynecology*. 8th edition. Los Altos, CA: Lange Medical Publishers, 1983.

Berkowitz, Richard L., MD, MPH, Donald R. Coustan, MD, and Tara K. Mochizuki, Pharm.D, JD. *Handbook for Prescribing Medications During Pregnancy*. 2nd edition. Boston: Little, Brown and Company, 1986.

Briggs, Gerald G., B.Pharm., Roger K. Freeman, MD., and Sumner J. Jaffe, MD. *A Reference Guide to Fetal and Neonatal Risk, Drugs in Lactation and Pregnancy*. Second edition. Baltimore: Williams and Wilkins, 1986.

Brody, Steven A., MD, and Kent Ueland, MD, eds. *Endocrine Disorders in Pregnancy*. Norwalk, CT: Appleton and Lange, 1989.

Burrow, Gerard N., MD, and Thomas F. Ferris, MD. *Medical Complications During Pregnancy*. 2nd edition. Philadelphia: W. B. Saunders Company, 1982.

Clark, Steven L., MD., Jeffrey P. Phelan, MD., and David B. Cotton, MD., eds. *Critical Care Obstetrics*. Oradell, NJ: Medical Economics Books, 1987.

Creasy, Robert K., MD, and Robert Resnick, MD. *Maternal Fetal Medicine, Principles and Practice*. Philadelphia: W. B. Saunders Company, 1984.

Danforth, David N., and James R. Scott, eds. *Obstetrics and Gynecology*. 5th edition. Philadelphia: J. B. Lippincott Company, 1986.

Dorland's Illustrated Medical Dictionary. 27th edition. Philadelphia: W. B. Saunders Company, 1988.

Friedman, Emanuel A., MD, ScD, David B. Acker, MD, and Benjamin P. Sachs, MB, BS, DPH, eds. *Obstetrical Decision Making*. 2nd edition. Toronto: B. C. Decker, 1987.

Gabbe, Steven G., MD., Jennifer R. Niebyl, MD, and Joe Leigh Simpson, MD, eds. *Obstetrics: Normal and Problem Pregnancies*. New York: Churchill Livingstone, 1986.

Katz, Michael, MD, Pamela Gill, RN, MSN, and Judith Turiel, EdD, eds.

Preventing Preterm Birth: A Parent's Guide, San Francisco: Health Publishing Company, 1988.

Mishell, Daniel R., Jr., MD, Thomas H. Kirschbaum, MD, and C. Paul Morrow, MD, eds. *1988 Year Book of Obstetrics and Gynecology.* Chicago: Year Book Medical Publishers, Inc., 1988.

Niswander, Kenneth R., MD, ed. *Manual of Obstetrics, Diagnosis and Therapy.* 3rd edition. Boston: Little, Brown and Company, 1987.

Pernoll, Martin L., MD, and Ralph C. Benson, MD, eds. *Current Obstetric and Gynecologic Diagnosis and Treatment 1987.* Norwalk, CT: Appleton and Lange, 1987.

Physician's Guide to Insulin-Dependent (type I) Diabetes: Diagnosis and Treatment. Alexandria, VA: American Diabetes Association, Inc., 1988.

Physician's Guide to Non-Insulin-Dependent, (type II) Diabetes: Diagnosis and Treatment. 2nd edition. Alexandria, VA: American Diabetes Association, Inc., 1988.

Powers, Margaret A., MS, RD, CDE, ed. *Nutrition Guide for Professionals: Diabetes Education and Meal Planning.* Alexandria, VA: American Diabetes Association and The American Dietetic Association, 1988.

Pritchard, Jack A., MD, Paul C, MacDonald, MD, and Norman F. Gant, MD. *Williams Obstetrics.* 18th edition. Norwalk, CT: Appleton and Lange, 1989.

Queenan, John T., MD, and John C. Hobbins, MD, eds. *Protocols for High Risk Pregnancies.* 2nd edition. Oradell, NJ: Medical Economics Books, 1987.

Riulin, Michael E., MD, John C. Morrison, MD, and G. William Bates, MD. *Manual of Clinical Problems in Obstetrics and Gynecology.* Boston: Little, Brown and Company, 1982.

Thomas, Clayton L., MD, MPH, FA, ed. *Taber's Cyclopedic Medical Dictionary.* 16th edition. Philadelphia: Davis Company, 1989.

Willson, Robert, MD, Elsie Reid Carrington, MD. *Obstetrics and Gynecology.* 8th edition. St. Louis: C. V. Mosby Company, 1987.

Wynn, Ralph M., MD. *Obstetrics and Gynecology: The Clinical Core.* 4th edition. Philadelphia: Lea and Febiger, 1988.

Journals:

Arias, Fernando, MD, PhD. "Cervical Cerclage for the Temporary Treatment of Patients with Placenta Previa."*Obstetrics and Gynecology,* vol. 70, number 4 (April 1988): 545–548.

Ayers, Jonathan W. T., MD, and George W. Morley, MD. "Surgical Incision for Cesarean Section." *Obstetrics and Gynecology,* vol. 70, number 5 (November 1987): 706–708.

Blickstein, I., MD, Z. Shoham-Schwartz, MD, and M. Lancet, MD. "Growth Discordancy in Appropriate for Gestational Age, Term Twins." *Obstetrics and Gynecology,* vol. 72, number 4 (October 1988): 582–584.

Blickstein, I., MD, Z. Shoham-Schwartz, MD, M. Lancet, MD, and R. Borenstein, MD. "Characterization of the Growth-Discordant Twin." *Obstetrics and Gynecology,* vol. 70, number 1 (July 1987): 11–15.

Bottoms, Sidney F, MD, Robert A. Welch, MD, Ivan E. Zador, PhD, and Robert J. Sokol, MD. "Clinical Interpretation of Ultrasound Measurements in Preterm Pregnancies with Premature Rupture of Membranes." *Obstetrics and Gynecology,* vol. 69, number 3, part 1 (March 1987): 358–362.

Brown, Haywood L., MD, Joseph M. Miller, Jr., MD, Harvey A. Gabert, MD, and Grace Kissling, PhD. "Ultrasonic Recognition of the Small-for-Gestational-Age Fetus." *Obstetrics and Gynecology,* vol. 69, number 4 (April 1987): 631–635.

Cardwell, Michael S., MD, Phillip Caple, MD, and C. Leslie Baker, MD. "Triplet Pregnancy with Delivery on Three Separate Days." *Obstetrics and Gynecology,* vol. 71, number 3, part 2 (March 1988): 448–449.

Catalano, Patrick M., MD, Ira M. Bernstein, MD, Robert R. Wolfe, PhD, S. Srikanta, MD, Elaine Tyzbir, MS, and Ethan A. H. Sims, MD. "Subclinical Abnormalities of Glucose Metabolism in Subjects with Previous Gestational Diabetes." *American Journal of Obstetrics and Gynecology,* vol. 155, number 6 (December 1986): 1255–1262.

Condon, John T., MB, BS, FRANZCP. "Predisposition to Psychological Complications After Stillbirth: A Case Report." *Obstetrics and Gynecology,* vol. 70, number 3, part 2 (September 1987): 495–497.

Cox, David N., PhD, Bernd K. Wittmann, MD, Melanie Hess, MSW, A. G. Ross, RN, John Lind, PhD, and Sandi Lindahl, RDMS. "The Psychological Impact of Diagnostic Ultrasound." *Obstetrics and Gynecology,* vol. 70, number 5 (November 1987): 673–676.

Cox, Susan M., MD, M. Lynne Williams, RN, and Kenneth J. Leveno, MD. "The Natural History of Preterm Ruptured Membranes: What to Expect of Expectant Management." *Obstetrics and Gynecology,* vol. 71, number 4 (April 1988): 558–562.

Duff, Patrick, MD, Karen Southmayd, MD, and John A. Read, MD. "Outcome of Trial of Labor in Patients with a Single Previous Low Transverse Cesarean Section for Dystocia." *Obstetrics and Gynecology,* vol. 71, number 3, part 1 (March 1988): 380–384.

Evans, Mark I., MD, John C. Fletcher, PhD, Ivan E. Zador, PhD, Burritt W. Newton, MD, Mary Helen Quigg, MD, and Curtis D. Struyk, MD. "Selective First-Trimester Termination in Octuplet and Quadruplet Pregnancies: Clinical and Ethical Issues." *Obstetrics and Gynecology,* vol. 71, number 3, part 1 (March 1988): 289–296.

Flamm, Bruce L., MD, Janice R. Goings, CNM, Norma-Jean Fuelberth, MD, Edward Fischermann, MD, Charles Jones, MD, and Edward Hersh, MD. "Oxytocin During Labor After Previous Cesarean Section: Results of a Multicenter Study." *Obstetrics and Gynecology,* vol. 70, number 5 (November 1987): 709–712.

Gilstrap III, Larry C., MC, John C. Hauth, MC, Gary D. V. Hankins, MC, and Amy Beck, MEd. "Twins: Prophylactic Hospitalization and Ward Rest at Early Gestational Age." *Obstetrics and Gynecology,* vol. 69, number 4 (April 1987): 578–581.

Grimes, David A., MD. "A Simplified Device for Intraoperative Autotransfusion." *Obstetrics and Gynecology,* vol. 72, number 6 (December 1988): 947–950.

Hage, Marvin L., MD, Michael J. Helms, William E. Hammond, PhD, and Charles B. Hammond, MD. "Changing Rates of Cesarean Delivery: The Duke Experience, 1978–1986." *Obstetrics and Gynecology,* vol. 72, number 1 (July 1988): 98–101.

Hatjis, Christos G., MD, Melissa Swain, RN, Lewis H. Nelson, MD, Paul J. Meis, MD, and J. M. Ernest, MD. "Efficacy of Combined Administration of Magnesium Sulfate and Ritodrine in the Treatment of Premature Labor." *Obstetrics and Gynecology*, vol. 69, number 3, part 1 (March 1987): 317–322.

Herbert, William N. P., MD, Helen G. Owen, RN, and Myra L. Collins, MD, PhD. "Autologous Blood Storage in Obstetrics." *Obstetrics and Gynecology*, vol. 72, number 2 (August 1988): 166–170.

Herron, M. A., RN, and J. T. Parer, MD, PhD. "Transabdominal Cerclage for Fetal Wastage Due to Cervical Incompetence." *Obstetrics and Gynecology*, vol. 71, number 6, part 1 (June 1988): 865–868.

Jauniaux, Eric, MD, Nabih Elkazen, MD, Fernand Leroy, MD, PhD, Paul Wilkin, MD, PhD, Frederic Rodesch, MD, PhD, and Jean Hustin, MD, PhD; "Clinical and Morphologic Aspects of the Vanishing Twin Phenomenon." *Obstetrics and Gynecology*, vol. 72, number 4 (October 1988): 577–581.

Kettel, L. Michael, MD, D. Ware Branch, MD, James R. Scott, MD. "Occult Placental Abruption After Maternal Trauma." *Obstetrics and Gynecology*, vol. 71, number 3, part 2 (March 1988): 449–453.

Kovacs, Bruce, MD, Bejan Shahbahrami, MS, Lawrence D. Platt, MD, and David E. Comings, MD. "Molecular Genetic Prenatal Determination of Twin Zygosity." *Obstetrics and Gynecology*, vol. 72, number 6 (December 1988): 954–956.

Krushall, Margot S., MD, Susan Leonard, RN, and Henry Klapholz, MD. "Autologous Blood Donation During Pregnancy: Analysis of Safety and Blood Use." *Obstetrics and Gynecology,* vol. 70, number 6 (December 1987): 938–941.

Laurin, Jan, MD, Goran Lingman, MD, Karel Marsal, MD, and Per-Hakan Persson, MD. "Fetal Blood Flow in Pregnancies Complicated by Intrauterine Growth Retardation." *Obstetrics and Gynecology*, vol. 69, number 6 (June 1987): 895–902.

Leikin, Enid, MD, James H. Jenkins, MD, and William L. Graves, PhD. "Prophylactic Insulin in Gestational Diabetes." *Obstetrics and Gynecology*, vol. 70, number 4 (October 1987): 587–592.

Levine, Michael G., MD, and Debra Esser, MD. "Total Parenteral Nutrition for the Treatment of Severe Hyperemesis Gravidarum: Maternal Nutritional Effects and Fetal Outcome." *Obstetrics and Gynecology*, vol. 72, number 1 (July 1988): 102–107.

Lock, Dennis R., MD, Adi Bar-Eyal, MSC, Hillary Voet, PhD, and Zecharia Madar, PhD. "Glycemic Indices of Various Foods Given to Pregnant Diabetic Subjects." *Obstetrics and Gynecology*, vol. 71, number 2 (February 1988): 180–183.

MacGregor, Scott N., DO, Rudy E. Sabbagha, MD, Ralph K. Tamura, MD, Bruce W. Pielet, MD, and Seth L. Feigenbaum, MD, MPH. "Differing Growth Patterns in Pregnancies Complicated by Preterm Labor." *Obstetrics and Gynecology*, vol. 72, number 6 (December 1988): 834–837.

Mackenzie, William E., MB, MRCOG, Deborah S. Holmes, PhD, and John R. Newton, MD, FRCOG. "Spontaneous Abortion Rate in Ultrasonigraphically Viable Pregnancies." *Obstetrics and Gynecology*, vol. 71 (January 1988): 81–83.

Main, Denise M., MD, Michael Katz, MD, Grace Chiu, PhD, Suzanne Campion, BSN, and Steven G. Gabbe, MD. "Intermittant Weekly Contraction Monitoring to Predict Preterm Labor in Low-Risk Women: A Blinded Study." *Obstetrics and Gynecology,* vol. 72, number 5 (November 1988): 757–761.

Mimouni, Francis, MD, Menachem Miodovnik, MD, Tarig A. Siddigi, MD, Michael A. Berk, MD, Charlotte Wittekind, RN, and Reginald C. Tsang, MBBS. "High Spontaneous Premature Labor Rate in Insulin Dependent Diabetic Pregnant Women: an Association with Poor Glycemic Control and Urogenital Infection." *Obstetrics and Gynecology,* vol. 72 (August 1988): 175–180.

Neilson, J. P., MD, MRCOG, D. A. A. Verkuyl, MRCOG, C. A. Crowther, MRCOG, and C. Bannerman, MRCP. "Preterm Labor in Twin Pregnancies: Prediction by Cervical Assessment." *Obstetrics and Gynecology,* vol. 72, number 5 (November 1988): 719–723.

Nisell, Henry, MD, Nils-Olov Lunell, MD, and Birgitta Linde, MD. "Maternal Hemodynamics and Impaired Fetal Growth in Pregnancy Induced Hypertension," *Obstetrics and Gynecology,* vol. 71, number 2 (February 1988): 163–166.

Papiernik, Emile, MD, Jean Bouyer, PhD, Kristine Yaffe, BS, Gerard Winisdorffer, MD, Dominique Collin, MD, and Jean Dreyfus, MD. "Women's Acceptance of a Preterm Birth Prevention Program." *American Journal of Obstetrics and Gynecology,* vol. 155, number 5 (November 1986): 939–946.

Parazzini, Fabio, MD, Carlo La Vecchia, MD, Eva Negri, ScD, Gabriela Cecchetti, MD, and Luigi Fedele, MD. "Epidemiologic Characteristics of Women with Uterine Fibroids: A Case-Control Study." *Obstetrics and Gynecology,* vol. 72, number 6 (December 1988): 853–857.

Rosendahl, Henrik, MD, and Seppo Kivinen, MD, PhD. "Routine Ultrasound Screening for Early Detection of Small-for-Gestational-Age Fetuses." *Obstetrics and Gynecology,* vol. 71, number 4 (April 1988): 518–521.

Sachs, Benjamin P., MB, BS, DHP, John Yeh, MD, David Acker, MD, Shirley Driscoll, MD, Dick A. J. Brown, MD, John F. Jewett, MD. "Cesarean Section-Related Maternal Mortality in Massachusetts, 1954–1985." *Obstetrics and Gynecology,* vol. 71, number 3, part 1 (March 1988): 385–388.

Sachs, David A., MD, Salim Abu-Fadil, MD, Gerald J. Karten, MD, Alan B. Forsythe, PhD, and James R. Hackett, BA. "Screening for Gestational Diabetes with the One-Hour 50g Glucose Test." *Obstetrics and Gynecology,* vol. 70, number 1 (July 1987): 89–93.

Shiono, Patricia H., PhD, Donald McNellis, MD, and George G. Rhoads, MD, MPH. "Reasons for the Rising Cesarean Delivery Rates: 1978–1984." *Obstetrics and Gynecology,* vol. 69, number 5 (May 1987): 696–700.

Sibai, Baha M., MD, Adel El-Nazer, MD, and Antonio Gonzalez-Ruiz, MD. "Severe Preeclampsia-Eclampsia in Young Primigravid Women: Subsequent Pregnancy Outcome and Remote Prognosis." *American Journal of Obstetrics and Gynecology,* vol. 155, number 5 (November 1986): 1011–1016.

Spinnato, J. A., MD. "Infrequency of Pulmonary Immaturity in an Indigent Population with Preterm Premature Rupture of the Membranes." *Obstetrics and Gynecology,* vol. 69, number 6 (June 1987): 942–944.

Spinnato, Joseph A., MD, David C. Shaver, MD, Eileen M. Bray, RN, and Jeffrey Lipshitz, MD. "Preterm Premature Rupture of the Membranes with Fetal Pulmonary Maturity Present: A Prospective Study." *Obstetrics and Gynecology,* vol. 69, number 2 (February 1987): 196–201.

Storlazzi, Evelina, MD, Anthony M. Vintzileos, MD, Winston A. Campbell, MD, David A. Nochimson, MD, and Paul J. Weinbaum, MD. "Ultrasonic Diagnosis of Discordant Fetal Growth in Twin Gestations." *Obstetrics and Gynecology,* vol. 69, number 3, part 1 (March 1987): 363–367.

Tierson, Forrest D., PhD, Carolyn L. Olsen, PhD, and Ernest B. Hook, MD. "Nausea and Vomiting of Pregnancy and Association with Pregnancy Outcome." *American Journal of Obstetrics and Gynecology,* vol. 155, number 5 (November 1986): 1017–1022.

Toth, Miklos, MD, Steven S. Witkin, PhD, William Ledger, MD, and Howard Thaler, PhD. "The Role of Infection in the Etiology of Preterm Birth." *Obstetrics and Gynecology,* vol. 71, number 5 (May 1988): 723–726.

Wood, Paul L., MBChB, MRCOG, and Brian H. Durham, PhD, MPHil, FIMLS. "Change in Plasma Cystyl Amniopeptidase (Oxytocinase) Between 30–34 Weeks' Gestation As a Predictor of Pregnancy-Induced Hypertension." *Obstetrics and Gynecology,* vol. 72, number 6 (December 1988): 850–852.

Yarkoni, Shaul, MD, E. Albert Reese, MD, Theodore Holford, PhD, Theresa Z. O'Connor, MPH, and John C. Hobbins, MD. "Estimated Fetal Weight in the Evaluation of Growth in Twin Gestations: A Prospective Longitudinal Study." *Obstetrics and Gynecology,* vol. 69, number 4 (April 1987): 636–639.

INDEX